Endocannabinoids: Molecular, Pharmacological, Behavioral and Clinical Features

Editor

Eric Murillo-Rodríguez

Laboratory of Molecular and Integrative Neurosciences
School of Medicine, Health Sciences Division
Anahuac University Mayab
Merida 97310
Yucatan, Mexico

Co-Editors

Emmanuel S. Onaivi

William Paterson University,
USA

Nissar A. Darmani

Western University of Health Sciences,
USA

Edward Wagner

Western University of Health Sciences,
USA

Bentham Science Publishers
Executive Suite Y - 2
PO Box 7917, Saif Zone
Sharjah, U.A.E.
subscriptions@benthamscience.org

Bentham Science Publishers
P.O. Box 446
Oak Park, IL 60301-0446
USA
subscriptions@benthamscience.org

Bentham Science Publishers
P.O. Box 294
1400 AG Bussum
THE NETHERLANDS
subscriptions@benthamscience.org

CONTENTS

About the eBook

The endocannabinoid system comprises at least two G-protein-coupled receptors (the cannabinoid CB_1 and CB_2 receptors) activated by marijuana's psychoactive principle Δ^9-tetrahydrocannabinol (THC) and the endogenous ligands known as endocannabinoids. The apex of endocannabinoid research seems to have been reached with the clinical development, and in some cases also the marketing, of synthetic or natural pharmaceuticals targeting this signalling system, which followed the understanding of its physiological and pathological role in several conditions, a role that was investigated first in rodent experimental models and then in humans.

We particularly take an interest in Manuscripts that report relevance of the endocannabinoid system. Original reports or Reviews describing the results of experimental evidence about the neurobiological role of the endocannabinoid system would be a great interest. Main topics include, but are not limited to:

*The genetics of cannabinoid CB_1 and CB_2 receptors and their tissue distribution, their splicing variants and polymorphisms, and the possible implications of all this in determining different behaviours as well as various pathological conditions and the addiction to substances of abuse.

*Pharmacological approaches describing the potential use in the central nervous system disorders of endocannabinoid-based drugs, such as cannabinoid receptor agonists and antagonists, inhibitors of endocannabinoid inactivation processes, and even plant cannabinoids other than THC and with a molecular mechanism of action.

*The role of the endocannabinoid system in several neurological and neuropsychiatric conditions, such as epilepsy.

Key feature: Cannabinoid receptor genes, arachidonic acid, homeostasis, drugs of abuse, neurogenesis, epilepsy.

INTENDED AUDIENCE/READERSHIP

The areas of interest would include genetics, molecular biology, biochemistry, pharmacology. Contributions may involve clinical, preclinical, or basic research.

FOREWORD

For me, personally, the year 2013 has a special significance. Exactly 50 years ago I published my first paper on cannabinoids. At that time, in 1963, research on the constituents of Cannabis sativa had mostly come to a stop. Although investigation on cannabis in its various forms –hashish, marijuana, bhang – had been reported over a century, its psychoactive constituent(s) had not been isolated in a pure form and its structure – or possibly structures – was unknown. And yet, there was no research going on in either North America or the UK – the major research countries at the time. The major reason for this neglect was possibly legal. Cannabis was an illicit substance and was not readily available to scientists. And even if it were obtained legally, research with it would have been impossible in an academic laboratory, due to strict security regulations for work with such substances. Luckily I was not aware of these problems. Through the research institute I worked at the time – the Weizmann Research Institute – I obtained 5kg of confiscated hashish from the police, who apparently were also unaware of the international agreements on cannabis. First, my colleagues, the late Yuval Shvo, Yehiel Gaoni and I reisolated cannabidiol, a non-psychoactive constituent. This compound had been obtained previously by Lord Todd, a Nobel Prize winner, and by Roger Adams but its structure had not been elucidated. By use of then modern methods – NMR and mass spectrometry – we established its structure and published the results in 1963 – 50 years ago. At this point I asked for a grant from the US National Institute of Health (NIH). My application never went beyond the administrative office. Their answer was that cannabis use was not an American problem. Would I, they wrote, apply with a more relevant topic. Nevertheless Yehiel Gaoni and I went ahead and by 1964 had isolated several cannabinoids – a term I coined several years later – and had elucidated their structures. Dr. Habib Edery and Yona Grunfeld, colleagues at a nearby biological research station, tested these constituents for psychoactivity in monkeys. Only one compound caused such activity. At that time we called the compound delta-1-tetrahydrocannabinol, but later it was renamed delta-9 –tetrahydrocannabiol (Δ^9-THC) and many thousands of publications on it have been published. Suddenly NIH decided that cannabinoid research is a relevant topic for research. A prominent NIH pharmacologist flew over, took with him the entire supply of pure

THC and for the next few years most of the research on this compound in the US was done with it. And NIH has supported my work ever since.

Over the next 2 decades we, and many other groups, worked on the chemistry, biochemistry, pharmacogy and even some clinical effects of the cannabinoids. We learned how the cannabinoids are formed in the body, how they are metabolized and what effects they cause *in vitro* and *in vivo*. Some clinical work was also published. THC was approved as a drug for enhancement of appetite (mostly in cancer and AIDS patients) and for prevention of vomiting and nausea in patients undergoing cancer chemotherapy. But, surprisingly, the mechanism of THC action remained unclear. It was believed that it had something to do with possible action on lipid membranes due to its lipophilic properties. In the mid-1980's Allyn Howlett's group showed that a specific receptor exists. Stimulation of this receptor, known now as the CB1 receptor today, leads to the well known marijuana effects. Later a second receptor, CB2, was discovered in the immune system. We assumed that these receptors are stimulated by endogenous constituents and went ahead looking for them. As THC is a lipid, we assumed that the endogenous constituents are also lipophilic compounds, In 1992 we isolated the first such endocannabinoid and named it anandamide. Later a second endocannabinoid, 2-AG, was identified. The present, outstanding eBook describes in considerable detail the enormous amount of research done on the endocannabinoids, the endocannabinoid receptors, the unique endocannabinoid signaling system and the advances in the clinic.

Where is endocannabinoid research going now? I shall try to put forward several areas, which I believe will lead to major advances:

LIPID SIGNALING THROUGH THE CB2 RECEPTOR AS A MAJOR PROTECTIVE SYSTEM

Pal Pacher and I have speculated in a recent review that "The mammalian body has a highly developed immune system which guards against continuous invading protein attacks and aims at preventing, attenuating or repairing the inflicted damage. It is conceivable that through evolution analogous biological protective systems have evolved against nonprotein attacks. There is emerging evidence that lipid endocannabinoid signaling through CB2 receptors may represent an example/part of such a protective system" Indeed over the last few years numerous groups have reported protective action through the CB2 receptors in numerous physiological systems. We can expect this trend to continue.

INVOLVEMENT OF THE ENDOCANNABINOID SYSTEM IN THE REGULATION OF PROGENITOR/STEM CELLS

Over the last few years several groups have shown that endocannabinoid signaling is involved in progenitor/stem cell development, thus leading to regulation of their proliferation, differentiation and survival. In view of the importance of stem cells in human health and disease, we should expect to see a major research effort in this fascinating field.

PHYSIOLOGICAL ACTIONS OF ENDOCANNABINOID-LIKE CONSTITUENTS

Many dozens of fatty acid amides of ethanol amines and amino acids, as well as esters of fatty acids with glycerol (endocannabinoid-like compounds) are present in the brain and possibly in other organs. Those that have been investigated have been shown to cause various physiological effects – lowering of pain, vasodilation, anti-osteoporotic and anti-cancer activity. It is quite possible that this type of compounds may represent a valuable treasure throve of physiological mediators.

Linda Parker and I have speculated that "If subtle chemical disparity is one of the causes for the variability in personality—an area in psychology that is yet to be fully understood—we may have to look for a large catalog of compounds in the brain with distinct CNS effects. Is it possible that the above-described large cluster of chemically related anandamide-type compounds in the brain is related to the chemistry of the human personality and the individual temperamental differences? It is tempting to assume that the huge possible variability of the levels and ratios of substances in such a cluster of compounds may allow an infinite number of individual differences, the raw substance which of course is sculpted by experience. If this intellectual speculation is shown to have some factual basis, it may lead to major advances in molecular psychology". Will the endocannabinoid system be the key to this yet unexplored niche of science?

R. Mechoulam
Hebrew University
Medical Faculty
Institute for Drug Research
Jerusalem
Israel

PREFACE

Cannabinoids are a group of terpenophenolic compounds present in Cannabis.

(*Cannabis sativa L*). The broader definition of cannabinoids refers to a group of substances that are structurally related to delta-9-tetrahydrocannabinol (Δ9-THC) or that bind to cannabinoid receptors.

Before the 1980's, it was often speculated that cannabinoids produced their physiological and behavioral effects *via* nonspecific interaction with cell membranes, instead of interacting with specific membrane-bound receptors. The discovery of the first cannabinoid receptors in the 1980s helped to resolve this debate. These receptors are common in animals, and have been found in mammals, birds, fish, and reptiles. There are currently two known types of cannabinoid receptors, termed CB_1 and CB_2.

The cannabinoid system has been around for over 600 million years…even before the dinosaurs!! The cannabinoid system is present in species such as hydra, mollusks, and insects, leading to speculation on the physiological importance of such a system preserved throughout evolution. To date, the presence in the central nervous system of specific lipids that bind naturally to the CB_1/CB_2 cannabinoid receptors has been documented. Pharmacological experiments have shown that injection of endogenous cannabinoids or endocannabinoids modulates diverse neurobiological functions, such as learning and memory, feeding, pain perception and sleep generation.

The system of endogenous cannabinoids is present in several species, including humans, leading to speculation regarding the neurobiological role of the endocannabinoid system in diverse functions. Hence, I thought it was time to bring out an editorial eBook on the subject containing advanced and up-to-date scientific information on this special and exclusive topic. I expect that such a eBook is likely to attain global circulation among students, teachers and researchers alike.

Fortunately, in response to our appeal, a number of leading scientists in the field across the globe agreed to contribute to the eBook. Thus, this eBook deals with various aspects of the endocannabinoid system, from phenomena to molecular processes. I am sincerely grateful to all the contributors for their scientific contribution.

Eric Murillo-Rodríguez
Laboratorio de Neurociencias Moleculares e Integrativas
Escuela de Medicina, División Ciencias de la Salud
Universidad Anáhuac Mayab
Mérida 97310
Yucatán, México

ACKNOWLEDGEMENTS

I would like to acknowledge and extend my heartfelt gratitude to the following persons who have made the completion of this eBook possible:

Our Dean, P. Rafael Pardo Hervás L.C, for his vital support.

Dr. Narciso Acuña González, our Vice Dean for Academic Affairs, for his understanding and support.

Dr. Manuel Echeverría y Eguiluz, Dean of the School of Medicine for his constant encouragement.

Most especially to my family and friends.

Eric Murillo-Rodríguez

List of Contributors

Nissar A. Darmani, Department of Basic Medical Sciences, College of Osteopathic Medicine of the Pacific, Western University of Health Sciences, Pomona, CA 91766, USA

Seetha Chebolu, Department of Basic Medical Sciences, College of Osteopathic Medicine of the Pacific, Western University of Health Sciences, Pomona, CA 91766, USA

Miriam Melis, Department of Biomedical Sciences, University of Cagliari, Monserrato (CA), Italy

Anna L. Muntoni, C.N.R. Neuroscience Institute-Cagliari, University of Cagliari, Monserrato (CA), Italy

Marco Pistis, Department of Biomedical Sciences, University of Cagliari, Monserrato (CA), Italy

Hiroki Ishiguro, Yamanashi University, Japan

Claire M. Leonard, William Paterson University, Wayne NJ 07470, USA

Susan Sgro, William Paterson University, Wayne NJ 07470, USA

Emmanuel S. Onaivi, Department of Biology, William Paterson University, Wayne NJ 07470 and NIDA-IRP, Baltimore MD 21224, USA

Dow P. Hurst, Center for Drug Discovery, Department of Chemistry and Biochemistry, University of North Carolina at Greensboro, Greensboro, NC 27402, USA

Jagjeet Singh, Center for Drug Discovery, Department of Chemistry and Biochemistry, University of North Carolina at Greensboro, Greensboro, NC 27402, USA

Patricia H. Reggio, Department of Chemistry and Biochemistry, UNC Greensboro, Greensboro, NC 27402, USA

Amanda Borgquist, Department of Basic Medical Sciences, College of Osteopathic Medicine of the Pacific, Western University of Health Sciences, Pomona, CA 91766, USA

Edward J. Wagner, Department of Basic Medical Sciences, College of Osteopathic Medicine, Western University of Health Sciences, 309 E. Second Street, Pomona, CA 91766, USA

Andrew J. Hill, The School of Chemistry, Food and Nutritional Sciences and Pharmacy, The University of Reading, Whiteknights, Reading, Berkshire, RG53SA, UK

Thomas D. M. Hill, The School of Chemistry, Food and Nutritional Sciences and Pharmacy, The University of Reading, Whiteknights, Reading, Berkshire, RG53SA, UK

Benjamin J. Whalley, The School of Chemistry, Food and Nutritional Sciences and Pharmacy, The University of Reading, Whiteknights, Reading, Berkshire, RG53SA, UK

2

CHAPTER 1

Cannabinoid Receptor Gene Variations in Neuropsychiatric Disorders

Hiroki Ishiguro[1], Claire M. Leonard[2], Susan Sgro[2] and Emmanuel S. Onaivi[2,3,*]

[1]Yamanashi University, Japan, [2]William Paterson University, Wayne NJ 07470, USA and [3]NIDA-NIH Baltimore MD 21224, USA

Abstract: The ubiquitous cannabinoid receptors (CBRs) – probably the most abundant binding sites in the CNS - are known to be involved in a number of neuropsychiatric disturbances. CBRs are coded in human chromosomes 1 and 6 and activated by endocannabinoids, phytocannabinoids and marijuana use (medical/recreational use). The components of the endocannabinoid system (ECS) include *CNR1 and CNR2* genes encoding these CBRs (CB1Rs and CB2Rs), endocannabinoids (eCBs), and their synthesizing and degradation enzymes are major targets of investigation for their impact in neuropsychiatry. Hence we have continued to study the influence of CBR variants in neuropsychiatric disorders. Many studies have shown that *CNR1* and *FAAH* single nucleotide polymorphisms (SNPs) may contribute to drug addiction, depression, eating disorders, schizophrenia, and multiple sclerosis. But little attention has been paid to the neuronal and functional expression of CB2Rs in the brain and their role in neuropsychiatric disorders has been much less well characterized. Indeed our studies provided the first evidence for neuronal CNS effects of CB2Rs and their possible role in drug addiction, eating disorders, psychosis, depression and autism spectrum disorders (ASDs). In the current ongoing studies many features of CBR gene structures, SNPs, copy number variations (CNVs), CpG islands, microRNA regulation and the impact of CBR gene variants in neuropsychiatry and where possible in rodent models have been assessed. Although *CNR1* gene has more CpG islands than *CNR2* gene, both have CPG islands less than 300 bases, but they may be regulated by DNA methylation. MicroRNA binding to the 3′ untranslated region of the *CNR1* gene with two polyadenylation sites may also potentially regulate CB1R expression. *CNR1* gene has 4 exons and there are 135 SNPs reported in more than 1% of the population with no common SNP that changes amino acids of CB1R currently known or reported. A copy number variant (CNV) which is 19.5kb found in 4 out of 2026 people covers exons 3 and 4 and codes amino acid that could alter the expression of CB1Rs. *CNR2* has 4 exons with CB2A with 3 exons and CB2B with 2 exons; and there are about 100 SNPs found in more than 1% of the population, which include common cSNPs that change amino acids of the CB2R, including R63Q, Q66R and H316Y. CNVs in Asian and Yoruba population

*Address correspondence to Emmanuel S. Onaivi: Department of Biology, William Paterson University, Wayne NJ 07470 and NIDA-IRP, Baltimore MD 21224, USA; Tel: +1 973-720-3453; Fax: +1 973-720-2338; Email: eonaivi@intra.nida.nih.gov; onaivie@wpunj.edu

Eric Murillo-Rodríguez, Emmanuel S. Onaivi, Nissar A. Darmani & Edward Wagner (Eds.)

have been reported. We also report on the identification of novel human and rodent CB2R isoforms, their differential tissue expression patterns and regulation by CBR ligands. Our findings also indicate increased risk of schizophrenia, depression, drug abuse, and eating and autism spectrum disorders in low CB2R function. Therefore, studying the CBR genomic structure, its polymorphic nature, subtype specificity, its variants and associated regulatory elements that confer vulnerabilities to a number of neuropsychiatric disturbances may provide deeper insight in unraveling the underlining mechanisms. Thus, understanding CBR variants and other components of the ECS may provide novel targets for the effects of cannabinoids in neuropsychiatry. *Support* R15DA032890 and WPUNJ.

Keywords: Cannabinoid, cannabinoid receptors, cannabinoid receptor genes, *CNR1*, *CNR2*, endocannabinoids, polymorphism, variants, CNVs, SNPs, cannabis, drug addiction, neuropsychiatric disorders.

INTRODUCTION

The discovery that specific genes codes for cannabinoid receptors (CBRs) that are activated by marijuana use, and that the human body makes its own marijuana-like substances - endocannabinoids [1], that also activate CBRs has provided surprising new knowledge about cannabinoid genomic and proteomic profiles. Our new remarkable understanding indicates that the cellular, biochemical and behavioral responses to marijuana, which remains one of the most widely used and abused drugs in the world, are coded in our genes and chromosomes. With increasing new information from the decoding of the human genome, many aspects of genetic risk factors in marijuana use including age of initiation, continuation and problem use undoubtedly will interact with environmental factors such as availability of marijuana along with the individual's genotype and phenotype. These remarkable advances in understanding the biological actions of marijuana, cannabinoids and endocannabinoids, are unraveling the genetic basis of marijuana use with implication in human health and disease. The two well characterized cannabinoid CB1 and CB2 receptors are encoded by *CNR1* and *CNR2* genes that have been mapped to human chromosome 6 and 1 respectively (Figs. **1** and **2**). A number of polymorphisms in cannabinoid receptor genes have been associated with human disorders including osteoporosis [2, 3], attention deficit hyperactivity disorder (ADHD) [4], post-traumatic stress disorder (PTSD) [4], drug dependency [5], obesity [6, 7] and depression [5, 8] and other neuropsychiatric disorders as discussed in this manuscript. Thus, because of the ubiquitous distribution and role of the endocannabinoid system in the regulation of a variety of normal human physiology, drugs that are targeted to different aspects of this system are already benefiting cancer subjects and those with AIDs and metabolic syndromes [7]. In the coming era of personalized medicine, genetic variants and haplotypes in *CNR1* and *CNR2* genes associated with obesity or addiction phenotypes may help identify specific targets in conditions of endocannabinoid dysfunction. Our previous investigations had defined a number of features of the *CNR1* gene's structure, regulation and variation [9], but many features of *CNR2* gene structure, regulation and variation still remain poorly defined. However, we and others have now demonstrated and reported that variants of the *CNR1* gene are associated with a number of disorders and substance abuse vulnerability in diverse ethnic groups including, European-American, African-American and Japanese subjects [9]. Most strikingly, variants of *CNR* genes co-occur with other genetic variations and share biological susceptibility that underlies comorbidity in most neuropsychiatric disturbances [10]. Thus, emerging evidence indicates that the endocannabinoid system exerts a powerful modulatory action on retrograde signaling associated with inhibition of synaptic transmission [11]. Interestingly a role for variations in *CNR1* gene has been associated with striatal responses to happy but not to disgust faces [12] with implication that functional variation of *CNR1* genotypes may be associated with disturbances of the brain involving emotional and social stimuli, such as autism [12] and depression [13, 14]. Here we review and present additional data that focuses on these recent advances in cannabinoid genomics and the surprising new fundamental roles that the ECS plays in the genetic basis of marijuana use and cannabinoid pharmacotherapeutics. The powerful influence of cannabinoid induced retrograde signaling modulates GABAergic and glutamatergic systems indicate that the main excitatory and inhibitory systems are in part under the influence of the endocannabinoid system. Thus, the genetic basis of compulsive marijuana use may involve interaction of *CNR* genes with other genes and environmental factors. As with other dependences with genetic risk factors, the risk for marijuana use is likely to be the result of *CNR* genes and other genes and environmental factors, each contributing a small fraction of the overall risk [15]. Additional evidence is provided for the complex *CNR1* and *CNR2* gene structures and their associated regulatory elements. In the current ongoing studies many features of CNR gene structures, SNPs, CNVs, CPG islands microRNA regulation and the impact of CNR gene variants in neuropsychiatry and where possible in rodent models have been assessed. Although *CNR1* gene has more CPG islands than *CNR2* gene, both have CPG islands less than 300 bases, but they may be regulated by DNA methylation. MicroRNA binding to the 3′ untranlated region of the *CNR1* gene with two polyadenylation sites may also potentially regulate CB1R expression. *CNR1* gene has 4 exons and there are 135 SNPs reported in more than 1% of the population with no common SNP that changes amino acids of CB1R currently known or reported. A copy number variant (CNV) which is 19.5kb found in 4 out of 2026 people covers exons 3 and 4 and codes amino acid that could alter the expression of CB1Rs. *CNR2* has 4 exons with CB2A with 3 exons and CB2B with 2 exons; and there are about 100 SNPs found in more than 1% of the population, which include common cSNPs that change amino acids of the CB2R, including R63Q, Q66R and H316Y. CNVs in Asian and Yoruba population have been reported. Therefore, studying the CBR genomic structure, its polymorphic nature, subtype specificity, their variants and associated regulatory elements that confer vulnerabilities to a number neuropsychiatric disturbance may provide deeper insight in unraveling the underlining mechanisms, as discussed below. Thus, understanding the ECS in the human body and brain will contribute to elucidating this natural regulatory mechanism in health and disease.

VARIATIONS IN CANNABINOID RECEPTOR GENES IN NEUROPSYCHIATRIC DISORDERS

While the expression of CBRs in humans varies according to ethnicity and gender [16], variations in other mammalian species are also notable. Therefore a number of confounding factors and disparities arise in different studies due to the variations in human CBRs dependent on gender and ethnicity. A number of variations have been found in genes associated with the ECS including those encoding the CBRs, and those involved in the synthesizing enzymes of endocannabinoids including diacylglycerol lipase alpha (DAGLA) and metabolizing enzymes like fatty acid amide hydrolase (FAAH). There are a number of reported mutations in the genes associated with the ECS that lead to altered mRNA stability and transcription rate with modification of the encoded proteins. These functional variations have been associated in a number of studies and meta-analysis with neuropsychiatric disturbances (Table **1**). We and others have reported that the human CB1R have a number of splice variants, which may in part account for the myriad behavioral effects of smoking marijuana. Up to five isoforms including the canonical or long, and short isoforms are known to be produced by alternative splicing of the *CNR1* transcript [9]. Some effects of marijuana and other cannabinoids may include actions at CB2Rs that have received much less attention than CB1Rs. However, we and others have now identified and characterized glial and neuronal CB2Rs in the brain. Nonetheless, many features of the *CNR2* gene structure, regulation and variation remain poorly characterized compared to the *CNR1*. In humans the *CNR2* gene is reported to consist of a single translated exon flanked by 5' and 3' untranslated regions and a single untranslated exon [3], Fig. **1**. Most regions of the *CNR2* gene are highly conserved, but the human has glutamine at position 63 instead of arginine [3, 17] and another SNP H316Y has been reported and linked to autoimmune disorders [3, 17]. There has been little or no data on the role of CB2Rs in neuropsychiatric disorders. However in neurological disorders associated with inflammation, the expression of CB2Rs has been reported in limited populations of microglial including plaque-associated glia in Alzheimer's disease brains [18, 19]. Indeed our studies provide the first evidence for a role of CB2Rs in depression and substance abuse [5, 14, 20, 21]. We and others have identified splice variants of the human CB1Rs and CB2Rs but have thus far been poorly characterized for functional specificity apart from the broad roles associated with CB1R and CB2R subtypes. Alternative splicing of RNAs appears to be more common than previously thought in people, and can generate a variety of proteins, with most genes producing at least two variants. The characterization of CBR variants will add validity to the functional evidence for the existence of multiple cannabinoid receptor subtypes. It has been demonstrated *in vitro* that amino-terminal processing of the hCB1R may involve rapid N-terminal truncation in the cytoplasm prior to translocation to the endoplasmic reticulum membrane. It was suggested that such a truncation process might be a way to create a novel type of CB1R isoforms but exactly how the truncated CB1R may be formed and how the processing is regulated remain to be determined [22]. In comparison to the monoaminergic system, the application of modern techniques to cannabinoid research is new. For example molecular cloning has revealed the presence of serotonin (5-hydroxytryptamine; 5-HT) receptor subtypes, which can be subdivided in seven subfamilies [23] and 15 serotonin (5-HT) receptor subtypes and growing. New knowledge on cannabinoid post-transcriptional and post-translational modifications, such as alternate splicing and perhaps RNA editing may indicate formation of multiple proteins that could unravel specific mechanisms associated with numerous behavioral and physiological effects of marijuana use. The cloning and sequencing of *CNR1* gene from 62 species have also been reported [24] and await full characterization. As predicted here the identification and characterization of these putative CBR isozymes and different elements of the ECS may reveal novel targets for medication development. However the limitless signaling capabilities and the endless complexity of the cannabinoid system require continuous intensive investigation. Specific genetic variants and polymorphisms in multiple genes including variations in the ECS genes have been associated with neuropsychiatric and other pathophysiology of human diseases [25]. It is to be noted that depending on the nature of classification, other CBRs exists. The vanilloid receptor 1 (VRI), the site at which capsaicin in hot chili peppers acts, is a site that anandamide is a full agonist. As anandamide is a partial agonist at the CBRs, some have suggested that VR1be classified as a CBR subtype...may be CB3. In fact the endocannabinoid that is a full agonist at the CBRs is 2-arachidonyl glycerol (2-AG), [26-28]. Another putative CBR, GPR55 has been suggested as a CBR that increases intracellular calcium and inhibits M current [29]. However, using a strategy for defining cannabinoid receptor functional fingerprints from mutagenesis and molecular recognition literature data, it was noted that hGPR55 does not appear to share similar fingerprint with the hCB1R and hCB2R [30]. While this could not be considered as a proof to exclude GPR55 from the CBR family, the data from other studies strongly suggests that GPR55 is a specific functional receptor for lysophosphatidylinositol receptor [31, 32]. Thus far, it appears that GPR55 is quite distinct from other GPCRs and represents an intriguing and unique therapeutic target whose functional receptor requires further validation and characterization [31]. The implication of variations in other putative CBRs genes will certainly contribute to unraveling the genetic basis of the ECS in neuropsychiatric disorders. We are mainly concerned here with the variations associated with *CNR* genes. However, a number of putative endocannabinoids have been identified and anandamide and 2-AG are better characterized. These endocannabinoids are known to act as retrograde messengers and are released on demand and undergo enzymatic hydrolysis. While 2-AG is metabolized by monoglyceride lipase (MGL) and cyclooxygenase-2 (COX2), anandamide is metabolized by fatty acid amide hydrolase (FAAH) and N-acylethanolamine acid amidase (NAAA). The *FAAH1* gene is located on Human chromosome 1p35-34 and *FAAH2* gene recently identified has been mapped to chromosome Xp11.21 or Xp11.1, while *MGL* gene is on 3q21.3.

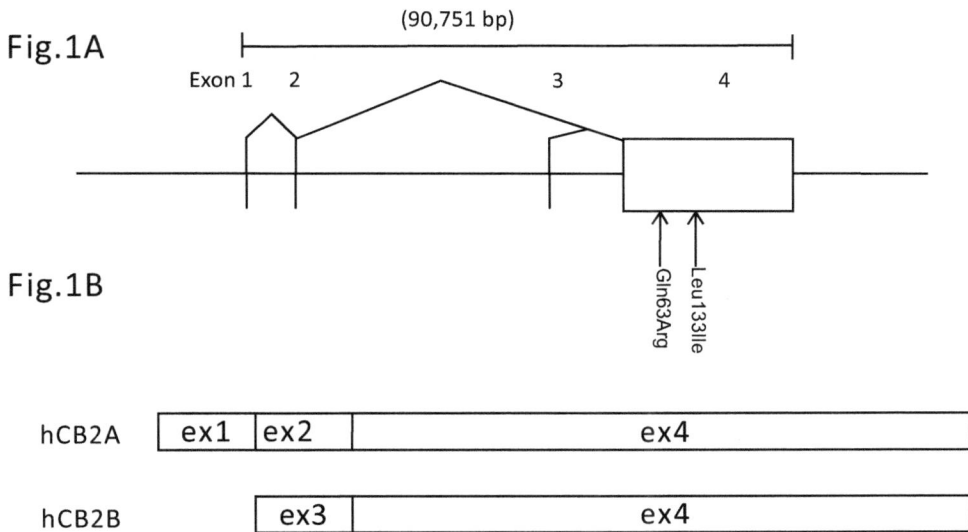

Figure 1: Human CB2 (*CNR2*, 1p36.1) genomic structure and alternative spliced transcripts: A, The gene size is marked in bp; vertical bars represent exons; triangles represent splicing patterns; arrows represent nonsynonymous single nucleotide polymorphisms (SNPs). B, CB2R subtypes, hCB2A and hCB2B alternatively spliced variants are shown under the gene structure.

The results of studies conducted thus far on the polymorphisms and haplotype blocks in endocannabinoid metabolizing enzymes and neuropsychiatric disorders appear to vary due to disparities and confounding factors associated with ethnicity, gender and phenotypes of the population studied [33, 34]. Firm conclusions on the role(s) of variations and polymorphisms in endocannabinoid metabolizing enzymes in neuropsychiatry and their diagnostic value and use in pharmacogenomics needs more study.

CNR1 and *CNR2* Gene Variations in Neuropsychiatric Disorders

CBRs and especially CB1Rs have been described as one of the most abundant binding sites in the human brain and many studies have focused on the *CNR1* gene variants in neuropsychiatric disturbances. Hence *CNR1* gene is a candidate for association and linkage studies not only in the effects of substance abuse and addiction but also with other neuropsychiatric disorders. However, polymorphisms in *CNR2* gene in neuropsychiatry gained less attention as CB2Rs were previously thought to be mainly expressed in immune cells and not expressed in neurons contrary to new research [5, 14, 21 35, 36-40]. To date many *CNR1* variants have been studied and implicated in different populations for their impact on a number of neuropsychiatric disorders including substance abuse and addiction, depression, schizophrenia, anxiety, ADHD, PTSD, impulsivity, neurological disorders including Alzheimer's, Parkinson's Huntington's, Multiple Sclerosis, Amyotrophic lateral sclerosis and more (Table **1**). The FAAH mutant P129T is well known and its strong association with problem drug use received much attention (Sipe JC *et al.* Proc Natl Acad Sci USA 99, 8394–9, 2002). Earlier studies on *CNR1* gene variations were on the triplet repeat polymorphism – the $(AAT)_n$ repeats and on the nonsynonymous 1359A>G polymorphism (rs1049353). For the $(AAT)_n$ triplet repeat polymorphism, and with other variants studied, caution is required as neuropsychiatric disorders appear to vary due to disparities and confounding factors associated with ethnicity, gender and phenotypes of the population studied [33, 34]. These initial studies found associations of these variants with schizophrenia, P300 event related potentials and substance dependence [41-45].

In our previous mapping of the *CNR1* gene locus [9], we conducted association studies between polymorphisms and haplotype-specific expression patterns in three human populations. Common human *CNR1* variants assessed in this study reveal patterns of linkage disequilibrium in European- and in African-American populations. It was also shown that a 5'*CNR1* 'TAG' haplotype displays significant allelic frequency differences between substance abusers and controls in European-American, African-American and Japanese samples [9]. In a review and meta-analysis of study conducted on three of the most studied *CNR1* gene

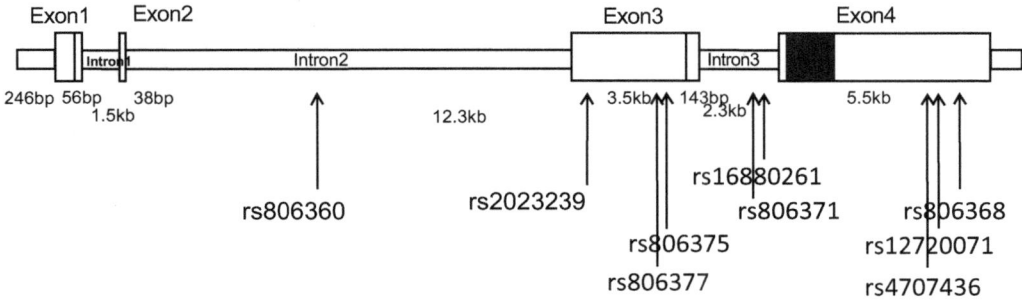

Genetic structure of *CNR1* transcripts

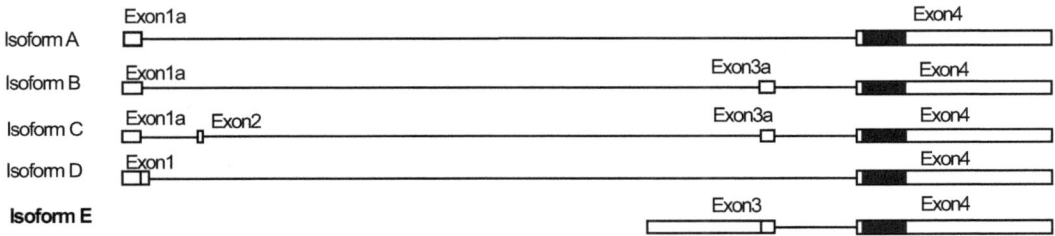

Figure 2: *CNR*1 gene structure showing 4 exons with some introns. A number of ESTs have been identified and some of the SNPs discussed and in Table **1** are shown. The CNR1 gene is in human chromosome 6q15. The currently identified structures of *CNR1* isoforms are indicated.

polymorphisms rs1049353, rs806379 and the (AAT)$_n$ in addictive disorders, it was reported that only the (AAT)$_n$ repeats (n$\geq$16) in the Caucasian population were significantly associated with substance dependence [46]. However, specifically the rs1049353 SNP in the *CNR1* gene was found to be associated with heroin addiction only in Caucasian population [47]. While some polymorphisms in the *CNR1* gene have been associated with some aspects of drug abuse and addiction such as the (AAT)$_n$ triplet repeat, rs64546774, rs1049353 and rs806368 (Table **1**), many other polymorphisms were not replicable probably due to various confounding and co-morbidity factors in the different studies. As CB2Rs was previously thought to be expressed in immune cells and referred to as peripheral CB2Rs, the functional neuronal expression and its variants were less investigated for roles in neuropsychiatric disorders. Indeed our studies from mice to human subjects provided the first evidence for a role of CB2Rs in depression, eating disorders, autism substance abuse [5, 14, 20, 21] and other neuropsychiatric disorders. *CNR2* has 4 exons with CB2A with 3 exons and CB2B with 2 exons;

and there are about 100 SNPs found in more than 1% of the population, which include common cSNPs that change amino acids of the CB2R, including R63Q, Q66R and H316Y. CNVs in Asian and Yoruba population have been reported. Association studies were also performed between polymorphisms in *CNR2* gene and schizophrenia [48], eating disorders [49], depression [1, 5, 14, 35], and alcoholics [20, 34] in two independent case-control populations. We also report on the identification of novel human and rodent CB2R isoforms, their differential tissue expression patterns and regulation by CBR ligands. There are associations between polymorphisms of *CNR2* gene and the neuropsychiatric disorders investigated. Our findings also indicate increased risk of schizophrenia, depression, drug abuse, and eating and autism spectrum disorders in low CB2R function and polymorphisms in *CNR2* gene associated with disease type, ethnicity and gender. In an Italian population using a case control study, the association of bipolar disorder was investigated with three missense SNPs of *CNR2* gene [50]. Genetic association between bipolar disorder and 524A>C polymorphism was reported and the investigators suggested that the CB2R may play a role in bipolar disorders. With the significant association of marijuana use and cannabinoids in modulating the physiological effects of the ECS, the *CNR1* gene has been investigated in not only in food intake and the current obesity epidemic worldwide, but also in a number of neuropsychiatric problems. Many studies have also demonstrated *CNR1* gene polymorphisms and haplotype blocks to investigate a number of parameters associated with eating disorders and obesity [25, 33]. Human *CNR1* gene polymorphisms associated with eating disorders are presented in Table **1**. Marijuana and cannabinoid induced psychoactivity is well documented in animal and human studies and both *CNR1* and *CNR2* gene polymorphisms have been associated with psychosis, multiple sclerosis, depression, attention deficit hyperactivity disorders (ADHD) and bipolar disorders (Table **1**). We and others have studied haplotype blocks in both the *CNR1* and *CNR2* genes in human population and disease and addiction vulnerability [9, 34, 51].

Cannabinoid Receptor (*CNR*) Gene Copy Number Variations (CNVs)

Copy number variation (CNV) is a structural variation in the genome when the number of copies of a gene(s) varies in the population and this is a source of diversity and uniqueness between the genomes of individual humans [52].

Normally in the human genome, we inherit one copy from each parent, but the copy number varies from two to several copies for some genes. Following the completion of the human genome sequence, recent evidence indicates that chunks of DNA and gene(s) can vary in copy-number (with duplications and/or deletions) and in some rare instances the gene(s) may not be expressed. Such CNVs may have functional implications in gene dosage imbalances by loss or gain in the level of gene expression [53, 54], and contribute to various complex human diseases. When CNVs alter the dose of genes critical for normal brain development and adult brain functioning they may cause severe disorders such as autism and schizophrenia [55]. But the vast majorities of most CNVs are harmless and impact human health when they alter gene expression or change gene dosage [55]. Significant advances have been made in mapping gene variations due to single nucleotide polymorphisms (SNPs) which were previously thought to be the most prevalent form of genetic variations. With advances in genomic technologies, analyses of CNVs of individual human genomes have been identified as a major cause of structural variations in those genomes that are more than the changes caused by SNPs [53]. In deed the HapMap project shows that CNVs encompass more nucleotide content per genome than SNPs, underscoring CNV's significance to genetic diversity [54]. It is important to study CNVs that encompass genes involving duplication and deletion of sequences and their role in human health, disease, pharmacotherapeutic and pharmacogenomic responses. It turned out that CNVs are an important form of human genetic variation, contributing more than SNPs to the number of bases differing between human genomes [56, 57]. While *CNR1* and *CNR2* SNPs have been associated with a number of neuropsychiatric disorders (Table **1**), it is still unclear to what extent *CNR* gene CNVs are involved in neuropsychiatric disorders. Numerous CNVs have now been identified with various genome analysis platforms [52]. In our studies many features of *CBR* gene structures, SNPs, CNVs, CPG islands microRNA regulation and the impact of *CNR* gene variants in neuropsychiatry and where possible in rodent models are assessed. A copy number variant (CNV) which is 19.5kb found in 4 out of 2026 people covers exons 3 and 4 and codes amino acid that could alter the expression of CB1Rs. For example CNVs in Asian and Yoruba population have been reported. In our preliminary *CNR2* gene CNV studies, we analyzed one of the CNV regions located in intron of the *CNR2* gene in a human population of Japanese alcoholics DNA samples in comparison to non-alcoholic controls. The CNVs in CNR2 gene region were confirmed to be relatively common in 10 out of 420 Japanese people [data not published]. It was difficult to make a conclusion from the high CNVs of the *CNR2* gene in alcoholics, and more alcoholic DNA samples and samples.

Table 1: Genetic Polymorphisms of Cannabinoid Receptor Genes (*CNR* Genes).

CB1 Two allele DNA polymorphism	Associated with *CNR1* gene [22].
CNR1 rs16880261	Associated with cannabis dependence [65]
CNR1 rs4707436	Associated with endocannabinoid effects [65]
CNR1 rs806377	Associated with endocannabinoid effects [65, 66]
CNR1 rs1049353	Associated with addictive disorders [46, 65, 67]
CNR1 rs2023239	Associated with endocannabinoid effects [65, 67, 68]
CNR1 rs12720071	Associated with endocannabinoid effects [65, 67]
CNR1 rs806375, rs806371, rs806368	Associated with drug addiction [69, 70]
1359 G/A *CNR1* variant	Associated with Alcohol dependence [45, 71]
1359 G/A *CNR1* variant	Not associated with Tourette syndrome [42]
1359 G/A *CNR1* variant	Not associated with Alcohol Withdrawal tremens [72]
1359 G/A *CNR1* variant	Associated with weight loss [73, 74]
3813 A/G and 4895 A/G variant	Associated with obesity in men [75]
CNR1 SNPs	Not association in obesity in German Children [76]
CNR1 SNPs	Associated with obesity and BMI [77-80]
CNR1, *FAAH*, *DRD2* gene	Associated with comorbidity of alcoholism & antisocial [81]
(*DRD2* is dopamine D2 receptor)	
(AAT)n repeat of *CNR1* gene.	Conflicting associations with drug dependence [7, 82-85]
CNR1 variants, SNPs, 'TAG' haplotype	Associated with polysubstance abuse [9]
CNR1 SNPs	Not associated with polysubstance abuse [87]
CNR1 SNPs	Associated with cannabis dependence [65, 88-90]
CBR haplotype	Associated with fewer cannabis dependence symptoms in adolescents [66, 91, 92]
CNR1 SNPs	Associated with alcohol and nicotine dependence [93, 94]
CNR1 SNPs	No association with anorexia nervosa [76, 95]
CNR1 (AAT)n repeats	Associated with restricting and binging/purging anorexia nervosa [96]
CNR1 (AAT)n repeats	Associated with depression in Parkinson's disease [97]
CNR1 SNPs	Associated to striatal responses to facial exp [12]

Table 1: contd….

(AAT)n repeats	Association with ADHD in alcoholics [98, 99]
CNR1 SNP haplotype	Risk factor for ADHD and PTSD [98]
1359 G/A *CNR1* variant	Associated with schizophrenia [44]
(AAT)n repeats	Not associated with schizophrenia [100, 101] and mood disorders [102].
(AAT)n repeats	Associated with schizophrenia [103].
(AAT)n repeats	Associated with hebephrenic schizophrenia [104, 105]
CNR1 variants	Associated with depression and anxiety [13]
CNR1 variants and (AAT)n repeats	Associated with impulsivity [106]
1359 G/A CNR1 tag SNP	Associated with antipsychotic response but not schizophrenia [107].
CNR1 SNPs	No association with cognitive impairment in MS [108]
CB2 *CNR2* SNPs and haplotypes	Associated with human Osteoporosis [17]
CNR2 SNPs	Not associated with myocardial infarction or cardiovascular risk factors [109]
CNR2 SNPs	Associated with bone mass [110]
CNR2 (Q63R) SNP	Risk factor for autoimmune disorders [3].
CNR2 (Q63R) but not (H316Y)	Associated with alcoholism and depression [20].
CNR2 (rs41311993)	Associated with Bipolar disorder [50]

from other neuropsychiatric disorders and in other ethnic populations should be analyzed to understand and determine the nature of elevated copy numbers of *CNR2* gene in neuropsychiatric disease risk. Whether the larger *CNR2* gene CNVs in Japanese alcoholics compared to non-alcoholics are associated with the disease is unknown and the phenotypic effects are often unclear and unpredictable, with larger CNVs [53, 54]. However the bigger the CNV, the more likely it will cause a change in gene dosage [55]. Therefore, the underlying pathogenic mechanism for the larger *CNR2* gene CNV obtained in the sample analyzed in the alcoholics is currently unknown.

Consequences of *CNR1* and *CNR2* Variants

Many *CNR* gene SNPs and their role in predisposing to disease have been well documented and studied (Table **1**), but studies on *CNR* gene CNVs have been less studied and our understanding of the functional impact of CNVs in neuropsychiatry is still limited [56]. Many studies have focused on analysis of regions in the human genome that vary in copy number in specific disorders, but others have focused on analysis on regions that the copy number never seems to vary in the general population [56]. With such a strategy, significant associations between some copy number stable regions have been identified in some patients with intellectual disability or autism, but not in controls [56]. It was therefore proposed that copy number stable regions can be used to complement maps of known CNVs to facilitate interpretation of patient data [56]. Overall some CNVs which may either be inherited or caused by *de novo* mutations, have been shown to explain some of the genetic contribution to common diseases and may also explain rare uncharacterized disorders [56, 58]. Other factors associated with consequences of CNVs include whether the copy number variant changes the sequence or relative location of specific segments of genomic DNA that act as enhancers or suppressors of gene expression [57]. The higher number of *CNR* gene CNVs and the length of the *CNR1* trinucleotide, AAT repeats may be associated with aberrant *CNR* gene expression and probably modifies cannabinoid induced biological function. CNVs which are highly prevalent form of genomic variation can also depend on the phenotypic and cellular context, and on the environmental background [57, 58]. For example CNVs in chromosome 6q14.1 and 5q13.2 have been reported to be associated with alcohol dependence [59]. The endocannabinoid system is involved in neuropsychiatric disorders and CB1Rs appear to be the most abundant binding receptor protein in many brain regions. A number of *CNR1* gene SNPs (Table **1**) are involved in many neuropsychiatric conditions. *CNR1* and *CNR2* gene polymorphisms are also associated with the effects of drugs of abuse and addiction and withdrawal process. The clinical consequences of CNV in the coding and non-coding *CNR* gene sequences associated with human phenotypes and disorders are unknown, but with new microarray and sequencing technologies, the (epi)genetic contributions to *CNR2* gene CNV can be determined. With advances in genomic technologies and the analysis and identification of *CNR* gene CNVs may uncover the relationship between *CNR* gene CNVs to phenotype and disease. Significant progress in understanding the nature of CNVs in the human genome has been achieved, but not yet extended to *CNR* gene CNVs apart from our pilot study described above. Yet accumulating evidence suggests the importance of CNVs in the etiology of neuropsychiatric disorders [60]. More studies are needed to determine the role and contribution of *CNR* gene CNV to conditions of endocannabinoid system disorders. We do not know if *CNR* gene CNVs will affect the entire subtype *CNR* genes and function and whether this may be a factor with marijuana use as medicine or in the biological effects after smoking marijuana and the propensity for its addictive potential in humans. But precise and accurate data from new genomic technologies will facilitate not only *CNR* gene CNVs but also other structural variants in individual genomes to disease susceptibilities and drug responses [61, 62]. Many CNVs have been reported to affect complex diseases including, autism, schizophrenia, bipolar disorder, obesity, Crohn's disease, neurological disorders, cardiovascular disease, nicotine metabolism and tobacco-related diseases and more [62]. Ultimately creating animal models of neuropsychiatric disorders that reflect human CNV will provide insight into human neuropsychiatric disorders that will contribute to novel drug screening for these disorders [63]. Great potential exists for CNVs along with other genomic variants including SNPs to explain and predict disorders and traits in the future, but great challenges exist for understanding the relationship between genomic changes and the phenotypes that might be predicted and may be treated or prevented [64].

SUMMARY, CONCLUSIONS AND FUTURE PERSPECTIVES

We now know that CNVs and other variants of the human genome are more prevalent than SNPs that have been well studied and analyzed and have been linked to human disorders. With many thousands of SNPs in the human genome, and some associated with CNRs, it appears their contributions to the genetic basis of complex diseases are relatively small effects. This has created the possibility of other genomic variants, epigenetic, and other nongenetic contributions to complex human diseases. For the endocannabinoid system many SNPs for both CB1 and CB2 receptors have been identified and characterized in a number of neuropsychiatric disorders. Our preliminary data indicated high CNVs in the *CNR2* gene in Japanese alcoholic patients compared to controls. It was difficult to make a conclusion from the high CNVs of the *CNR2* gene in alcoholics, and more alcoholic DNA samples and samples from other neuropsychiatric disorders and in other ethnic populations should be analyzed to understand and determine the nature of elevated copy numbers of *CNR2* gene in neuropsychiatric disease risk. Numerous CNVs have now been identified with various genome analysis platforms. Whether the larger *CNR2* gene CNVs in Japanese alcoholics compared to non-alcoholics are associated with the disease is unknown and the phenotypic effects are often unclear and unpredictable, with larger CNVs [53, 54]. However the bigger the CNV, the more likely it will cause a change in gene dosage [55]. Therefore, the underlying pathogenic mechanism for the larger *CNR2* gene CNV obtained in the sample analyzed in the alcoholics is currently unknown. While *CNR1* and *CNR2* SNPs have been associated with a number of neuropsychiatric disorders (Table **1**), it is still unclear to what extent *CNR* gene CNVs are involved in neuropsychiatric disorders. Thus it is important to study CNVs that encompass genes involving duplications and deletions of sequences and their role in human health, disease, pharmacotherapeutic and pharmacogenomic responses.

ACKNOWLEDGEMENTS

We thank Dr. Qing-Rong Liu for our collaboration and pivotal work on cannabinoid receptor gene structures and revision of *CNR2* gene features and for helpful comments and suggestions. ESO, SS, and CML are supported by WPUNJ and ESO is also supported by NIH grant DA032890. We are forever indebted to Norman Schanz and Dr. Robert Benno for laboratory animal support and the Dean Dr. Ken Wolf for support of student workers for the maintenance of research animals.

CONFLICT OF INTEREST

The author(s) confirm that no conflict of interest in this chapter.

REFERENCES

[1]   Onaivi ES, Sugiura T, DiMarzo V, eds. Endocannabinoids: The brain and body's marijuana and beyond. Boca Raton: CRC Press, Taylor and Francis Group, 2006.
[2]   Karsak M, Cohen-Solal M, Freudenberg *et al*. Cannabinoid receptor type 2 gene is associated with human osteoporosis. Human Molecular Genetics 2005; 14: 3389-3396.
[3]   Sipe JC, Arbour N, Gerber A, *et al*. Reduced endocannabinoid immune modulation by a common cannabinoid 2 (CB2) receptor gene polymorphism: possible risk for autoimmune disorders. J Leukoc Biol 2005; 78: 231-238.
[4]   At L, Ogdie MN, Jarvelin MR, *et al*. Association of the cannabinoid receptor gene (CNR1) with ADHD and post-traumatic stress disorder. Am J Med Genet B Neuropsychiatr Genet 2008; 147: 1488-1489.
[5]   Onaivi ES, Ishiguro H, Gong J-P, *et al*. Discovery of the presence and functional expression of cannabinoid CB2 receptors in brain. Ann N Y Acad Sci 2006; 1074: 514-536.

[6]   Cota D, Marscicano G, Lutz B, *et al.* Endogenous cannabinoid system as a modulator of food intake. International J Obesity 2003; 27: 289-301.

[7]   Jesudason D, Wittert G. Endocannabinoid system in food intake and metabolic regulation. Curr Opin Lipidol 2008; 19: 344-348.

[8]   Serra G, Fratta, W. A possible role for the endocannabinoid system in the neurobiology of depression. Clinical Practice and Epidemiology in Mental Health 2007; 325: 1-11.

[9]   Zhang PW, Ishiguro H, Ohtsuki T, *et al.* Human cannabinoid receptor 1:5' exons, candidate regulatory regions, polymorphisms, haplotypes and association with polysubstance abuse. Molecular Psychiatry 2004; 9: 916-931.

[10]   Palomo T, Kostrzewa RM, Beninger RJ, *et al.* Genetic variation and sgared biological susceptibility underlying comorbidity in neuropsychiatry. Neurotox Res. 2007; 12: 29-42.

[11]   Lovinger DM. Presynaptic modulation by endocannabinoids. Handb Exp Pharmacol 2008; 184: 435-477.

[12]   Chakrabarti B, Kent L, Suckling J, *et al.* Variations in the human cannabinoid receptor (*CNR1*) gene modulate striatal responses to happy faces. Eur J Neurosc 2006; 23: 1944-1948.

[13]   Domschke K, Dannlowski U, Ohrmann P, *et al.* Cannabinoid receptor 1 (*CNR1*) gene: Impact on anti-depressant treatment response and emotion processing in major depression. Eur Neuropsychopharmacology 2008; 18: 751-759.

[14]   Onaivi ES, Ishiguro H, Gong J-P, *et al.* Brain neuronal CB2 cannabinoid receptors in drug abuse and depression: From mice to human subjects. 2008; PLoS one 3: e1640.

[15]   Tyndale RF. Genetics of alcohol and tobacco use in humans. Ann Med 2003; 35; 94-121.

[16]   Onaivi ES, Chaudhuri G, Abaci AS *et al.* Expression of cannabinoid receptors and their gene transcripts in human blood cells. Prog Neuropsychopharmacol Biol Psychiatry 1999; 23: 1062-1077.

[17]   Karsak M, Cohen-Solal M, Freudenberg *et al.* Cannabinoid receptor type 2 gene is associated with human osteoporosis. Human Molecular Genetics 2005; 14: 3389-3396.

[18]   Nunez E, Benito C, Pazo MR *et al.* Cannabinoid CB2 receptors are expressed by perivascular microglia cells in the human brain: an immunohistochemical study. Synapse 2004; 53: 208-213.

[19]   Pazos MR, Nunez E, Benito C, *et al.* Role of the endocannabinoid system in Alzheimers's disease: new perspectives. Life Sci 2004; 75: 1907-1915.

[20]   Ishiguro H, Iwasaki S, Teasenfitz L, *et al.* Involvement of cannabinoid CB2 receptor in alcohol preference in mice and alcoholism in humans. The Pharmacogenomics J 2007: 7: 380-385.

[21]   Onaivi ES. Neuropsychobiological evidence for the functional presence and expression of cannabinoid CB2 receptors in the brain. Neuropsychobiology 2006; 54: 231-246.

[22]   Nordstrom R, Andersson H. Amino-terminal processing of the human cannabinoid receptor 1. J Receptor Signal Transduction 2006; 26: 259-267.

[23]   Gerhardt CC, van Heerikhuizen H. Functional characteristics of heterologously expressed 5-HT receptors. Eur J Pharmacol 1997; 334: 1-23.

[24]   Murphy WJ Elzirik E Johnson WE, *et al.* Molecular phylogenetics and origins of placental mammals. Nature 2001; 409: 614-618.

[25]   Vasileiou I, Fotopoulou G, Matzourani M. Evidence for the involvement of cannabinoid receptors' polymorphisms in the pathophysiology of human diseases. Expert Opin Ther Targets 2013; (ahead of print).

[26]   Gonsiorek W, Lunn C, Fan X *et al*. Endocannabinoid 2-Arachidonyl glycerol is a full agonist through human type 2 cannabinoid receptor: Antagonism by anandamide. Mol Pharmacology 2000; 57: 1045-1050.

[27]   Sugiura T, Kishimoto S, Oka S, *et al*. Biochemistry, pharmacology and physiology of 2-arachidonyl glycerol, an endogenous cannabinoid receptor ligand. Prog Lip res 2006; 45: 405-446.

[28]   Sugiura T, Kodaka T, Nakane S, *et al*. Evidence that cannabinoid CB1 receptor is a 2-arachidonyl glycerol receptor. J Biol Chem 1999; 274: 2794-2801.

[29]   Lauckner JE, Jensen JB, Chen H-Y *et al*. GPR55 is a cannabinoid receptor that increases intracellular calcium and inhibits M current. Proc Natl Acad Sci USA 2008; 105: 2699-2704.

[30]   Petitet F, Donlan M, Michel A. GPR55 as a new cannabinoid recptor: still a long way to prove it. Chem Biol drug Des 2006; 67: 252-253.

[31]   Henstridge CM, Balenga NAB, Ford LA *et al*. The GPR55 ligand L-α-lysophosphatidylinositol promotes RhoA-dependent Ca $^{2+}$ signaling and NFAT activation. The Faseb J 2008; 23: 183-193.

[32]   Oka S, Nakajima K, Yamashita A, *et al*. Identification of GPR55 as a lysophosphatidyinositol receptor. Biochem and Biophysical Res Com 2007; 362: 928-934.

[33]   Lopez-Moreno JA, Echeverry-Alzate V, Buhler K-M. The genetic basis of the endocannabinoid system and drug addiction in humans. J Psychopharmacol 2012; 26: 133-143.

[34]   Iwasaki S, Ishiguro H, Higuchi S, Onaivi ES, Arinami T. Association study between alcoholism and endocannabinoid metabolic enzyme genes encoding fatty acid amide hydrolase and monoglyceride lipase in a Japanese population. Psychiatric Genetics 2007; 17: 215-220.

[35]   Onaivi ES, Ishiguro H, Gong J-P *et al*. Functional expression of brain neuronal CB2 cannabinoid receptors are involved in the effects of drugs of abuse and in depression. Ann NY Acad Sci 2008; 1139: 434-449.

[36]   Onaivi ES. Endocannabinoid system, pharmacogenomics and response to therapy. Pharmacogenomics 2010; 11: 907-910.

[37]   Onaivi ES, Ishiguro H, Gu S, Liu QR. CNS effects of CB2 cannabinoid receptors: beyond neuro-immuno-cannabinoid activity. J Psychopharmacol 2012; 26: 92-103.

[38]   Onaivi ES. Commentary: Functional neuronal CB2 cannabinoid receptors in the CNS. Curr Neuropharmacol 2011; 9: 205-208.

[39]   Ishiguro H, Carpio O, Horiuchi Y, Shu A, Higuchi S, Schanz N, Benno R, Arinami T, Onaivi ES. A nonsynonymous polymorphism in cannabinoid CB2 receptor gene is associated with eating disorders in humans and food intake is modified in mice by its ligands. Synapse 2010; 64: 92-96.

[40]   Liu QR, Pan CH, Hishimoto A, Li CY, Xi ZX, Llorente-Berzal A, Viveros MP, Ishiguro H, Arinami T, Onaivi ES, Uhl GR. Species differences in cannabinoid receptor 2 (CNR2 gene): identification of novel human and rodent CB2 isoforms, differential tissue expression and regulation by cannabinoid ligands. Genes Brain Behav 2009; 8: 519-30.

[41]   Comings DE. Genetic factors in drug abuse and dependence. NIDA Res Monogr 1996; 159: 16-48.

[42]   Gadzicki D, Müller-Vahl KR, Heller D *et al*. Tourette syndrome is not caused by mutations in the central cannabinoid receptor (CNR1) gene. Am J Med Genet B Neuropsychiatr Genet 2004; 127: 97-103.

[43]   Johnson JP, Muhleman D, MacMurray J, *et al*. Association between the cannabinoid receptor gene (CNR1) and the P300 event-related potential. Mol Psychiat 1997; 2: 169-171.

[44]   Leroy S, Griffon N, Bourdel MC, *et al*. Schizophrenia and the cannabinoid receptor type 1 (CB1): Association study using a single-base polymorphism in coding exon 1. Am J Med Genet 2001; 105:749-752.

[45]   Schmidt LG, Samochowiec J, Finckh U *et al*. Association of a CB1 cannabinoid receptor gene (CNR1) polymorphism with severe dependence. Drug and Alcohol Dependence 2002; 65: 221-224.

[46]   Benyamina A, Kebir O, Blecha L, Reynaud M, Krebs M-O. CNR1 gene polymorphisms in addictive disorders: a systematic review and meta-analysis. Addiction Biology 2011; 16: 1-6.

[47]   Proudnikov D, Kroslak T, Sipe JC, Randesi M, Li D, Hamon S, Ho A, Ott J, Kreek MJ. Association of polymorphisms of the cannabinoid receptor (*CNR1*) and fatty acid amide hydrolase (*FAAH*) genes with heroin addiction: impact of lonf repeats of *CNR1*. The Pharmacogenomics Journal 2010; 10: 232-242.

[48]   Ishiguro H, Horiuchi Y, Ishikawa M *et al*. Brain cannabinoid CB2 receptor in schizophrenia. Biol Psychiatry 2010; 67: 974-982.

[49]   Ishiguro H, Carpio O, Horiuchi Y, Shu A, Higuchi S, Schanz N, Benno R, Arinami T, Onaivi ES. A nonsynonymous polymorphism in cannabinoid CB2 receptor gene is associated with eating disorders in humans and food intake is modified in mice by its ligands. Synapse 2010; 64: 92-96.

[50]   Minocci D, Massei J, Martino A *et al*. Genetic association between bipolar disorder and 524A>C (Leu133Ile) polymorphism of CNR2 gene, encoding for CB2 cannabinoid receptor. J Affective Disorders 2011; 134: 427-430.

[51]   Hillard CJ, Weinlander KM, Stuhr KL. Contributions of endocannabinoid signaling to psychiatric disorders in humans: Genetic and biochemical evidence. Neuroscience 2012; 204: 207-229.

[52]   Zhang F, Gu W, Hurles ME, Lupski JR. Copy number variation in human health, disease, and evolution. Annual Rev Genomics and Human Genetics 2009; 10: 451-481.

[53]   Kloppocki E, Mundlos S. Copy-number variations, noncoding sequences, and human phenotypes. Annual Rev Genomics and Human Genetics 2011; 12: 53-72.

[54]   Stankiewicz P, Lupski JR. Strructural variation in the human genome and its role in disease. Ann Rev Med 2010; 61: 437-455.

[55]   Clair DS. Structural and copy number variants in the human genome: implications for psychiatry. B J Psychiatry 2013; 202: 5-6.

[56]   Johannsson ACV Feuk L. Characterization of copy number-stable regions in the human genome. Hum Mutat 2011; 32: 947-955.

[57]   Conrad DF, Pinto D, Redon R *et al*. Origins and functional impact of copy number variation in the human genome. Nature 2010; 464: 704-712.

[58]   Wain LV, Armour JAL, Tobin MD. Genomic copy number variation, human health, and disease. Lancet 2009; 374: 340-350.

[59]   Lin P, Hartz SM, Wang J-C *et al*. Copy number variations in 6q14.1 and 5q13.2 are associated with alcohol dependence. Alcohol Clin Exp Res 2012; 36: 1512-1518.

[60]   Horev G, Ellegood J, Lerch JP *et al*. Dosage-dependent phenotypes in models of 16p11.2 lesions found in autism. PNAS 2011; 108: 17076-17081.

[61] Kaname T. A commentary on implication of gene copy number variation in health and disease. J Human Genetics 2012; 57: 79-80.

[62] Almal SH, Padh H. Implications of gene copy-number variation in health and diseases. J Human Genetics 2012; 57: 6-13.

[63] Nomura J, Takunmi T. Animal models of psychiatric disorders that reflect human copy number variation. Neural Plasticity 2012; ID 589524.

[64] Lee C, Scherer SW. The clinical context of copy number variation in the human genome. Expert Rev Mol Med 2012; 12: e8.

[65] Agrawal A, Wetherill L, Dick DM *et al.* Evidence for association between polymorphisms in the cannabinoid receptor 1 (CNR1) gene and cannabis dependence. Am J Med Genet Part B. 2009; 150B: 736-740.

[66] Hopfer CJ, Lessem JM, Hartman CA *et al.* A genome-wide scan influencing adolescent cannabis dependence symptoms: evidence for linkage on chromosomes 3 and 9. Drug Alchol Depend. 2007; 89: 34-41.

[67] Dinu IR, Popa S, Bicu Mihaela, Mota E, Mota M. The implication of CNR1 gene's polymorphism in the modulation of endocannabinoid system effects. Rom J Intern Med 2009; 47: 9-18.

[68] Filbey FM, Schacht JP, Myers US, Chavez RS, Hutchison KE. Individual and additive effects of the CNR1 and FAAH genes on brain response to marijuana use. Neuropsychopharmacology 2010; 35: 967-975.

[69] Corley RP, Zeiger JS, Crowley T *et al.* Association of candidate genes with antisocial drug dependence in adolescents. Drug Alcohol Depend 2008; 96: 1-2.

[70] Zuo L, Kranzler HR, Luo X *et al.* Interaction between two independent CNR1 variants increases risk for cocaine dependence in European Americans: a replication study in a family-based sample and population based sample. Neuropsychopharmacology 2009; 36: 1504-1513.

[71] Gadzicki D, Muller-Vahl K, Stuhrmann M. A frequent polymorphism in the coding exon of the human cannabinoid receptor (CNR1) gene. Molecular and Cellular Probes 1999; 13: 321-323.

[72] Preuss UW, Koller G, Zill P, *et al.* Alcoholism related phenotypes and genetic variants of the CB1 receptor. Eur Arch Psychiatry Clin Neurosci 2003; 253: 275-280.

[73] Aberle J, Fedderwitz I, Klages N, *et al.* Genetic variation in two proteins of the endocannabinoid system and their influence on body mass index and metabolism under low fat diet. Horm Metab Res 2007; 39: 395-397.

[74] Aberle J, Flitsch J, Beck NA *et al.* Genetic variation may influence obesity only under conditions of diet: analysis of three candidate genes. Molecular Genetics and Metabolism. 2008; 95: 188-191.

[75] Russo P, Strazzulo P, Cappuccio DA *et al.* Genetic variations at the endocannabinoid type 1 receptor gene (CNR1) are associated with obesity phenotype in men. J Clinical Endocrinology & Metabolism 2007; 92: 2382-2386.

[76] Muller TD, Reichwald K, Bronner G *et al.* Lack of association of genetic variants in genes of the endocannabinoid system with anorexia nervosa. Child Adolesc Psychiatry Health 2008; 2: 33.

[77] Benzinou M, Chevre JC, Ward KJ, *et al.* Endocannabinoid receptor 1 gene variations increase risk for obesity and modulate body mass index in European populations. Hum Mol Genet 2008; 17: 1916-1921.

[78] Gazzero P, Caruso MG, Notarnicola M, *et al.* Association between cannabinoid type-1 receptor polymorphism and body mass index in a southern Italian population. Int J Obes 2007; 31:908-912.

[79] Jaeger JP, Mattevi VS, Callegri-Jacques SM *et al.* Cannabinoid type-1 receptor gene polymorphisms are associated with central obesity in a Southern Brazilian population. Disease Markers 2008; 25: 67-74.

[80] Peeters A, Beckers S, Mertens I, *et al.* The G1422A variant of the cannabinoid receptor gene (CNR1) is associated with abdominal adiposity in obese men. Endocrine 2007; 31: 138-141.

[81] Hoenicka J, Ponce G, Jimenez-Arriero MA, *et al.* Association in alcoholic patients between psychopathic traits and the additive effect of allelic forms of CNR1 and FAAH endocannabinoid genes, and the 3' region of the DRD2 gene. Neurotox Res 2007; 11: 51-60.

[82] Ballon N, Leroy S, Roy C *et al.* (AAT)n repeat in the cannabinoid receptor gene (CNR1): association with cocaine addiction in an African-Caribbean population. Pharmacogenomics J 2006; 6: 126-130.

[83] Comings DE, Muhleman D Gade R *et al.* Cannabinoid receptor gene (CNR1): association with IV drug use. Mol Psychiat 1997; 2: 161-168.

[84] Covault J, Gelernter J, Kranzler H. Association study of cannabinoid receptor gene (CNR1) alleles and drug dependence. Mol Psychiat 2001; 6: 510-502.

[85] Heller D, Schneider U, Seifert J, *et al.* The cannabinoid receptor gene (CNR1 is not affected in German i.v. drug users. Addict Biol 2001; 6: 183-187.

[86] Zuo L, Kranzler HR, Luo Z *et al.* CNR1 variation modulates risk for drug and alcohol dependence. Biol Psychiatry. 2007; 62: 616-626.

[87] Herman AI, Kranzler HR, Cubells JF *et al.* Association study of the CNR1 gene exon 3 alternative promoter region polymorphisms and substance abuse. Am J Med Genet B Neuropsychiatr Genet. 2006; 141B: 499-503.

[88] Agrawal A, Lynskey MT. Are there genetic influences on addiction: evidence from family, adoption and twin studies? Addiction 2008; 103: 1069-1081.

[89] Agrawal A, Lynskey MT. The genetic epidemiology of cannabis use, abuse and dependence. Addiction 2006; 101: 801-812.

[90] Agrawal A, Morley KI, Hansell NK *et al.* Autosomal linkage analysis for cannabis use behaviors in Australian adults. Drug and Alchol Dependence 2008; 98: 185-190.

[91] Hopfer CJ, Stallings MC, Hewith JK *et al.* Family transmission of marijuana use, abuse, and dependence. J. Am. Acad. Child Adolesc. Psychiatry 2003; 42: 834-841.

[92] Hopfer CJ, Young SE, Purcell S *et al.* Cannabis receptor haplotype associated with fewer cannabis dependence symptoms in adolescents. Am J MedGenet B Neuropsychiatr Genet 2006; 141: 895-901.

[93] Chen X, Williamson VS, An SS *et al.* Cannabinoid receptor 1 gene association with nicotine dependence. Arch Gen Psychiatry 2008; 65: 816-824.

[94] Hutchison KE, Haughley H, Niculescu M *et al.* The incentive salience of alcohol: Translating the effects of genetic variant in CNR1. Arch Gen Psychiatry 65; 841-850.

[95] Muller TD, Reichwald K, Wermter A-K, *et al.* No evidence for an involvement of variants in the cannabinoid receptor gene (CNR1 in obesity in German children and adolescents. Molecular Genetics and Metabolism 2007; 90: 429-434.

[96]   Siegfried Z, Kanyas K, Latzer Y *et al.* Association study of cannabinoid receptor gene (CNR1) alleles and anorexia nervosa: differences between restricting and binging/purging subtypes. Am J Med Genet B Neuropsychiatr Genet 2004; 125: 126-130.

[97]   Barrero FJ, Ampuero I, Morales B, *et al.* Depression in Parkinson's disease is related to a genetic polymorphism of the cannabinoid receptor gene (CNR1). Pharmcogenomics J 2005; 135-141.

[98]   Lu AT, Ogdie MN, Jarvelin MJ, *et al.* Association of the cannabinoid receptor gene (CNR1) with ADHD and post-traumatic stress disorder. Am J Med Genet Part B 2008; 147B: 1488-1494.

[99]   Ponce G, Hoenicka J, Rubio G, *et al.* Association between cannabinoid receptor gene (CNR1) and childhood attention deficit/hyperactivity disorder in Spanish male alcoholic patients. Molecular Psychiatry 2003; 8: 466-467.

[100]   Li T, Liu X, Zhu Z-H, *et al.* No association between (AAT)n repeats in the cannabinoid receptor gene (CNR1) and heroin abuse in a Chinese population. Mol Psychiat 2000; **5**: 128-130.

[101]   Tsai SJ, Wang YC, Hong CJ. Association study of a cannabinoid receptor gene (CNR1) polymorphism and schizophrenia. Psychiatric Genet 2000; 10: 149-151.

[102]   Tsai SJ, Wang YC, Hong CJ. Association study between cannabinoid receptor gene (CNR1) and pathogenesis and psychotic symptoms of mood disorders. Am J Med Genet 2001; 105: 219-221.

[103]   Martinez-Gras I, Hoenicka J, Ponce G, *et al.* (AAT)n repeat in the cannabinoid receptor gene, CNR1: association with schizophrenia in a Spanish population. Eur Arch Psychiatry Clin Neurosci 2006; 256: 437-441.

[104]   Chavarria-Siles I, Contrras-Rojas J, Hare E, *et al.* Cannabinoid receptor 1 gene (CNR1) and susceptibility to a quantitative phenotype for hebephrenic schizophrenia. Am J Med Genet 2008; 147: 279-284.

[105]   Ujike H, Takaki M, Nakata K *et al.* CNR1, central cannabinoid receptor gene, associated with susceptibility to hebephrenic schizophrenia. Mol Psychiatry 2002; 7: 515-518.

[106]   Ehlers CL, Slutske WS, Lind PA, *et al.* Association between single nucleotide polymorphisms in the cannabinoid receptor gene (CNR1) and impulsivity in South west California Indians. Twin Research and Human Genetics 2007; 10: 805-811.

[107]   Hamdani N, Tabeze J-P, Ramoz N, *et al.* The *CNR1* gene as a pharmacogenetic factor for antipsychotics rather than a susceptibility gene for schizophrenia. Eur Neuropsychopharmacology 2008; 18: 34-40.

[108]   Woolmore JA, Stone MJ, Holley SL *et al.* Polymorphism of the cannabinoid 1 recpetor gene and cognitive impairment in multiple sclerosis. Multiple Sclerosis 2008; 14: 177-182.

[109]   Reinhard W, Stark K, Neureuther K, *et al.* Common polymorphisms in the cannabinoid CB2 gene (CNR2) are not associated with myocardial infarction and cardiovascular risk factors. Int J Mole Med 2008; 22: 165-174.

[110]   Yamada Y, Ando F, Shimkata H, *et al.* Association of candidate gene polymorphisms with bone mineral density in community-dwelling Japanese women and men. Int J Mole Med 2007; 19: 791-801.

Send Orders for Reprints at reprints@benthamscience.net

CHAPTER 2

The Role of Endocannabinoids and Arachidonic Acid Metabolites in Emesis

Nissar A. Darmani[*] and Seetha Chebolu

Department of Basic Medical Sciences, College of Osteopathic Medicine of the Pacific, Western University of Health Sciences, Pomona, CA 91766, USA

Abstract: Research in the last decade has well established that Δ^9-THC and related synthetic direct-acting cannabinoid $CB_{1/2}$ receptor agonists (such as WIN55,212-2, CP55,940) possess broad-spectrum antiemetic efficacy against diverse emetogens *via* activation of CB_1 receptors. We now extend the antiemetic efficacy of these $CB_{1/2}$ agonists against 20-hydroxyPGE$_2$ and arachidonoyl-2-chloroethylamide (ACEA). Increasing evidence in more recent years also suggests that chronic use of large doses of Δ^9-THC in humans can induce intractable vomiting referred to as the cannabinoid hyperemesis syndrome. This chapter discusses the antiemetic/proemetic potential of endocannabinoids such as anandamide, virodhamine, NADA and 2-AG as well as that of synthetic indirect-acting cannabimimetic agents that increase endogenous endocannabinoid tissue levels either by inhibiting their metabolism {such as FAAH and MAGL inhibitors (*e.g.* AA-5-HT/URB597 and JZL184, respectively)} or by blocking their reuptake (*e.g.* OMDM1, VDM11, AM404). To date published findings indicate that exogenous administration of either 2-AG or anandamide can lead to both antiemetic and proemetic effects depending upon the laboratory conditions used and/or the emetic models utilized. Furthermore, lack of full dose-response studies in most emesis models further confounds a firm conclusion. Likewise, available data indicate that the well-studied FAAH inhibitor URB597 and the above reuptake blockers can prevent vomiting induced by some but not all tested emetogens, and at large doses they can be emetic by themselves. It appears that while the antiemetic efficacy of exogenously-administered endocannabinoids (as well as that of drugs that increase their endogenous levels) is due to activation of CB_1- or CB_1/TRPV1-receptors, *e.g.* 2-AG or anandamide, respectively, their emetic potential reside in their tendency to be rapidly metabolized to the proemetic agent arachidonic acid and its downstream emetic metabolites such as prostaglandins (*e.g.* PGE$_2$, 20-hydroxyPGE$_2$ and PGF$_{2\alpha}$), leukotrienes (*e.g.* LTC$_4$ and LTD$_4$) and/or 20-HETE. In fact some analogs of anandamide such as ACEA (a selective CB_1 agonist) that are more rapidly metabolized are proemetic, while its more stable congeners (methanandamide or ACPA) lack emetic activity. Thus, exogenously-administered endocannabinoids and drugs that enhance their tissue levels can be antiemetic under certain conditions but unlike Δ^9-THC they generally lack broad-spectrum antiemetic efficacy.

*Address coresspondence to Nissar A. Darmani: Western University of Health Sciences, College of Osteopathic Medicine of the Pacific, Department of Basic Medical Science, Pomona, CA91766, USA; Tel: (909) 469 5654; Lab Tel: (909) 469 5218; Fax: (909) 469 5698; E-mail: ndarmani@westernu.edu

Eric Murillo-Rodríguez, Emmanuel S. Onaivi, Nissar A. Darmani & Edward Wagner (Eds.)

Keywords: Emesis, cannabinoids, Δ^9-THC, virodhamine, ACEA, CP55,940, WIN55,212-2, Prostaglandin $F_{2\alpha}$, Prostaglandin E_2, 20-hydroxy- prostaglandin E_2, Prostaglandin G_2, 20-HETE, Area postrema, nucleus tractus solitarius.

INTRODUCTION

The discovery of delta-9-tetrahydrocannabinol (Δ^9-THC) in the early 1960s as the major psychoactive component of cannabis plant was a significant landmark in establishing how cannabis exerts its pharmacological effects [1]. Subsequent milestones in understanding the cellular actions of Δ^9-THC were: i) the cloning and further identification of its two G protein-coupled receptors in 1990 and 1993, called the cannabinoid CB_1 and CB_2 receptors, and ii) the discovery of endogenous cannabinoid receptor ligands (endocannabinoids) arachidonoyl-ethanolamide (AEA) in 1992, and 2-arachidonoylglycerol (2-AG) in 1995. Δ^9-THC, many of its synthetic analogs (such as WIN55, 212-2 and CP55, 940) and the discussed endocannabinoids often do not distinguish between the CB_1 and CB_2 receptors, and therefore are termed herewith as $CB_{1/2}$ receptor agonists. When activated both cannabinoid receptors inhibit adenylyl cyclase and activate mitogen-activated protein kinase by signaling through Gi/o proteins. The CB_1 receptor also mediates activation of A-type and inwardly rectifying potassium currents, inhibition of N- and P/Q-type calcium currents, as well as signals through Gs proteins. Cannabinoid CB_1 receptors are found mainly at the terminals of central and peripheral neurons, where they usually inhibit the ongoing release of a number of different excitatory and inhibitory neurotransmitters. CB_2 receptors are located predominantly in immune cells, and when activated, modulate immune cell migration and cytokine release both outside and within the brain. Although more recently other putative endocannabinoids have been described (*e.g.* noladin ether, N-arachidonoyl-dopamine (NADA) and virodhamine), only 2-AG and anandamide are currently considered to be of physiological importance. Moreover, its full agonist efficacy combined with μM basal abundance in the brain and other tissues, strongly suggest that 2-AG, rather than anandamide, is the true endogenous ligand for both CB_1 and CB_2 receptors [2]. Indeed, anandamide and NADA behave as agonists of both CB_1 and the transient potential vanilloid-1 (TRPV1) receptors, whereas virodhamine appears to be a potential endogenous antagonist of the CB_1 receptor [3]. Moreover, though

NADA is present at low (< 1 pmol/g) levels in some brain regions, neither noladin ether nor virodhamine are present in the rodent CNS at concentrations above detection levels in sensitive assay systems [3].

2-AG appears to be the primary lipid-derived retrograde signaling molecule that is synthesized upon demand in postsynaptic neurons. Subsequent to its liberation to presynaptic terminals, 2-AG activates presynaptic CB_1 receptors to inhibit the release of both excitatory and inhibitory neurotransmitters [4]. Anandamide may also act *via* presynaptic TRPV1 receptor as a retrograde messenger. As discussed later, arachidonic acid (AA) is a downstream metabolite of both endocannabinoids, and its free form can be metabolized by diverse enzymes to produce several dozen different compounds. Although initially AA was also viewed as a retrograde messenger, but more recent studies indicate that a number of its downstream products, such as some PGs, act on corresponding presynaptic receptors to inhibit neurotransmitter release [4].

In the past two decades significant strides have been made in understanding the biochemical pharmacology of anandamide and 2-AG. However, other putative endocannabinoids have not been studied at such depth. Likewise, the gastrointestinal pharmacology of eicosanoids, including AA and its downstream products, remain to be fully explored. In the context of emesis, it is well established that where tested, structurally diverse phytocannabinoids (*e.g.* Δ^9-THC; Δ^8-THC; cannabidiol) and direct-acting synthetic cannabinoids (*e.g.* CP55,940; HU-2010; WIN55,212-2; nabilone; levonantradol; nonabine) possess broad-spectrum antiemetic efficacy, *via* stimulation of cannabinoid CB_1 receptor, against diverse emetogens in several vomit competent-species including humans [6-10]. However, as will be discussed later, Δ^9-THC and related agents may also induce vomiting under some conditions by themselves. The broad-spectrum antiemetic potential of both exogenously-administered endocannabinoids and indirect cannabinoid agonists which increase the endogenous levels of 2-AG and/or anandamide (*i.e.* inhibitors of their metabolism and/or reuptake) are under investigation. Thus far, only a few of such agents have been tested and the scant published findings are not always consistent in terms of their anti- and/or proemetic potential across both the tested classes of agents employed and the emesis models used. On the other hand, the emetic potential of some of the tested agents downstream of endocannabinoids, particularly those of AA-derived eicosanoids, such as certain prostaglandins and leukotrienes, are more consistent. The purpose of this chapter is to: i) review published findings regarding the emetic/antiemetic potential of the well-established endocannabinoids 2-AG and anandamide and some of their downstream eicosanoid products, ii) present some of the author's new data concerning the emetic potential of the putative endocannabinoids virodhamine and noladin ether, as well as representatives of AA-related eicosanoids such as some prostaglandins (*e.g.* PGE_2; $PGF_{2\alpha}$; 20-hydroxy$PGF_{2\alpha}$; PGG_2; PGH_2), prostacyclins (*e.g.* PGI_2), hydroxyeicosatetraenoic acids (HETEs such as 20-HETE), hydroperoxy eicosattraenoic acids (HPETEs such as 5(S) HPETE), and epoxyeicosatetraenoic acids (EETs such as 5(6)EpETrE and ±11(12)EpETrE) in the least shrew model of emesis; iii) discuss the relative role of rapid metabolism in emetic efficacy of 2-AG, anandamide and some of their related products.

Interplay Between Endocannabinoid and Eicosanoid Biosynthetic and Metabolic Pathways

Although endocannabinoids and eicosanoids share a common lipid precursor pool, their synthesis, degradation, signaling and their putative pharmacological actions have often been discussed independently of each other. While endocannabinoid signaling can occur in the absence of eicosanoid pathway activation and *vice versa*, several findings [5] suggest possible cross-talk between these pathways. In fact: i) both pathways share a common precursor lipid pool, ii) the lipases that initiate both sets of pathways respond to some of the same second messengers, iii) some enzymes of the eicosanoid biosynthetic pathways (*e.g.* COX-2) can metabolize endocannabinoids as well as AA., iv) both anandamide and 2-AG are sources of free AA and related metabolites, v) some oxygenated endocannabinoid products (*e.g.* ethanolamide of $PGE_2 = PGE_2$-EA) that do not bind cannabinoid receptors have high affinity for prostanoid EP receptors, vi) some oxygenated endocannabinoids act at distinct receptors (*e.g.* $PGF_{2\alpha}$-EA). Such interactions have already been explored to some extent and the results suggest that some potential cross-talk occurs both in cultured cells and *in vivo* [5]. Furthermore, certain *in vivo* effects of Δ^9-THC are also dependent upon production of eicosanoids such as PGE_2 [11].

Endocannabinoid Synthesis and Metabolism

Although several routes exist for anandamide and 2-AG formation [2,5,12], the primary route of anandamide synthesis begins with the membrane phospholipid precursor, N-arachidonoylphosphatidylethanolamine (NAPE), which is formed by the transfer of AA from the sn-1 position of a donor phospholipid to phosphatidylethanolamine (PE) by N-acyltransferase (NAT) (Fig. **1**). Hydrolysis of this precursor by an N-acylphosphatidylethanolamine- hydrolyzing phospholipase D (NAPE-PLD) produces anandamide. Synthesis of 2-AG begins with activation of phospholipase C (PLC) which hydrolyzes phosphatidylinositol 4,5-bisphosphate (PIP_2), producing diacylglycerol (DAG) (Fig. **1**). When serving as an endocannabinoid, 2-AG is produced almost exclusively by the hydrolysis of DAG *via* sn-1-selective diacylglycerol lipases α and β. Once generated, 2-AG is primarily (over 85%) hydrolyzed by monoacylglycerol lipase (MAGL) to arachidonic acid and glycerol, and to a smaller extent by other lipases. Fatty acid amide hydrolase (FAAH) is the enzyme primarily responsible for the hydrolysis of anandamide to AA and ethanolamine. FAAH can also hydrolyze 2-AG to a minor extent. One can potentiate the activity of endocannabinoids by drugs that either block their reuptake (*e.g.* OMDM1; UCM-707), or inhibit their biotransformation such as inhibitors of FAAH (URB-597; arachidonoylserotonin) and MAGL (JZL184).

Eicosanoid Synthesis and Metabolism

Eicosanoids are 20-carbon signaling molecules derived from omega (ω)-3 and ω-6 essential free fatty acids, eicosapentaenoic acid, AA, or γ-linoleic acid. The eicosanoids may include prostaglandins (PGs), prostacyclins (PGIs), thromboxanes (TXs), and leukotrienes (LTs) [5] (Fig. **1**). AA is an ω-6 tetraunsaturated fatty acid that is a component of the mammalian cell membrane. A wide range of stimuli may trigger the activation of phospholipases A2 and C to generate intracellular AA from membrane phospholipid pools. Then, the free AA can be subject to oxidative metabolism by cyclooxygenase 1 and/or 2 (COX-1; COX-2) to form the endoperoxide PGH_2. Tissue-specific metabolism of PGH_2 by a group of PG synthases will yield the biologically active PGs (*e.g.* PGE_2, PGD_2, $PGF_{2\alpha}$), prostacyclin (PGI_2), and thromboxane A_2 (TxA_2). COX-2 may also

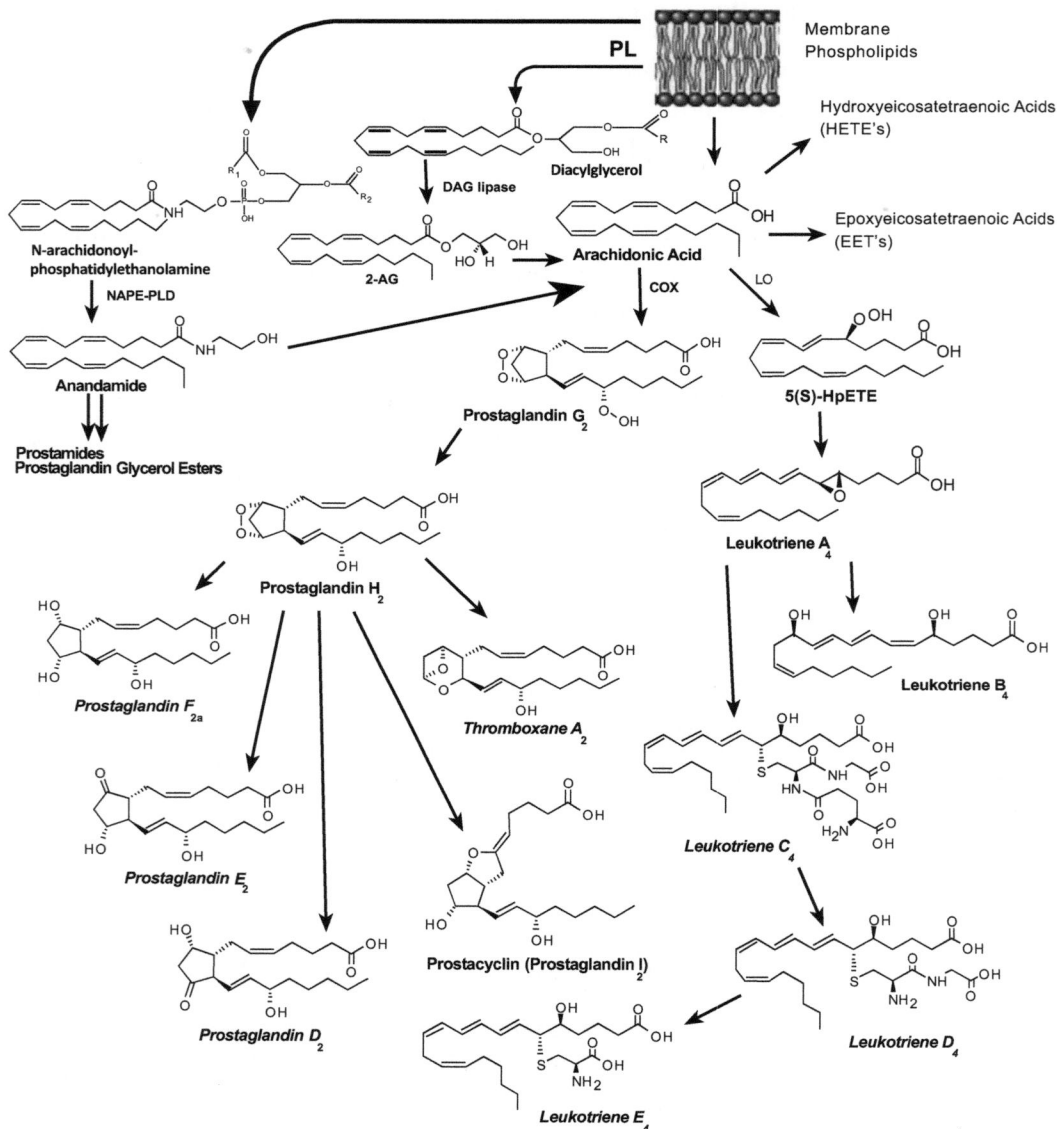

Figure 1: Biosynthesis of eicosanoids and endocannabinoids. In both cases, membrane phospholipids are enzymatically metabolized to produce the lipid-based eicosanoids and endocannabinoids. The endocannabinoids, anandamide and 2-arachidonoylglycerol, are produced from phospholipids *via* phospholipase (PL) activity. Both species can be metabolized back to arachidonic acid, or modified further to produce prostamides or prostaglandin glycerol esters. The other eicosanoids are produced *via* several different enzymes acting upon arachidonic acid, which is itself produced enzymatically from phospholipids. Several "families" of eicosanoids are produced from arachidonic acid, depending on the initial enzymatic pathway. The main

metabolites of two families with known emetogenic variants are depicted. The prostanoid (prostaglandin-related) family is produced *via* cyclooxygenase activity (COX), and the leukotriene family is produced *via* lipoxygenase (LO) activity. Dozens of related metabolites exist within each of these families, so for clarity only major emesis-related metabolites and their precursors are shown in detail. The cysteinyl leukotrienes, which have a glutathione-derived moiety which may allow cross-reactivity with cisplatin-transporting proteins, are the leukotrienes C4, D4, and E4. Abbreviations: 2-AG – 2-arachidonoylglycerol; COX – cyclooxygenases; LO – lipoxygenases; PL – phospholipases.

convert both anandamide and 2-AG to corresponding prostaglandin ethanolamides (PG-EAs) and prostaglandin glycerols (PG-Gs). The free AA may also be metabolized by several lipoxygenases (LOs) to yield hydroperoxyeicosatetraenoic acids (HPETEs). These compounds can be reduced to the corresponding hydroxyeicosatetraenoic acids (HETEs). Generation of LTs occurs when free AA is converted by 5-lipoxygenase (5-LO) to produce 5-hydroxyeicosatetraenoic acid to form leukotriene A_4 (LTA$_4$). This parent leukotriene can then be converted into LTB$_4$ or conjugated to the peptide glutathione to generate the parent cysteinyl leukotriene LTC$_4$. The latter can be stripped of a glutamic acid residue to form LTD$_4$, which can be stripped of its glycine residue to produce LTE$_4$. Furthermore, LTC$_4$ can be converted *via* carboxypeptidase activity to LTF$_4$. In addition, the free AA can be oxidized at each of its double bonds or at the ω-terminus by cytochrome P450 (CYPP450), leading to the epoxyeicosatrienoic acids (EETs) or HETEs.

Pathophysiology of Emesis

Vomiting (emesis) is a multi-neurotransmitter-mediated complex reflex. Emesis has developed to varying degrees in different species, which allows an animal to rid itself of ingested toxins. Not all animals are capable of vomiting and despite extensive research, the reflex is only partially characterized. This reflex can respond to a wide variety of toxic agents (*e.g.* chemotherapeutics such as cisplatin), bacterial or viral infection, diverse diseases, as well as other conditions (*e.g.* radiation, excessive motion). Fig. **2** outlines the established anatomical circuits and key features of the emetic reflex arc.

In the periphery emetogens may act directly in the gastrointestinal tract and/or indirectly by activating the central nervous system (CNS) emetic nuclei through stimulation of vagal afferents whose somata are in the nodose ganglion [6].

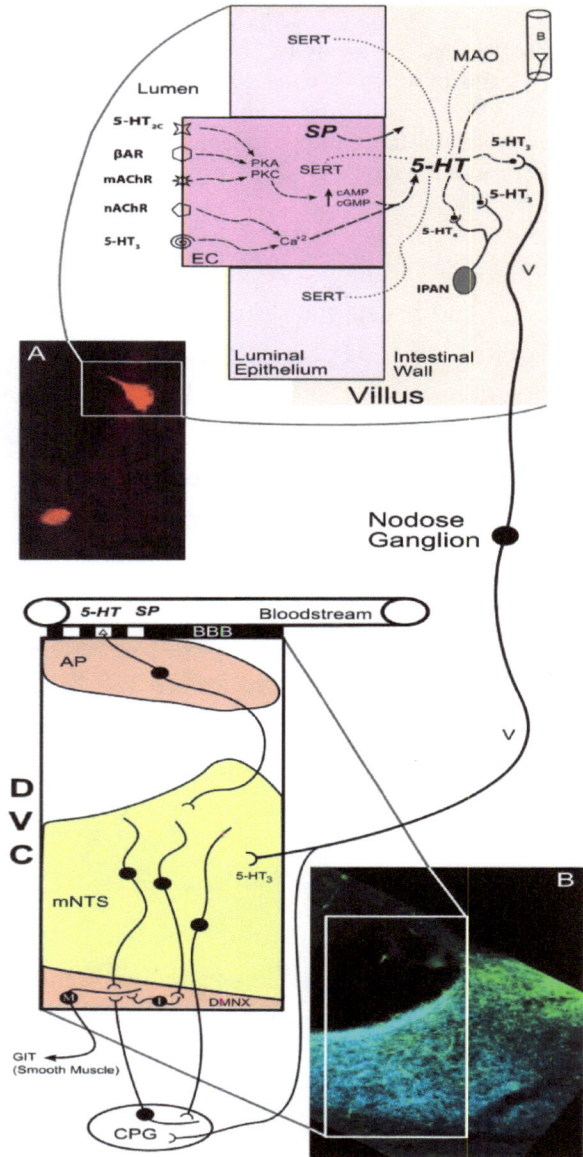

Figure 2: Key components of the brain-gut circuit mediating emesis. Emetogens such as cisplatin or bacterial enterotoxins induce acute vomiting by a powerful release of serotonin (5-HT) from enterochromaffin (EC) or mast cells embedded in the luminal epithelium. Photomicrograph A depicts a strip of least shrew luminal epithelium (boxed area) from a villus immunolabeled for 5-HT (red) to highlight EC cells. EC cells can also be stimulated to release 5-HT by a variety of luminal membrane-bound receptors, ultimately leading to stimulation of various second messenger systems and secretion of 5-HT (dashed lines in diagram). Secreted 5-HT can act locally *via* 5-

HT$_{3/4}$ receptors on vagal and intrinsic primary afferent neuron fibers in the intestinal wall, or may act distantly *via* the bloodstream to stimulate: 1) the enteric nervous system, and 2) possibly the dorsal vagal complex of the medulla. Likewise, SP can be released by cisplatin: 1) from EC cells where it can bind locally to specific neurokinin NK$_1$ receptors in the GIT, or on vagal afferents, or it can diffuse into the bloodstream and enter the brainstem to induce vomiting; 2) from vagal afferent terminals in the brainstem to cause emesis. Photomicrograph B depicts a coronal hemisection of the dorsal vagal complex (boxed area) of the least shrew, immunolabeled for SP (blue) and 5-HT (green). Vagal afferents projecting from the nodose ganglion to both the gut and brain, and area postrema neurons, accessing the bloodstream through the locally fenestrated blood-brain-barrier, enable rapid communication between the brain and gut. Vagal stimulation of the nucleus of the solitary tract (or serotonergic and/or tachykininergic stimulation of the area postrema) induces the emetic motor output of GIT smooth muscle *via* action on both motoneurons (M) and interneurons (I) of the dorsal motor nucleus of the vagus, while concomitant stimulation of the CPG area near the nucleus ambiguus coordinates related prodromal respiratory/salivatory activity (precursors to vomiting) with the actual act of vomiting. Abbreviations: 5-HT – serotonin; 5-HT# – serotonin receptor subtype; AP – area postrema; βAR – beta-adrenergic receptor; B – blood vessel; BBB – blood-brain barrier; CPG – central pattern generator area; DMNX – dorsal motor nucleus of the vagus; DVC – dorsal vagal complex; EC – enterochromaffin cell; GIT – gastrointestinal tract; IPAN – intrinsic primary afferent neuron; mAChR – muscarinic cholinergic receptor; MAO – monoamine oxidase; mNTS – medial subnucleus, nucleus of the solitary tract; nAChR – nicotinic cholinergic receptor; PKA/PKC – protein kinase A/C; SERT – serotonin reuptake transporter; V – vagal afferent nerve fiber.

Nodose neurons project extensively branched afferent fibers in both ascending and descending directions, such that the same neurons innervate both the brainstem dorsal vagal complex (DVC) and a segment within the enteric nervous system (ENS). The vagus contains afferent as well as efferent nerves and acts as a communication circuit between the brainstem and the gastrointestinal tract (GIT). A variety of emetogens (such as cisplatin, bacterial toxins, *etc.*) stimulate enterochromaffin cells (and/or enteric mast cells) to release serotonin (5-HT), substance P (SP) and possibly AA products such as prostaglandins and leukotrienes in the GIT [6,13]. The secreted serotonin and SP may act locally to stimulate their corresponding 5-HT$_3$- and NK$_1$- receptors present on vagal afferent terminals in the GIT, thus potentiating vagal afferent activity and subsequently the DVC emetic nuclei in the brainstem. Other proemetic signals such as prostanoids also increase vagal afferent activity and in fact PGE$_2$ receptors are present in nodose ganglionic cells. Vagal afferents are glutamatergic and appear to co-release SP, thus providing excitatory input to much of the emetic reflex arc. Absorbed or released emetogens may also act more distantly *via* the bloodstream to stimulate the DVC directly. In the CNS, both the DVC and a more ventrolaterally localized group of cells that make up the central pattern generator are key sites in the mediation of emesis. The DVC is a cluster of nuclei in the dorsomedial medulla comprising the area postrema (AP), the nucleus of the solitary tract (NTS), and the dorsal motor nucleus of the vagus (DMNX). The AP comprises the chemoreceptor trigger zone (CTZ), a circumventricular organ that allows bloodborne chemicals absorbed or secreted (*e.g.* SP) from the intestinal mucosa to bypass the blood-brain-barrier and stimulate the DVC directly. The medial NTS (mNTS) is the key integrative site for CNS modulation of the emetic reflex. It receives input from the AP, vagal afferents, the posterior paraventricular hypothalamic nuclei, and the serotonergic raphe nuclei. After integrating the central and peripheral signals relating to emesis or other GI activity, NTS neurons project to the DMNX as well as to the central pattern generator. Activation of the NTS during emesis results in a biphasic response. In the initial phase, glutamatergic neurons excite DMNX motor output neurons, producing a retroperistaltic contraction in the intestine and a strong stomach contraction. In the following phase, inhibitory NTS GABAergic projections and glutamatergic NTS projections that synapse onto DMNX inhibitory interneurons combine to suppress DMNX motor output, allowing relaxation of the gastric fundus and lower esophageal sphincter and opening of a physical path for expulsion of stomach contents. The DMNX motor neurons project to various parts of the GIT, including the stomach, lower esophageal sphincter, duodenum, and jejunum which completes the act of vomiting. Activity in the central pattern generator seems to be an important mediator of the emetic reflex as well as the prodromal signs of emesis such as salivation.

Presence of Endocannabinoid, Endovanilloid and Eicosanoid Signaling Markers in the Gut-Brain Emetic Circuit

Alteration in gastrointestinal motility is an important aspect of emesis. Although the brainstem plays an essential role in both the initiation and co-ordination of intestinal motility, most motility functions of the GIT are mediated by the local ENS [6,14]. It is well accepted that phytocannabinoids and endocannabinoids reduce intestinal smooth muscle contractility, GIT motility and peristaltic propulsion *via* prejunctional cannabinoid CB_1 receptors [6,14,15]. Both 2-AG and anandamide, as well as their biosynthetic enzymes, are present at relatively high levels in the GIT epithelium and the ENS. Furthermore, regional variations in endocannabinoid levels occur with 2-AG being higher in the ileum than the colon, and anandamide being considerably higher in the colon than the ileum [6,14,15]. Likewise, significant concentrations of both endocannabinoids and their synthetic and metabolic enzymes are present in the rat brainstem, including the DVC [6,14, 16,17]. Eicosanoids are also widely distributed in the GIT. In fact the mucosa and muscle layers of the gut are capable of generating the major downstream products of AA such as PGE_2, $PGF_{2\alpha}$, PGI_2 and thromboxanes [18,19]. Many of these prostanoids modulate intestinal motility, and deficiency of endogenous prostaglandins due to inhibition of COX enzymes by nonsteroidal anti-inflammatory drugs leads to gastrointestinal ulcers. Moreover, several different eicosanoids have been found to act in the ENS of the gut [6].

The CB_1 receptor is differentially distributed at terminal ends of diverse nerves in the ENS along the entire length of the GIT (with stomach and the colon being highly enriched) and controls normal gut motility [6,14,15]. To date, there is less evidence for CB_2 receptors being involved in the control of normal intestinal motility. Furthermore, CB_1 immunoreactivity is present on the cell bodies of the nodose ganglion, and the CB_1 receptor is largely transported to the peripheral terminals of the vagus nerve in the GIT [6]. Stimulation of vagal CB_1 receptors leads to reduction in vagal tone. While the brainstem as a whole appears to be relatively CB_1 receptor sparse, its NTS, AP and DMNX emetic nuclei in several species contain moderate but significant amounts of CB_1 receptors [6, 14]. Since anandamide also behaves as an endovanilloid agonist for TRPV1 receptor (see introduction), anandamide itself, as well as several AA products of lipoxygenases (12-(S)HPETE, 15(S)HPETE, LTB4 and N-arachidonoyldopamine) may produce added antiemetic activity *via* activation of this receptor [6]. TRPV1 receptors are found on vagal afferents, and the NTS, DMNX and AP nuclei of the DVC [6, 15].

As with CB_1 receptors, prostanoid EP_{1-4}, DP, IP and FP receptors as well as CysLT receptors are found in the ENS of the gut [6]. In addition, cellular localization studies indicate that the external muscle layers of the gut as well as ileal circular muscles exhibit EP_{1-3} receptors [20]. Moreover, not only does the enterochromaffin cell bear prostanoid EP_1, EP_4 and FP receptors, prostanoids can also potentiate nodose ganglionic vagal afferent activity [6]. Within the DVC, prostanoid EP_2, EP_3 and IP receptors are found in the NTS, while the AP expresses EP_4 receptors [6].

Role of Phytocannabinoids and Synthetic Direct-Acting Cannabinoids *versus* Synthetic Endocannabinoid Metabolic- and Reuptake-Inhibitors in Emesis

Phytocannabinoids and Synthetic Direct-acting Cannabinoids as Antiemetics

Prior to addressing the antiemetic/emetic potential of endocannabinoids and agents that increase their tissue levels, it is essential to briefly describe the antiemetic/emetic potential of phytocannabinoids and the direct-acting synthetic cannabinoid $CB_{1/2}$ agonists. The antiemetic potential of cannabis use in Western medicine against acute-phase chemotherapy-induced nausea and vomiting (CINV) in cancer patients began in mid 1970s and early 1980s [21-23]. The antiemetic action of the marijuana plant mainly resides in its major psychoactive component, Δ^9-THC {(-) *trans*-delta-9-tetrahydrocannabinol} and to a lesser extent to its closely related but less psychoactive (Δ^8-THC) and nonpsychoactive (cannabidiol) components. The antiemetic efficacy of synthetic cannabinoids such as levonantradol, nonabine, nabilone (Cesamet) and Δ^9-THC (dronabinol = Marinol) in cancer patients has also been investigated. Both marinol and cesamet are available in the clinic for the prevention of acute CINV. Meta-analysis of 30 CINV clinical trials in cancer patients indicates that Δ^9-THC possesses significant antiemetic activity and appears to be a superior antiemetic relative to conventional nonselective dopamine D_2 receptor antagonists [24]. However, combinations of these antiemetics were no more effective than each agent being tested alone [23]. Likewise, the more selective D_2 receptor antagonist sulpride was unable to potentiate the antiemetic efficacy of Δ^9-THC against the acute-phase of cisplatin-induced vomiting in the least shrew model of emesis [25]. To date, no extensive clinical trials comparing the antiemetic potential of such cannabinoids with the currently used antiemetics against the immediate (*e.g.* 5-HT$_3$ antagonists)- or delayed-phase (NK$_1$ receptor antagonists) CINV is available. Only one published double-blind, placebo-controlled clinical trial has compared the efficacy and tolerability of dronabinol (Δ^9-THC) and the 5-HT$_3$ antagonist ondansetron, against delayed CINV over a 5 day period [26]. The results indicate both agents were similarly effective against delayed emesis and the combination therapy was no more effective than either antiemetic tested alone. A more recent dose-response study in the least shrew demonstrated that combination of low doses of Δ^9-THC (0.25 and 0.5 mg/kg) and tropisetron (0.025-0.25) were more efficacious in reducing the frequency of emesis than each dose given individually [27]. However, larger doses of these antiemetics failed to exhibit such interaction, and relative to their tested individual doses, none of the combined doses provided significantly greater total emesis protection. These findings are not too surprising since not only Δ^9-THC but also anandamide as well as other synthetic $CB_{1/2}$ agonists, reduce 5-HT$_3$ receptor-mediated current [6, 27]. Thus, the limited basic and clinical findings suggest that Δ^9-THC does not potentiate the antiemetic efficacy of dopamine D_2- and 5-HT$_3$-receptor antagonists against CINV.

Although the advent of "setron" 5-HT$_3$ receptor antagonists in the 1980s led to the cessation of further antiemetic research in the clinic, the discovery of the cannabinoid receptors, their endogenous ligands, drugs that increase tissue levels of endocannabinoids *via* inhibition of their uptake or metabolism, combined with the introduction of new animal models of emesis, have rekindled a renaissance in the field of cannabinoid antiemetic research. The first published manuscript suggesting that the antiemetic efficacy of Δ^9-THC is *via* activation of cannabinoid CB_1 and not CB_2 receptors was in the least shrew [28]. Δ^9-THC and its direct-acting analogs such as WIN55-212-2, CP55,994 and HU-210, behave as broad-spectrum agonist antiemetics in a CB_1 receptor antagonist-sensitive manner against diverse centrally- and peripherally-acting emetogens in several animal models of emesis. These emetogens include: SR141716A [28], cisplatin-induced immediate [29-34] and delayed emesis [34,35]; serotonin (5-HT), its precursor 5-hydroxytryptophan (5-HTP), as well as the selective (*e.g.* 2-methylserotonin)- and nonselective (*e.g.* 5-HT)-5-HT$_3$ receptor agonists [36]; the dopamine precursor L-DOPA and dopaminergic $D_{2/3}$ receptor selective (quinpirole, quinelorane, 7-(OH) DPAT)- and nonselective (apomorphine)-agonists [37,38]; 2-AG [39]; AA [39]; radiation [40]; SP [41]; morphine or morphine-6-glucuronide [42,43]; motion [44], lithium [45] and staphylococcal enterotoxin [46]. The current chapter expands the antiemetic efficacy of Δ^9-THC and related direct-acting cannabinoids against 20-hydroxyPGE$_2$ (Fig. **7**), and the selective CB_1 receptor agonist arachidonoyl-2-chloroethylamide (ACEA) which can be metabolized by FAAH to the emetic agent arachidonic acid [1] (Fig. **3**).

The broad-spectrum antiemetic nature of phytocannabinoids and direct-acting synthetic CB_1 agonists against diverse centrally- and/or peripherally-acting emetogens implies that such agents may affect several emetic loci in GIT/DVC circuit and/or a final shared point in this circuit. Significant evidence supports the first possibility since both central [32,34] and peripheral mechanisms [36] contribute to the antiemetic efficacy of such cannabinoids. Indeed, Δ^9-THC pretreatment strongly suppresses cisplatin-induced Fos expression in the AP, NTS and DMNX during acute phase [32,34] and at relatively lower degrees during delayed emesis [34]. In the periphery Δ^9-THC-related agents act on prejunctional CB_1 receptors and reduce both smooth muscle intestinal contractility and peristaltic propulsion, which may affect emesis [3,6,9,10,14]. In addition, such agonists inhibit transient lower esophageal sphincter relaxation in several emetic species *via* CB_1 receptor activation, which can prevent reflux of gastric content into the esophagus [47].

Phytocannabinoids and Synthetic Direct-acting Cannabinoids as Vomit Inducers

Δ^9-THC and related clinically used agents are often used on a subacute basis as prophylactic agonist antiemetics for the prevention of nausea and vomiting caused by chemotherapeutics. Cannabis-induced hyperemesis is a recently recognized syndrome associated with chronic large doses of cannabis use. It is characterized by repeated cyclical vomiting and learned compulsive hot water bathing behavior [48]. Although it was considered rare, recent international publications of numerous case reports suggest the contrary. Basic and clinical studies suggest that chronic exposure to Δ^9-THC may not be necessary for the induction of emesis. In fact, acute intravenous injection of a crude marijuana extract in a single volunteer [49], or acute oral administration of dronabinol (Δ^9-THC) in 3-30% of patients, have been shown to cause nausea, vomiting, diarrhea or crampy abdominal pain [50-53]. Indeed, a relatively recent systematic review of adverse effects of medical cannabinoids in clinical trials has revealed that while 19-64% of patients experienced CNS events, 28-40% of them also experienced adverse gastrointestinal side-effects [54]. If the discussed acute symptoms also represent components of cannabis hyperemesis syndrome, then chronic exposure to cannabinoids is not a necessary prerequisite for the induction of vomiting, but may be needed for the intensification and cyclic nature of hyperemesis. Published results from animal models of emesis support the latter proposal since acute intravenous or intraperitoneal administration of Δ^9-THC can produce vomiting in naive dogs [55] or in 20-30% of naïve least shrews [34], while severe emesis is observed when Δ^9-THC-dependent chronically-exposed dogs were given a small dose of the CB_1 antagonist, rimonabant (SR141716A) [56]. The recent use of synthetic cannabinoids (*e.g.* JWH-018 and HU-210) spiked in herbal products sold as "spice", is a relatively recent phenomenon in Europe. Use of spice and related products is also becoming popular in the USA. Increasingly, use of such agents is associated with nausea and emesis [57,58]. Overall, these basic and clinical findings suggest that in a number of emetic species including humans, acute administration of Δ^9-THC or related products (JWH-018) in susceptible individuals can induce emesis, whereas chronic Δ^9-THC exposure can cause severe hyperemetic syndrome. Even more intriguing, relatively larger doses of the CB_1 receptor-selective inverse agonist/antagonist SR141716A produces dose-dependent emesis in the least shrew [28], ferrets [59] and cannabinoid-dependent dogs [56], while at lower doses (0.05-0.2 mg/kg) it causes nausea and vomiting in 4-14% of humans [60]. The latter effects of SR141716A are thought to be due to inverse agonism and/or its ability to cause substantial release of emetic neurotransmitters such as serotonin and dopamine [61]. Reason(s) for Δ^9-THC causing emesis in some drug naïve and apparently normal individuals, but not in all patients or test animals, still remain to be fully explained. However, possible pharmacokinetic and pharmacodynamics mechanisms have been suggested [48].

Exogenously-administered Endocannabinoids as Anti- and Proemetic Agents

Only a few putative endocannabinoids have been systematically tested across available emesis models to allow a firm conclusion as to whether exogenously-administered endocannabinoids possess emetic and/or antiemetic properties. Furthermore, published studies have often utilized only one or two endocannabinoid doses which further prevent any robust conclusion. Intraperitoneal administration of the endocannabinoid 2-AG (0, 0.25, 1, 2.5, 5, 10 and 20 mg/kg) in the least shrew has been shown to induce dose-dependent emesis with significant vomiting occurring at 1 mg/kg, and 100% of animals vomiting at the 5 mg/kg dose [39]. To the best of the author's knowledge no such dose-response study has been carried out in any other emesis model. The induced emesis in the least shrew is probably due to rapid metabolism of 2-AG by MAGL enzyme [2] to AA since the latter agent is a potent emetogen by itself, and the emetic efficacy of both 2-AG and AA can be fully blocked by the COX inhibitor, indomethacin [39]. Indirect support for the latter conclusion comes from the ability of the MAGL inhibitor JZL184 to prevent LiCl-induced vomiting in house musk shrews [62]. Surprisingly, JZL184 was ineffective in the conditioned gaping model of nausea-like behavior in rats [62]. The emetic effect of 2-AG in least shrew and the antiemetic efficacy of JZL184 in the house musk shrew were only partially reversed by selective CB_1 receptor antagonists/inverse agonists SR141716A and AM251, respectively. Although the emetic potential of exogenously administered 2-AG was not studied in house musk shrew, administration of exogenous 2-AG (and also surprisingly AA) was shown to attenuate, in a dose-dependent manner, the frequency of LiCl-induced gaping in rats. While AM251 failed to reverse the inhibitory effect of 2-AG on gaping, indomethacin prevented the inhibitory effects of both 2-AG and its metabolite AA on gaping. In addition, when JZL184 was co-administered to prevent metabolism of exogenously administered 2-AG, the inhibitory effect of 2-AG against LiCl-induced gaping became sensitive to AM251. Moreover, the emetic potential of exogenous 2-AG in the ferret has not yet been fully investigated and the available data indicate that by itself 2-AG lacks emetic activity in this species at 0.5 and 2 mg/kg (i.p.) doses, but exhibits antiemetic activity against morphine-6-glucuronide at 2 mg/kg [63]. However, lack of emetic potential of 2-AG in ferrets should not be too surprising, since unlike in shrews, peripheral administration of serotonin or SP does not produce vomiting in ferrets [6]. Overall, these findings suggest that when 2-AG is exogenously-administered by itself, it is rapidly metabolized in both least shrews and rats, and the discussed effects in both species are due to AA and downstream metabolites [39]. In fact the chemotherapeutic agent cisplatin not only can increase brainstem and gut tissue levels of well-known emetogens such as dopamine, serotonin and SP, but also increases brain levels of 2-AG in the least shrew [64].

The emetic/antiemetic potential of exogenously-administered anandamide appears to be less controversial. In a wide dose-response (0, 2.5, 5, 10 and 20 mg/kg, i.p.) study in the least shrew, anandamide only caused significant emesis at its 10 mg/kg [39]. Moreover, in the ferret anandamide lacks direct emetic activity but was shown to potentiate vomiting caused by morphine-6-glucuronide (M6G) [65]. Lack of full emetic efficacy of anandamide could be explained by its endovanilloid agonist activity at TRPV1 receptors, and by its relatively slower metabolism [6]. In fact, the TRPV1 receptor can also be targeted by the burning component of chili peppers, capsaicin, as well as by resiniferatoxin, which can produce both pro- and anti-emetic effects in least shrews [Darmani, unpublished findings] and house musk shrews [66], but can be an antiemetic in ferrets [67]. Likewise, exogenous anandamide has pro-emetic activity in least shrews by itself [39] and possesses antiemetic efficacy against vomiting caused both by 2-AG in the least shrew [39] and by M6G in ferrets [42]. Complete lack of pro-emetic activity of the metabolically more stable synthetic analog of anandamide, methanandamide, is also consistent with for a more gradual degradation of anandamide [6,39]. Furthermore, our recent findings demonstrate that another analog of anandamide, arachidonoyl-2-chloroethylamide (ACEA), which behaves as a selective CB_1 receptor agonist and undergoes rapid metabolism by FAAH [1], can also produce intense and dose-dependent emesis in least shrews (Fig. **3A, 3B**). In fact a significant increase in percentage of shrews vomiting relative to vehicle-treated controls occurred at the 5 mg/kg dose (i.p.), and 100% emesis in shrews was achieved at 10 mg/kg dose of ACEA. Thus, ACEA appears to be slightly less potent than 2-AG in producing emesis [39]. On the other hand, another anandamide analog arachidonoylcyclopropamide (ACPA), which is also thought to be a CB_1 receptor-selective agonist and a substrate for FAAH [1], failed to produce emesis in the least shrew. This new finding suggests that ACPA is probably metabolized at a much lower rate.

As with anandamide, another putative endocannabinoid, *N*-arachidonoyldopamine (NADA), stimulates both CB_1 and TRPV1 receptors and attenuates M6G-induced emesis in the ferret [65]. Exogenously-administered NADA was an effective antiemetic at 2 mg/kg (i.p.), and at this dose, by itself, failed to induce vomiting. However, the emetic/antiemetic potential of NADA has not been fully explored either in other species or against other emetogens. Another putative novel endocannabinoid is virodhamine which consists of arachidonic acid and ethanolamine joined by an ester linkage [68]. Virodhamine behaves as a partial

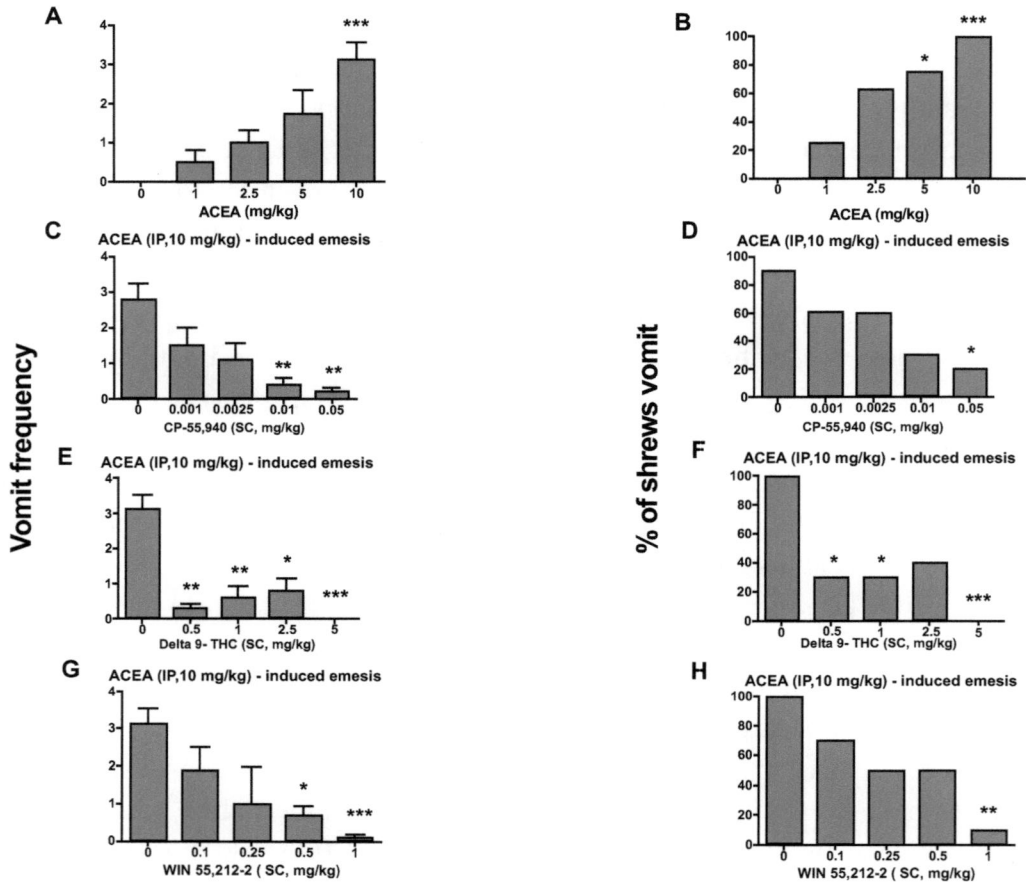

Figure 3: Dose-response emetic effects of varying doses (0, 1, 2.5, 5 and 10 mg/kg, i.p., n = 8 per group) of the hydrolyzable CB_1 receptor selective agonist ACEA (arachidonoyl-2-chloroethylamide) in the least shrew (Graphs A and B). The mean frequency of emesis (±S.E.M.) and the percent of shrews vomiting were recorded during a 30 min observation period immediately post ACEA injection. The antiemetic dose-response effects of three structurally different cannabinoid $CB_{1/2}$ receptor agonists CP55,940 (0, 0.001, 0.0025, 0.01 and 0.05 mg/kg, ip., n = 10 per group; depicted in graphs C and D); Δ^9-THC (0, 0.5, 1, 2.5 and 5 mg/kg, ip., n = 8-10 per group; depicted in graphs E and F), and WIN55,212-2 (0, 0.1, 0.25, and 1 mg/kg, ip., n = 8-10 per group; depicted in graphs G and H) against emesis caused by a 10 mg/kg intraperitoneal dose of ACEA are also shown. The $CB_{1/2}$ agonists were injected into different groups of shrews 30 min prior to ACEA administration and the induced emetic parameters were recorded for 30 min post ACEA injection. Frequency data are presented as mean (±S.E.M.). Significantly different from corresponding vehicle control (0 mg/kg) at P < 0.05 (*), P < 0.01 (**) and P < 0.001 (***). These experiments and statistical analyses were performed in accord with our published protocols [39].

agonist with *in vivo* antagonist activity at the CB_1 receptor, but with full agonist activity at the CB_2 receptor. Our new findings demonstrate that exogenously administered virodhamine produces vomiting in the least shrew in a dose-dependent fashion (Fig. **4A, 4B**). However, a significant number of vomits and percentage (70-90%) of animals exhibiting emesis were observed at its 10 and 20 mg/kg (i.p.) doses. Thus, relative to both 2-AG and ACEA, virodhamine appears to be a less potent and not a fully efficacious emetogen. Again the chemical structure of virodhamine suggests that its downstream metabolites are probably emetogenic. The possible antiemetic potential of lower doses of virodhamine against various emetogens has not been investigated. Since the possibility of the CB_2 receptor contributing towards antiemetic efficacy of cannabinoids has been suggested [63], and virodhamine is a full agonist of CB_2 receptors,

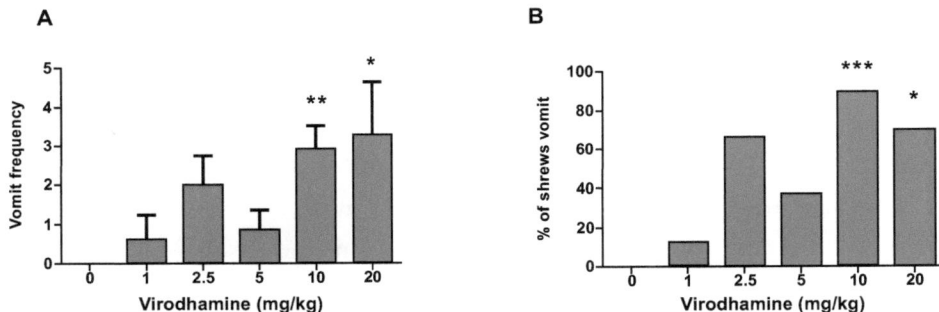

Figure 4: Emetic dose-response effects of the putative endocannabinoid virodhamine (0, 1, 2.5, 5, 10 and 20 mg/kg, i.p., n = 8-10 per group) in the least shrew. Graph A depicts the mean increase in the frequency of vomiting (±S.E.M.), while graph B shows the increase in the percentage of shrews vomiting. Emesis parameters were recorded for 30 min post injection. Significantly different from vehicle control (0 mg/kg) at $P < 0.05$ (*) and $P < 0.01$ (**). For experimental details and statistical analyses see [39].

activation of the latter receptors could be important in its antiemetic potential. However, the majority of findings rule against the functional contribution of CB_2 receptors in emetic circuits.

Endocannabinoid Metabolic- and Reuptake-inhibitors as Antiemetic/ Proemetic Agents

With conventional neurotransmitter systems (such as serotonin), clinically useful agents have often been developed to increase neurotransmitter tissue concentration either *via* the inhibition of their reuptake (*e.g.* serotonin reuptake inhibitors) or metabolism (*e.g.* monoamine oxidase inhibitors) so as to prolong their synaptic function (*e.g.* antidepressants). Likewise, endocannabinoid reuptake blockers and enzyme inhibitors are being developed to extend duration of action and potentiate their function [69]. A number of FAAH (*e.g.* AA-5-HT, URB597) and MAGL (*e.g.* JZL184) inhibitors as well as some endocannabinoid reuptake blockers (OMDM1, VDM11, AM404) have already been tested for their antiemetic potential in several emesis and nausea-like models. However, as with the use of exogenously administered endocannabinoids, the antiemetic/proemetic nature of some of these agents can be contradictory, and unlike phytocannabonoids or direct-acting synthetic CB_1 agonists, they lack broad-spectrum antiemetic efficacy. For example, the FAAH inhibitor URB597, either alone or in combination with exogenously administered anandamide, attenuates M6G-induced emesis in the ferret [63,65], and nicotine- as well as cisplatin-induced vomiting in house musk shrews [70], and reduces indices of nausea in rats [71,72] in a CB_1 receptor-dependent manner. On the other hand, URB597 has been shown to lack antiemetic efficacy against apomorphine in both ferrets [73] and least shrews [64], and against cisplatin- and 2-AG-induced vomiting in the latter species [64]. Another tested FAAH inhibitor AA-5-HT, also lacks antiemetic efficacy against these emetogens in the least shrew [64]. More importantly, in the least shrew both URB597 and AA-5-HT at doses greater than 10 mg/kg (i.p.) induce significant emesis by themselves. The emetic potential of such doses of URB597 and AA-5-HT has not yet been tested in other species. The MAGL inhibitor JZL184 selectively prevents metabolism of 2-AG and thus increases its tissue levels in rodents as well as in house musk shrews [62]. JZL184 was shown to attenuate vomiting caused by LiCl in the house musk shrew which was partially reversed by the selective CB_1 antagonist AM251. However, in the latter study JZL184 was ineffective against lithium-induced nausea in rats. The reuptake blocker VDM11 elevates 2-AG but not anandamide levels in the ferret brain [63] and has been shown to attenuate vomiting caused by M6G in ferrets [63] and apomorphine-induced emesis in the least shrew [64]. However, VDM11 was not effective against both cisplatin- and 2-AG-induced emesis in the least shrew [64]. Its inability to suppress 2-AG-induced emesis stands to reason since 2-AG can still be metabolized by MAGL to AA and downstream metabolites to produce its emetic effects. Another reuptake blocker OMDM1 lacked antiemetic efficacy against all of the above discussed emetogens in the least shrew [54]. One more tested reuptake blocker is AM404, which also lacks efficacy against vomiting caused by apomorphine, copper sulfate and cisplatin (observed for 24 hours post cisplatin injection) in the ferret [74]. However, it did slightly attenuate emesis by 37% when post-cisplatin observation of vomiting was limited to the first six hours of injection. Thus, it appears that the antiemetic/emetic nature of both exogenously administered endocannabinoids and agents that increase their endogenous tissue concentrations depends on a balance between their beneficial effects in elevating their tissue levels *versus* unfavorable actions in their conversion to proemetic AA and downstream emetogenic metabolites.

Role of Downstream Endocannabinoid and AA Metabolites in Emesis

As discussed earlier, endocannabinoids can be converted to AA and these lipophilic agents can be further metabolized by diverse enzymes to about 100 different compounds. The pharmacology of many of these substances remains relatively unexplored. Thus, the task of evaluating their pro- and/or antiemetic properties is daunting, since animal models of emesis are quite expensive and few laboratories outside the drug industry can support their maintenance. As already discussed, the emetic potential of several endocannabinoids across a wide range of doses has been studied only in the least shrew. In this species, except for noladin ether, other tested putative endocannabinoids are either potently (2-AG and virodhamine) or weakly (anandamide) emetogenic. Their common metabolite AA is also a potent emetogen in the least shrew [39] and can induce symptoms of nausea in rats [62]. As a further corresponding example, human studies have shown that 2-AG activates blood platelets, mainly *via* its metabolite AA and not through a direct action on either cannabinoid CB_1 or CB_2 receptors [75]. Our published studies in the least shrew demonstrate that the multistep 5-LOX products of AA are diverse leukotrienes (LTA_4, LTB_4, LTC_4, LTD_4, LTE_4 and LTF_4), some of which can be potent emetogens, and their emetic efficacy exhibits a close structure-activity relationship. In fact the parent leukotriene LTA_4 lacks emetic activity and can either be converted into a non-emetogen LTB_4, or conjugated to the peptide glutathione to generate the parent cysteinyl leukotriene LTC_4 which is a potent emetic agent in the least shrew [75]. The latter can be stripped of a glutamic acid residue to form LTD_4 with an equal emetic potency, which can be stripped of its glycine residue to produce a weak emetogen LTE_4 (Fig. **1**). Furthermore, LTC_4 can be converted *via* carboxypeptidase to LTF_4, which lacks emetic activity. The LTC_4-induced vomiting was attenuated by both the leukotriene $CysLT_1$ antagonist pranlukast and the $CysLT_2$ partial agonist/antagonist Bayu9773 [76]. Fos tissue immunoreactivity, measured subsequent to LTC_4-induced vomiting to define its putative anatomical emetic substrates, was significantly increased in the enteric nervous system of the least shrew as well as in the NTS and DMNX but not in the AP of the DVC emetic nuclei in the brainstem, suggesting that both peripheral and central mechanisms are involved in the process of induced vomiting.

The 5 major types of prostanoid receptors include DP, EP, FP, IP and TP. Some of these receptors are further subdivided, particularly the EP receptor, namely EP_{1-4} receptors. As discussed earlier, the cyclooxygenase products of AA are diverse PGs. The clinical use of PGE_2 and $PGF_{2\alpha}$ and their analogs (*e.g.* misoprostol; sulprostone) in obstetric medicine is often associated with nausea and vomiting [77,78]. In the ferret only DP (*e.g.* BW245C)-, EP (*e.g.* PGE_2; misoprostol; sulprostone)- and FP (*e.g.* $PGF_{2\alpha}$)-receptor agonists induce vomiting [78]. In humans, administration of BW245 is also associated with nausea and gastrointestinal disturbance [79]. The thromboxane A2 mimetic U466619 produces vomiting *via* TP receptors in ferrets since this effect was attenuated by vapiprost [78]. These agonists also depolarized the isolated ferret vagus nerve preparation, which suggests activation of the vagus is a component of emetic action of these agents, with $PGF_{2\alpha}$, being both the least potent depolarizing agent and emetogen [78,80]. Their pro-emetic activity may also have a central component since both PGE_2 and $PGF_{2\alpha}$, as well as other PGs, excite the neurons of the area postrema in the canine DVC [81]. The induced emesis was blocked by $5-HT_3$ (ondansetron)- and NK_1 (CP99,994)-receptor antagonists which can also reverse the ability of serotonin and SP in exciting the vagus nerve [82-84]. However, bilateral vagotomy was ineffective in reducing prostanoid-induced emesis in the ferret [84], indicating involvement of other nerves (*e.g.* splanchnic) as well. There appear to be species differences in the emetic potential of prostanoids since in the house musk shrew only TP receptor agonists (*e.g.* U46619) consistently produced vomiting, and PGE_2 and $PGF_{2\alpha}$ lacked emetic activity up to 1 mg/kg [85]. Unlike the case of the ferret [84], bilateral vagotomy reduced U46619-induced vomiting in the house musk shrew [86]. The role of prostanoids causing emesis in the least shrew has not been fully evaluated. In the least shrew $PGF_{2\alpha}$ demonstrated dose-dependent (0, 0.25, 1, 5, 10, 20 mg/kg, i.p.), but bell-shaped, increases in both the frequency of emesis (Fig. **5A**) and the percentage of animals vomiting (Fig. **5B**). However, significant emesis in both emetic parameters was seen only at its 10 mg/kg dose. Its metabolite 20-

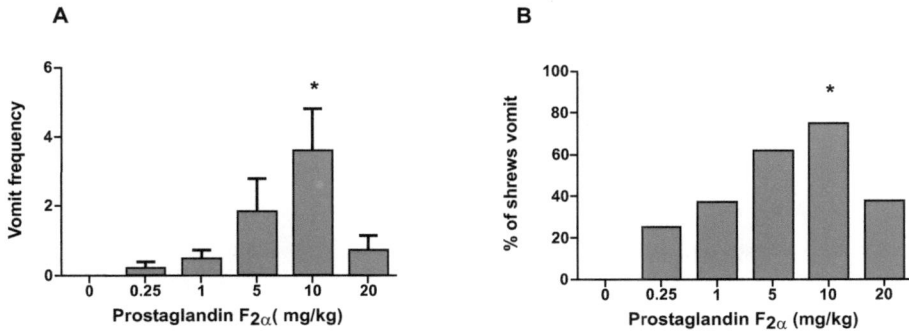

Figure 5: Emetic bell-shaped dose-response effects of prostaglandin $F_{2\alpha}$ ($PGF_{2\alpha}$) (0, 0.25, 1, 5, 10 and 20 mg/kg, i.p., n = 8 per group) in the least shrew. Graph A depicts the mean increase in the frequency of vomiting (±S.E.M.), while graph B shows the increase in the percentage of shrews vomiting. Emesis parameters were recorded for 30 min post injection. Significantly different from vehicle control (0 mg/kg) at $P < 0.05$ (*). For experimental details and statistical analyses see [39].

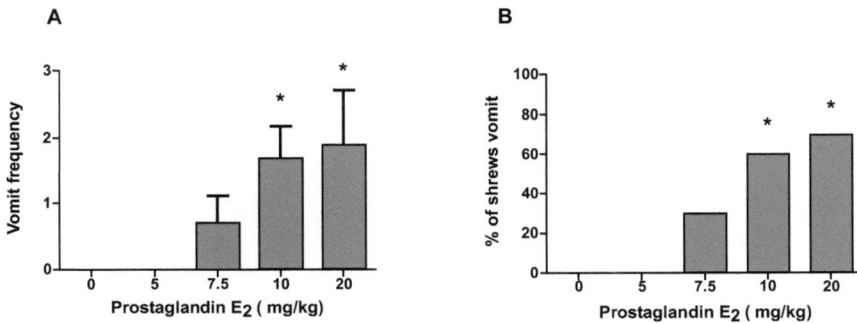

Figure 6: Emetic dose-response effects of prostaglandin E_2 (PGE_2) (0, 0.25, 1, 5, 10 and 20 mg/kg, i.p., n = 8-10 per group) in the least shrew. Graph A depicts the mean increase in the frequency of vomiting (±S.E.M.), while graph B shows the increase in the percentage of shrews vomiting. Emesis parameters were recorded for 30 min post injection. Significantly different from vehicle control (0 mg/kg) at $P < 0.05$ (*). For experimental details and statistical analyses see [39].

hydroxy$PGF_{2\alpha}$, failed to demonstrate consistent emetic efficacy in the least shrew even at larger doses. Moreover, its other metabolites, such as 13,14-dihydro-15-keto $PGF_{2\alpha}$; 15-keto $PGF_{2\alpha}$; and 19 (R) hydroxyl $PGF_{2\alpha}$ also had no emetic activity. As with $PGF_{2\alpha}$, in the least shrew intraperitoneal administration of PGE_2

caused dose-dependent emesis at large doses with significant effects at 10 and 20 mg/kg doses (Fig. **6A, 6B**). However, unlike with the discussed $PGF_{2\alpha}$ metabolite, biotransformation of PGE_2 to its 20-hydroxyPGE_2 product significantly potentiated its emetic efficacy since 100% of animals vomited at its 0.5 mg/kg dose (i.p.), and the induced effects were dose-dependent (Fig. **7A, 7B**).

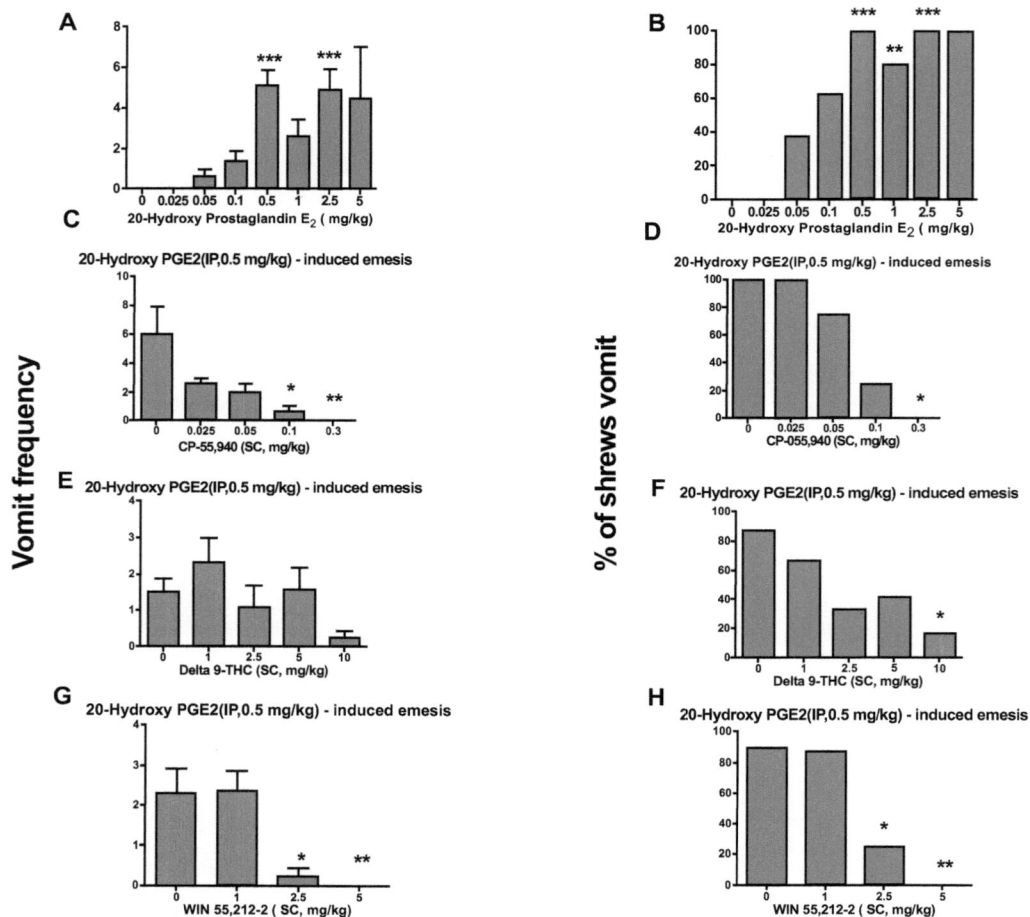

Figure 7: Dose-response emetic effects of varying doses (0, 0.025, 0.05, 0.1, 1, 2.5 and 5 mg/kg, i.p., n = 8-12 per group) of 20-hydroxyprostaglandin E_2 (20-hydroxyPGE_2) in the least shrew (Graphs A and B). The mean frequency of emesis (±S.E.M.) and the percent of shrews vomiting were recorded during a 30 min observation period immediately post 20-hydroxyPGE_2 injection. The antiemetic dose-response effects of three structurally different cannabinoid $CB_{1/2}$ receptor agonists CP55,940 (0, 0.025, 0.05, 0.1 and 0.3 mg/kg, ip., n = 8 per group; depicted in graphs C and D); Δ^9-THC (0, 1, 2.5, 5 and 10 mg/kg, ip., n = 8-12 per group; depicted in graphs E and F), and WIN55,212-2 (0, 1, 2.5 and 5 mg/kg, ip., n = 8-10 per group; depicted in graphs G and H) against emesis caused by an 0.5 mg/kg intraperitoneal dose of 20-hydroxyPGE_2 are also shown.

The $CB_{1/2}$ agonists were injected into different groups of shrews 30 min prior to 20-hydroxyPGE$_2$ administration and the induced emetic parameters were recorded for 30 min post 20-hydroxyPGE$_2$ injection. Frequency data are presented as mean ($\pm$S.E.M.). Significantly different from corresponding vehicle control (0 mg/kg) at P < 0.05 (*), P < 0.01 (**) and P < 0.001 (***). These experiments and statistical analyses were performed in accord with our published protocols [39].

Likewise, PGG$_2$ caused emesis in least shrews in a dose-dependent fashion with maximal emetic efficacy at 0.5 mg/kg (i.p.) (Fig. **8A, 8B**). Since no antagonist-inhibition data is available for the discussed emetic effects, one cannot assign a particular prostanoid receptor for their emetic activity. However, it is important to note that PGD$_2$, PGH$_2$ and PGI$_2$ as well as the tetranor PGFM failed to induce vomiting in least shrews at up to 5 mg/kg doses. CYPP450 hydroxylases generate the hydroxyeicosatetraenoic acid downstream products of AA (such as 16-, 17-, 18-, 19-, or 20-HETE) and 20-HETE is a major metabolite in the gut [87]. Furthermore, intraperitoneal injection of 20-HETE in the least shrew caused dose-dependent increases in both the frequency (Fig. **9A**), and percentage of animals vomiting (Fig. **9B**), with 100% efficacy at 2 mg/kg (Fig. **9B**). Epoxyeicosatrienoic acids such as$\pm$5(6)-EpETrE are produced from AA *via* CYPP450 epoxygenases and are involved in the regulation of inflammation, angiogenesis, cellular

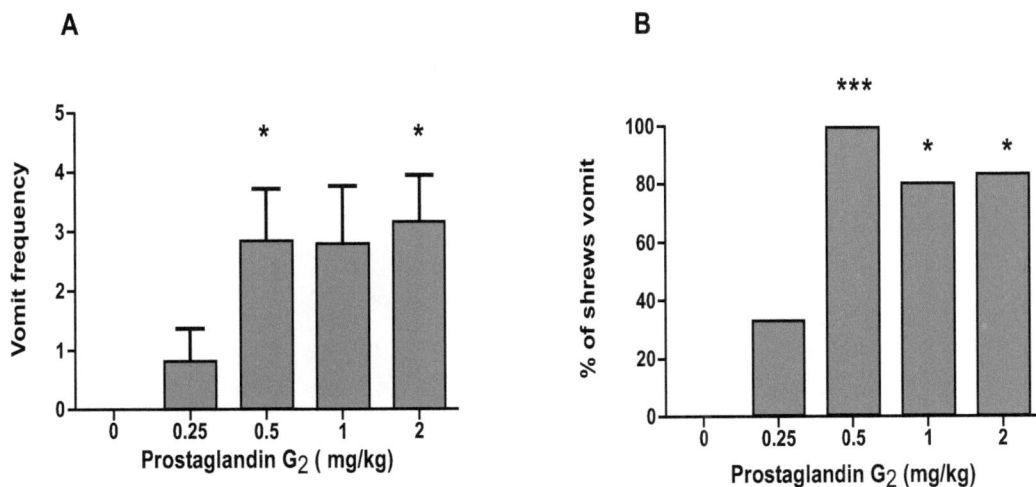

Figure 8: Emetic dose-response effects of prostaglandin G$_2$ (PGG$_2$) (0, 0.25, 0.5, 1 and 2 mg/kg, i.p., n = 6-9 per group) in the least shrew. Graph A depicts the mean increase in the frequency of vomiting ($\pm$S.E.M.), while graph B shows the increase in the percentage of shrews vomiting. Emesis parameters were recorded for 30 min post injection. Significantly different from vehicle control (0 mg/kg) at P < 0.05 (*) and P < 0.001 (***). For experimental details a statistical analyses see [39].

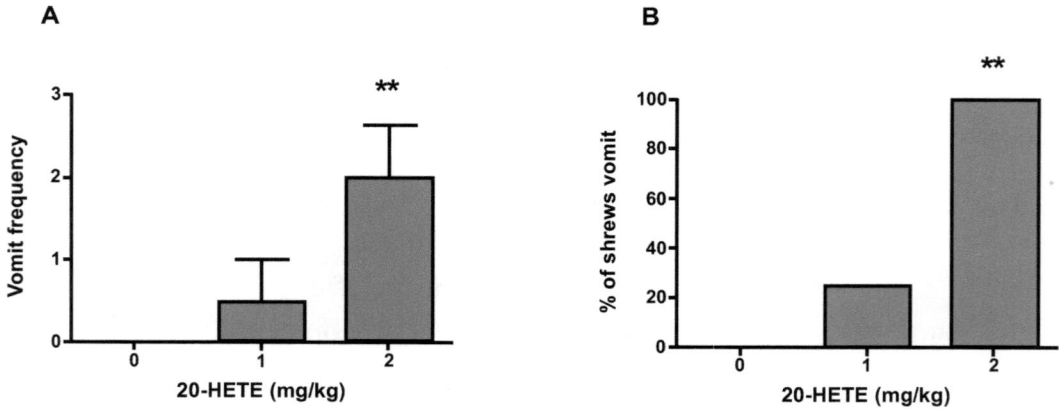

Figure 9: Emetic dose-response effects of 20-HETE (0, 1 and 2 mg/kg, i.p., n = 4-6 per group) in the least shrew. Graph A depicts the mean increase in the frequency of vomiting (±S.E.M.), while graph B shows the increase in the percentage of shrews vomiting. Emesis parameters were recorded for 30 min post injection. Significantly different from vehicle control (0 mg/kg) at P < 0.01 (**). For experimental details and statistical analyses see [39].

proliferation, ion transport and steroidogenesis [88]. We now report involvement of ±5(6)- EpETrE in emesis since it caused dose-dependent vomiting in the least shrew both in terms of emesis frequency (Fig. **10A**) and percentage of animals exhibiting vomiting (Fig. **10B**). Maximal emesis occurred at 0.5 and 1 mg/kg (i.p.) doses. However, other tested products of AA such as ±11(12)-EpETrE and 5(S)-HpETE lacked emetogenicity in the least shrew. Significant indirect evidence supports these findings since *S*. aureus enterotoxin B produces vomiting in monkeys which is associated in a time-dependent manner with increases in plasma concentration of several AA metabolites including $PGF_{2\alpha}$, Leukotriene B_4, and 5-HETE [89]. Such enterotoxins increase intestinal levels of serotonin in the house musk shrew and subsequently stimulate $5-HT_3$ receptors found on vagal afferents in the GIT to induce vomiting [90]. In fact the latter study has demonstrated that pretreatment with either an inhibitor of 5-HT synthesis (p-chlorophenylalanine), or a serotonergic neuronal neurotoxin (5,7-dihydroxytryptamine), or a $5-HT_3$ receptor antagonist (granisetron), or bilateral vagotomy, can attenuate the induced emesis. In addition, both the COX-2 inhibitor nabumetone and the nonspecific COX inhibitor indomethacin which prevent AA metabolism, also reduce serotonin release induced by cisplatin from ileal enterochromaffin cells [91]. Furthermore, indomethacin, can prevent 2-AG-

and AA-induced vomiting in the least shrew [39], and vomiting caused by cisplatin or lipopolysaccharide in piglets [92,93].

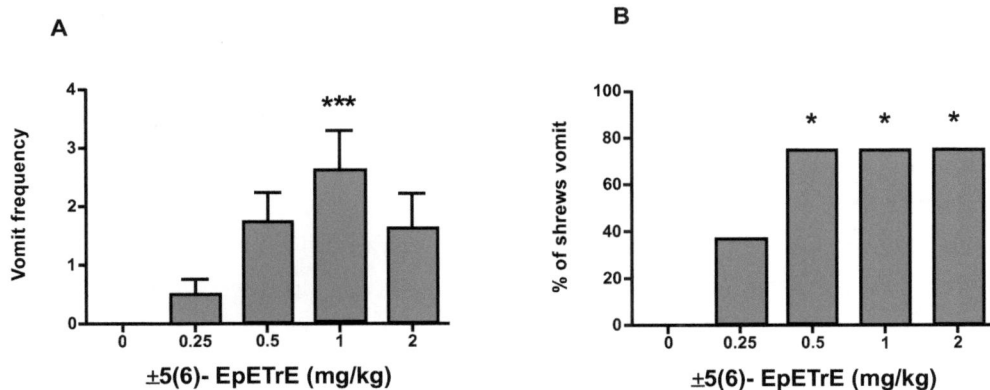

Figure 10: Emetic dose-response effects of ±5(6)EpETrE (0, 0.25, 0.5, 1 and 2 mg/kg, i.p., n = 8 per group) in the least shrew. Graph A depicts the mean increase in the frequency of vomiting (±S.E.M.), while graph B shows the increase in the percentage of shrews vomiting. Emesis parameters were recorded for 30 min post injection. Significantly different from vehicle control (0 mg/kg) at P < 0.01 (**). For experimental details and statistical analyses see [39].

Effect of Established Antiemetics Against Emesis Caused by Endocannabinoids and their Downstream Products

As discussed earlier, we already have shown that pretreatment with Δ^9-THC or related cannabinoids (WIN55,212-2 and CP55,994) attenuate 2-AG-induced vomiting in the least shrew in a dose-dependent fashion [39]. Likewise, and in line with this evidence, we now demonstrate the antiemetic efficacy of subcutaneously-administered cannabinoid $CB_{1/2}$ receptor agonists (Δ^9-THC, WIN55,212-2, and CP55, 940) against the emetic capacity of the previously discussed CB_1 receptor-selective agonist ACEA (10 mg/kg, i.p.), which is an anandamide analog but undergoes rapid metabolism to AA and its other downstream emetic metabolites (Fig. 3). The tested cannabinoids appear to behave as potent antiemetics (CP55,940 > WIN55,940 > Δ^9-THC) since over 90% of ACEA-induced emesis was prevented at their 1 mg/kg dose or less (Fig. **3C-3H**). These cannabinoids also prevented the ability of the highly emetogenic downstream metabolite of AA, 20-hdroxyPGE$_2$ (0.5 mg/kg, i.p.), in a dose-dependent fashion with a similar potency order (Fig. **7C-7H**). Moreover, WIN55,212-2 has been shown to prevent emesis in the house musk shrew caused by staphylococcal enterotoxin [90]. These findings further establish the broad-spectrum antiemetic nature of Δ^9-THC and its synthetic analogs. Furthermore, both 5-HT$_3$ (ondansetron)- and NK$_1$ (CP99,994)-receptor antagonist pretreatment can attenuate PGE$_2$-induced vomiting in the ferret [84], while only the NK$_1$ receptor antagonist CP122,721 prevented emesis caused by the prostanoid TP receptor antagonist U46619 in the house musk shrew [86]. Dexamethasone is one antiemetic that is often used in conjunction with a 5-HT$_3$- or an NK$_1$-receptor antagonist to protect against CINV [6]. Dexamethasone can also be used by itself as an antiemetic. Glucocorticoids such as dexamethasone seem to shift AA metabolism towards endocannabinoid synthesis to produce nongenomic anti-inflammatory effects [94] and probably vomit protection.

SUMMARY AND CONCLUSIONS

Studies in both humans and animal models of emesis suggest that Δ^9-THC and its synthetic direct-acting CB$_{1/2}$ receptor agonist analogs possess broad-spectrum antiemetic activity against diverse emetogens *via* the activation of cannabinoid CB$_1$ receptors present in the DVC and GIT emetic loci. Increasingly more recent reports reveal a complex enigma in that some patients suffer from severe nausea and intractable vomiting of unknown etiology following chronic use of large doses of Δ^9-THC. In addition, the current literature regarding the anti- and proemetic nature of endocannabinoids is equivocal. In fact published studies in diverse emesis models indicate that the antiemetic efficacy of exogenously-administered endocannabinoids, or the antiemetic potential of agents that raise the endogenous tissue concentrations of endocannabinoids *via* the blockade of either their metabolism or reuptake, depends on a balance between the beneficial effects in elevating their tissue levels *versus* unfavorable actions in converting them to proemetic AA and downstream emetogenic metabolites. Furthermore, unlike Δ^9-THC, such agents lack broad-spectrum antiemetic efficacy. The apparent lack of emetic potential of endocannabinoids in the commonly used emesis models such as the ferret and the house musk shrew probably stems from testing only a few doses of such agents, since in the least shrew full dose-response studies have often revealed both pro- and antiemetic activities. The latter situation mirrors the early 2000s publications regarding the emetic potential of the CB$_1$ antagonist/inverse agonist SR141716A, which was originally shown to induce dose-dependent emesis in least shrew [28] with no such activity in either the ferret [42,43] or the house musk shrew [44,45]. However, much later the emetic efficacy of SR141716A was confirmed in the ferret [95] but such validation has not been obtained in the house musk shrew.

ACKNOWLEDGEMENTS

The author would like to thank Professor Jeffrey Felton for his comments and proof reading the manuscript and Mrs. Nona Williamson for typesetting. The data was supported in part by NIH grant #RO1CA115331 and by WesternU/COMP startup funds.

CONFLICT OF INTEREST

The authors confirm that this chapter content has no conflicts of interest.

REFERENCES

[1]   Pertwee, RG, Howlett, AC, Abood, ME, Alexander, SPH, Di Marzo, V, Elphick, MR, Gresley, PJ, Hansen, HS, Kunos, G, Mackie, K, Mechoulam, R, Ross, RA. International union of basic and clinical pharmacology. LXXIX. Cannabinoid receptors and their ligands: beyond CB1 and CB2. Pharmacological Revs 2010; 62: 588-631.

[2]   Ueda, N, Tsuboi, K, Uyama, T, Ohnishi, T. Biosynthesis and degradation of the endocannabinoid 2-arachidonoylglycerol. Biofactors 2011; 37: 1-7.

[3]   Storr, MA, Sharkey, KA. The endocannabinoid system and gut-brain signaling. Current Opinion Pharmacol 2007; 7: 575-582.

[4]   Regehr, WG, Carey, MR, Best, AR. Activity-dependent regulation of synapses by retrograde messengers. Neuron 2009; 63: 154-170.

[5]   Rouzer, CA, Marnett, LJ. Endocannabioid oxygenation by cyclooxygenases, lipoxygenases, and cytochrome P450: cross-talk between the eicosanoid and endocannabinoid signaling pathways. Chemical Rev 2011; 111: 5899-5921.

[6]   Darmani, NA, Ray, AP. Evidence for a re-evaluation of the neurochemical and anatomical bases of chemotherapy-induced vomiting. Chemical Rev 2009; 109: 3158-3199.

[7]   Darmani, NA. Mechanisms of broad-spectrum antiemetic efficacy of cannabinoids against chemotherapy-induced acute and delayed vomiting. Pharmaceuticals 2010; 3: 2930-2955.

[8]   Parker, LA, Rock, EM, Limebeer, CL. Regulation of nausea and vomiting by cannabinoids. Br J Pharmacol 2011; 163: 1411-1422.

[9]   Abalo, R, Vera, G, Lopez-Perez, AE, Martinez-Vilaluenga, M, Martin-Fontelles, MI. The gastrointestinal pharmacology of cannabinoids: Focus on motility. Pharmacology 2012; 90: 1-10.

[10]   Izzo, AA, Sharkey, KA. Cannabinoids and the gut: new developments and emerging concepts. Pharmacology Therapeutics 2010; 126: 21-38.

[11]   Fairbaim, JW, Pickens, JT. The oral activity of delta-9-tetrahydrocannabinol and its dependence on prostaglandin E2. Br J Pharmacol 1979; 67: 379-385.

[12]   Di Marzo, V. Endocannabinoids: synthesis and degradation. Rev Physiol Biochem Pharmacol 2008; 160; 1-24.

[13]   Hu, DL, Zhu, G, Mori, F, Omoe, K, Okada, M, Wakabayashi, K, Kaneko, S, Shinagawa, K, Nakane, A. Staphylococcal enterotoxin induces emesis through increasing serotonin release in intestine and it is downregulated by cannabinoid receptor. Cell Microbiol 2007; 9: 2267-2277.

[14]   Darmani NA. Endocannabinoid and gastrointestinal function. In: Oniavi, ES, Sugiura, T, Di Marzo, V. Eds. Endocannabinoids: The brain and body's marijuana and beyond. CRC Press, 2005; pp 393-418.

[15]   Izzo AA, Sharkey KA. Cannabinoids and the gut: new developments and emerging concepts. Pharmacol Therap 2010; 126: 21-38.

[16]   Buczynski MW, Parsons LH. Quantification of brain endocannabinoid levels: methods, interpretation and pitfalls. Br J Pharmacol 2010; 160: 423-442.

[17]   Chen J, Paudel KS, Derbenev AV, Smith BN, Stincomb AL. Simultaneous quantification of anandamide and other endocannabinoids in the dorsal vagal complex of rat brainstem by CC-MS. Chromatographia 2009; 91: 1-7.

[18]   Dey, I, Lejeune, M, Chadee, K. Prostaglandin E2 receptor distribution and function in the gastrointestinal tract. Br J Pharmacol 2006; 149: 611-623.

[19]   Kim, JH, Choi, SJ, Yeum, CH, Yoon, PJ, Choi, S, Jun, JY. Involvement of thromboxane in the modulation of pacemaker activity of interstitial cells of Cajal of mouse intestine. Korean J Physiol Pharmacol 2008; 12: 25-30.

[20]   Shahbazian, A, Heinemann, A, Pesker, BA, Holzer, P. Differential motor effects of prostanoid (DP,EP, IP, TP) and leukotriene receptor agonists in the guinea-pig isolated small intestine. Br J Pharmacol 2002; 137: 1047-1054.

[21]   Darmani NA. Antiemetic actions of Δ^9-tetrahydrocannabinol and synthetic cannabinoids in chemotherapy-induced nausea and vomiting. In: Onaivi ES, ed. Biology of marijuana:from gene to behavior. London, UK, Taylor and Frances Books Ltd, 2002; pp. 356-389.

[22]   Parker LA, Rock EM, Limbeer CL. Regulation of nausea and vomiting by cannabinoids. Br J Pharmacol 2011; 163: 1411-1422.

[23]   Darmani NA. Mechanisms of broad-spectrum antiemetic efficacy of cannabinoids against chemotherapy-induced acute and delayed vomiting. Pharmaceuticals 2010; 3: 2930-2955.

[24]   Macado Rocha FC, Stefano SC, De Cassia Haiek R, Rosa Oliveira LMQ, Da Silveira DX. Therapeutic use of Cannabis Sativa on chemotherapy-induced nausea and vomiting among cancer patients: systematic review and meta-analysis. Eur J Cancer Care 2008; 17: 431-443.

[25]   Wang Y, McClanhan BA, Darmani NA. Interactions of Δ^9-THC with classically used antemetics against the acute phase of cisplatin-induced emesis. Soc Neuroscience Abs 2006, No 766.3.

[26]   Meiri E, Jhangiani H, Vredenburgh JJ, Barbato LM, Carter FJ, Yang H-M, Baranowski V. Efficacy of dronabinol alone and in combination with ondansetron *versus* ondansetron alone for delayed chemotherapy-induced nausea and vomiting. Curr Med Res Opin 2007; 23: 533-543.

[27]   Wang Y, Ray AP, McClanahan BA, Darmani NA. The antiemetic interaction of Delta-9-tetrahydrocannabinol when combined with tropisetron or dexamethasone in the least shrew. Pharmacol Biochem Behav 2009; 91: 367-373.

[28]   Darmani NA. Delta (9)-tetrahydrocannabinol and synthetic cannabinoids prevent emesis produced by the cannabinoid CB(1) receptor antagonist/inverse agonist SR141716A. Neuropsychopharmacology 2011; 24: 198-2003.

[29]   Darmani NA. Delta-9-tetrahydrocannabinol differentially suppresses cisplatin-induced emesis and indices of motor function *via* cannabinoid CB1 receptors in the least shrew. Pharmacol Biochem Behav 2001; 69: 239-249.

[30]   Darmani NA, Sim-Selley LJ, Martin BR, Janoyan JJ, Crim JL, Parekh B, Breivogel CS. Antiemetic and motor depressive actions of CP55,994: cannabinoid CB1 receptor characterization, distribution and G-protein activation. Eur J Pharmacol 2003; 459: 83-95.

[31]   Darmani NA. The cannabinoid CB1 receptor antagonist SR141716A reverses the antiemetic and motor depressant actions of WIN55,212-2. Eur J Pharmacol 2001; 430: 49-58.

[32]   Van Sickle MD, Oland LD, Ho W, Hillard CJ, Mackie K, Davison JS, Sharkey KA. Delta-9-tetrahydrocannabinol selectively acts on CB1 receptors in specific regions of dorsal vagal complex to inhibit emesis in ferrets. Am J Physiol Gastrointes Liver Physiol 2003; 285: G566-G576.

[33]   Kwiatkowska, M, Parker LA, Burton P, Mechoulam RA. A comparative analysis of the potential of cannabinoids and ondansetron to suppress cisplatin-induced emesis in Suncus murinus (house musk shrew). Psychopharmacology (Berl) 2004; 174: 437-440.

[34]   Ray AP, Griggs L, Darmani NA. Delta-9-tetrahydrocannabinol suppresses vomiting behavior and Fos expression in both acute and delayed phases of cisplatin-induced emesis in the least shrew. Behav Brain Res 2009; 196: 30-36.

[35]   Abrahamov A, Abrahamov A, Mechoulam R. An efficient new cannabinoid antiemetic in pediatric oncology. Life Sci 195; 56: 2097-2102.

[36]   Darmani NA, Johnson JC. Central and peripheral mechanisms contribute to the antiemetic actions of delta-9-tetrahydrocannabinol against 5-hydroxytryptophan-induced emesis. Eur J Pharmacol 2004; 488: 201-2012.

[37]   Darmani, NA, Crim, J, McClanahan, BA, Wang, Y. Δ^9-THC prevents emesis produced by L-DOPA in the least shrew. Soc Neuroscience Abs 2006, Abtract number 765.26.

[38]   Darmani, NA, Crim, JL. Delta-9-tetrahydrocannabinol differentially suppresses emesis *versus* enhanced locomotor activity produced by chemically diverse dopamine D2/D3 receptor agonists in the least shrew (Cryptotis parva). Pharmacol Biochem Behav 2005; 80: 35-44.

[39]   Darmani, NA. The potent emetogenic effects of the endocannabinoid, 2-AG (2-arachidonoylglycerol) are blocked by delta (9)-tetrahydrocannabinol and other cannabinoids. J Pharmacol Exp Therap 2002; 300: 34-42.

[40]   Darmani, NA, Janoyan, JJ, Crim, J, Ramirez, J. Receptor mechanism and antiemetic activity of structurally diverse cannabinoids against radiation-induced emesis in the least shrew. Eur J Pharmacol 2007; 563: 187-196.

[41]   Darmani, NA, Gerdes, D, Trinh, C. Structurally diverse cannabinoids prevent substance P-induced emesis *via* cannabinoid CB1 receptor in Cryptotis parva. The 15th annual symposium on the cannabinoids, Clearwater, FL, USA, 2005.

[42]   Van Sickle, MD, Oland, LD, Ho, W, Mackie, K, Davison, JS, Sharkey, KA. Cannabinoids inhibit emesis through CB1 receptors in the brain of the ferret. Gastroenterology 2001; 121: 767-774.

[43]   Simoneau, II, Hamza, MS, Mata, HP, Siegel, EM, Vanderah, TW, Porreca, F, Makriyannis, A, Malan, TP, Jr. The cannabinoid agonist WIN55,212-2 suppresses opioid-induced emesis in ferrets. Anesthesiology 2011, 94, 882-887.

[44]   Cluny, NL, Naylor, RJ, Whittle, BA, Javid, FA. The effects of cannabidiol and tetrahydrocannabinol on motion-induced emesis in Suncus murinus. Basic Clin Pharmacol Toxicol 2008; 103: 150-156.

[45]   Parker, LA, Kwiatkowska, M, Burton, P, Mechoulam, R. Effect of cannabinoids on lithium-induced vomiting in Suncus murinus. Psychopharmacology 2004; 171: 156-161.

[46]   Hu, DL, Zhu, G, Mori, F, Omoe, K, Okada, M, Wakabayashi, K, Kaneko, S, Shinagawa, K, Nakane, A. Staphylococcal enterotoxin induces emesis through increasing serotonin release in intestine and it is downregulated by cannabinoid receptor. Cell Microbiol 2007; 9: 2267-2277.

[47]   Beaumont, H, Jenson, J, Carlsson, A, Ruth, M, Lehmann, A, Boeckxstaens, G. Effect of delta-9-tetrahydrocannabinol, a cannabinoid receptor agonist, on the triggering of transient lower esophageal sphincter relaxations in dogs and humans. Br J Pharmacol 2009; 156: 153-162.

[48]   Darmani, NA. Cannabinoid-induced hyperemesis: a conundrum-from clinical recognition to basic science explanations. Pharmaceuticals 2010; 3: 2163-2177.

[49]   Vaziri, ND, Thomas, R, Sterling, M, Seiff, K, Pahl, MV, Davila, J, Wilson, A. Toxicity with intravenous injection of crude marijuana extract. Clin Toxicol 1981; 81: 353-366.

[50]   Martin, BR. The use of cannabinoids in patients with chronic illness. US Pharmacist 2002; 27: 61-70.

[51]   Frytak, S, Moertel, CG, O'Fallen, JR, Rubib, J, Creagen, ET, O'Connel, MJ, Schutt, AJ, Schwartan, NW. Delta-9-tetrahydrocannabinol as an antiemetic for patients receiving chemotherapy: a comparison with prochorperazine and placebo. Ann Intern Med 1979; 91: 825-830.

[52]   Noyes, R, Brunk, SF, Avery, DH, Carter, R. The analgesic properties of delta-9-tetrahydrocannabinol and codeine. Clin Pharmacol 1975; 18: 84-89.

[53]   Orr, LE, McKernan, JF. Antiemetic effect of Δ^9-tetrahydrocannabinol in chemotherapy-associated nausea and vomiting as compared to placebo and compazine. J Clin Pharmacol Ther 1980; 21: 76S-80S.

[54]   Wang, T, Collet, J-P, Shapiro, S., Ware, MA. Adverse effects of medical cannabinoids: a systematic review. CMAJ 2008;178: 1669-1678.

[55]   Shannon, HE, Martin, WR, Silcox, D. Lack of antiemetic effects of Δ^9-tetrahydrocannabinol in apomorphine-induced emein the dog. Life Sci. 197; 23: 49-54.

[56]   Lichtman, AH, Wiley, JL, LaVecchia, K.L, Neviaser, ST, Arthur, DB, Wilson, DM, Martin, BR. Effects of SR141716after acute or chronic cannabinoid administration in dogs. Eur J Pharmacol 1998; 357: 139-148.

[57]   Schneir, AB, Baumbacher, T. Convulsions associated with the use of a synthetic cannabinoid product. J Med Tox 2012; 8: 62-64.

[58]   Forrester, MB, Kleinschmidt, K, Schwarz, E, Young A. Synthetic cannabinoid exposure reported to Texas poison centers. J Addict Dis 2011; 30: 351-358.

[59]   Bergman, J, Delatte, MS, Paronis, CA, Vemuri, K, Thakur, GA, Makriyannis, A. Some effects of CB1 antagonists with inverse agonist and neutral biochemical properties. Phys Behav 2008; 93: 666-670.

[60]   Van Gaal, LF, Rissanin, AM, Scheen, AJ, Ziegler, O, Rossner, S. Effects of the cannabinoid-1 receptor blocker rimonabant on weight reduction and cardiovascular risk factors in overweight patients: 1-year experience from the RIO-Europe study. Lancet 2005; 365: 1389-1397.

[61] Darmani, NA, Janoyan, JJ, Kumar, N, Crim, JL. Behaviorally-active doses of the CB1 receptor antagonist SR141716A increase brain serotonin and dopamine levels and turnover. Pharmacol Biochem Behav. 2011; 22: 565-572.

[62] Sticht, MA, Long, JZ, Rock, EM, Limebeer, CL, Mechoulam, R, Cravatt, BF, Parker, LA. Inhibition of monacylglycerol lipase attenuates vomiting in Suncus murinus and 2-arachidonoyl glycerol attenuates nausea in rats. Br J Pharmacol 2012; 165: 2425-2435.

[63] Van Sickle, MD, Duncan, M, Kingsley, PJ, Mouihate, A, Urbano, P, Mackie, K, Stella, N, Makriyannis, A, Piomelli, D, Davison, JS, Marnett, LJ, Di Marzo, V, Pittman, QJ, Patel KD, Sharley. Identification and functional characterization of brainstem cannabinoid CB2 receptors. Science 2005; 310: 329-332.

[64] Darmani, NA, McClanahan, BA, Trinh, V, Petrosino, S, Valenti, M, Di Marzo, V. Cisplatin increases brain 2-arachidonoylglycerol (2-AG) and concomitantly reduces intestinal 2-AG and anandamide levels in the least shrew. Neuropharmacology 2005; 49: 502-513.

[65] Sharkey, KA, Cristino, L, Oland, LG, Van sicle, MD, Starowicz, K, Pittman, QJ, Guglielmotti, V, Davison, J, Di Marzo, V. Arvanil, anandamide and N-arachidonoyl-dopamine (NADA) inhibit emesis through cannabinoid CB1 and vanilloid TRPV1 receptors in the ferret. Eur J Neurosci 2007; 25: 2773-2782.

[66] Andrews, PL, Okada, F, Woods, AJ, Haiwara, H, Kakaimoto, S, Toyoda, M, Matsuki, N. The emetic and antiemetic effects of the capsaicin analog resiniferatoxin in Suncus murinus, the house musk shrew. Br J Pharmacol 2000; 130; 1247-1254.

[67] Andrews, PL, Bhandari, P. Resiniferatoxin, an ultrapotent capsaicin analogue, has antiemetic properties in the ferret. Neuropharmacology 1993; 32: 799-806.

[68] Porter, AC, Sauer, J-M, Knierman, MD, Becker, JW, Berna, MJ, Baq, J, Nomikos, GG, Carter, P, Bymaster, FP, Leese, AB, Felder, CC. Characterization of a novel endocannabinoid, virodhamine, with antagonist activity at the CB1 receptor. J Pharmacol Exp Therap 2002; 301: 1020-1024.

[69] Schicho, R, Storr, M. Alternative targets within the endocannabinoid system for future treatment of gastrointestinal diseases. Can J Gastroenterol 2011; 25: 377-383.

[70] Parker, LA, Limebeer CL, Rock, EM, Litt, DL, Kwiatkowska M, Oiomelli, D. The FAAH inhibitor URB-597 interferes with cisplatin- and nicotine-induced vomiting in Suncus murinus (house musk shrew). Physiol Behav 2009; 97: 121-124.

[71] Cross-Mellor, SK, Ossenkopp, K-P, Piomelli, D, Parker, LA. Effects of the FAAH inhibitor, URB597, and anandamide on lithium-induced taste reactivity responses: a measure of nausea in the rat. Psychopharmacology 2007; 190: 135-143.

[72] Rock, EM, Limebeer, CL, Mechoulam, R, Piomelli, D, Parker, LA. The effect of cannabidiol and URB597 on conditioned gaping (a model of nausea) elicited by lithium-paired context in the rat. Psychopharmacology 2008; 196: 389-395.

[73] Du Sert, NP, Ho, WSV, Rudd, JA, Andrews, PLR. Cannabinoid-induced reduction in antral pacemaker frequency: a telemetric study in the ferret. Neurogastroenterol Motil 2010; 22: 1257-e324.

[74] Chu, K-M, Ngan, P-P, Wai, M-K, Yeung, C-K, Andrews, PLR, de Sert, NP, Rudd, JA. Olvanil: a non-pungent TRPV1 activator has anti-emetic properties in the ferret. Neuropharmacology 2010; 58: 383-391.

[75] Keown, OP, Winterbum, TJ, Wainright, CL, Macrury, SM, Neilson, I, Barrett, F., Leslie, SJ, Megson, IL. 2-arachidonoylglycerol activates platelets *via* conversion to arachidonic

acid and not by direct activation of cannabinoid receptors. Br J Clin Pharmacol 2010; 70: 180-188.

[76] Chebolu, S, Wang, Y, Ray, AP, Darmani, NA. Pranlukast prevents cysteinyl leukotriene-induced emesis in the least shrew (Cryptotis parva). Eur J Pharmacol 2010; 628: 195-201.

[77] Ngo, TD, Park, MH, Shakur, H, Free, C. Comparative effectiveness, safety and acceptability of medical abortion at home and in a clinic: a systemic review. Bull World Health Organ 2011; 89: 360-370.

[78] Kan, KKW, Jones, RL, Ngan, M-P, Rudd, JA. Actions of prostanoids to induce emesis and defecation in the ferret. Eur J Pharmacol 2002; 453: 299-308.

[79] Scammell, T, Gerashchenko, D, Urade, Y, Onoe, H, Saper, C, Hayaishi, O. Activation of ventrolateral preoptic neurons by the somnogen prostaglandin D2. Proc Natl Acad Sci USA 1998; 95: 7754-7759.

[80] Kan, KKW, Jones, RL, Ngan, P-P, Rudd, JA. Excitatory action of prostanoids on the ferret isolated vagus nerve preparation. Eur J Pharmacol 2004; 491: 37-41.

[81] Briggs, DB, Carpenter, DO. Excitation of neurons in the canine area postrema by prostaglandins. Cell Mol Neurobiol 1986; 6: 421-426.

[82] Minami, M, Endo, T, Kikuchi, K, Ihira, E, Hirafuji, M, Hamaue, N, Monma, Y, Sakurada, T, Tan-no, K, Kisara, K. Antiemetic effects of sendide, a peptide tachykinin NK1 receptor antagonist, in the ferret. Eur J Pharmacol 1998; 363: 49-55.

[83] Minami, M, Endo, T, Ogawa, T, Nemoto, M, Hamaue, N, Hirafuji, M, Yoshiokawa, M, Nagahisa, A, Andrews, PL. Effects of CP-99,994, a tachykinin NK(1) receptor antagonist, on abdominal afferent vagal activity in ferrets: evidence for involvement of NK(1) and 5-HT(3) receptors. Eur J Pharmacol 2001; 428: 215-220.

[84] Kan, KKW, Rudd, JA, Wai, MK. Differential action of anti-emetic drugs on defecation and emesis induced by prostaglandin E2 in the ferret. Eur J Pharmacol 2006; 544: 153-159.

[85] Kan, KKW, Jones, RL, Ngan, M-P, Rudd, JA. Action of prostanoids on the emetic reflex of Suncus murinus (the house musk shrew). Eur J Pharmacol 2003; 477;: 247-251.

[86] Kan, KKW, Jones, RL, Ngan, M-P, Rudd, JA, Wai, MK. Emetic action of the prostanoid TP receptor agonist, U46619, in Suncus murinus (house musk shrew). Eur J Pharmacol 2003; 482: 297-304.

[87] Macica, C, Balazy, M, Falk, JR, Mioskowski, C, Carroll, MA. Characterization of cytochrome P-450-dependent arachidonic acid metabolism in rabbit intestine. Am J Physiol 1993; 265: G735-G74.1

[88] Irusta, G, Murphy, MJ, Perez, WD, Hennebold, JD. Dynamic expression of epoxyeicosatrienoic acid synthesizing and metabolizing enzymes in the primate corpus luteum. Mol Hum Reprod 2007; 13: 541-548.

[89] Jett, M, Brinkley, W, Neill, R, Gemski, P., Hunt, R. Staphylococcus aureus enterotoxin B challenge of monkeys: correlation of plasma levels of arachidonic acid cascade products with occurrence of illness. Infection Immunology 1990; 58: 3494-3499.

[90] Hu, D-L, Zhu, G, Mori, F, Omoe, K, Okada, M, Wakabayyashi, K, Kaneko, S, Shinsgawa, K, Nakane, A. Staphylococcal enteroxin induces emesis through increasing serotonin release in intestine and it is down-regulated by cannabinoid receptor 1. Cellular Microbiol 2007; 9: 2267-2277.

[91] Kudo, C, Minami, M, Hirafugi, M, Endo, t, Hamaue, N, Akita, K, Murakami, T,, Kawagichi, H. The effects of nabumatone, a cyclooxygenase-2 inhibitor, on cisplatin-

induced 5-hydroxytryptamine release from the isolated rat ileum. Res Commun Mol Pathol Pharmacol 2011; 110: 117-132.

[92]   Girod, V, Dapzol, J, Buovier, M, Grelot, L. The COX inhibitors indomethacin and meloxicam exhibit antiemetic activity against cisplatin-induced emesis in piglets. Neuropharmacology 2002; 42: 428-436.

[93]   Girod, V, Buovier, M, Grelot, L. Characterization of lipopolysaccharide-induced emesis in conscious piglets: effects of cervical vagotomy, cyclooxygenase inhibitors and a 5-HT(3) receptor antagonist. Neuropharmacology 2000; 39: 2329-2335.

[94]   Malcher-Lopes, R, Franco, A, Tasker, JG. Glucocorticoids shift arachidonic acid metabolism toward endocannabinoid synthesis: a non-genomic anti-inflammatory switch. Eur. J. Pharmacol 2008; 583: 322-339.

[95]   Salamone, JD, McLaughin, PJ, Sink, K, Makriyannis, A, Parker, LA. Cannabinoid CB1 receptor inverse agonists and neutral antagonists: effects on food intake, food-reinforced behavior and food aversions. Physiol Behav 2007; 91: 383-388.

CHAPTER 3

On the Cannabinoid Regulation of Energy Homeostasis: Past, Present and Future

Amanda Borgquist and Edward J. Wagner[*]

Department of Basic Medical Sciences, College of Osteopathic Medicine of the Pacific, Western University of Health Sciences, Pomona, CA 91766, USA

Abstract: The term "cannabinoid" refers to the class of 60 or so compounds found in the plant *Cannabis sativa*, of which Δ^9-tetrahydrocannabinol (THC) is the major bioactive constituent. In addition, endogenous cannabinoids such as anandamide and 2-arachidonyl glycerol are synthesized *de novo* from phospholipids *via* the enzymatic activities of phospholipases such as phospholipase (PL)C, PLD and diacylglycerol lipase. These compounds act to varying degrees at three subtypes of cannabinoid receptors: the CB1 and CB2 receptors, as well as GPR55. There is a wealth of evidence demonstrating that both endogenous and exogenous cannabinoids regulate energy homeostasis by increasing energy intake and decreasing energy expenditure. Based on our current understanding it is apparent that this occurs *via* complex interactions between the gut, liver, pancreas, brainstem, hypothalamus and limbic forebrain. Moreover, the regulatory effects of cannabinoids on energy balance are sexually differentiated and subject to the modulatory influences of steroid and peptide hormones. This chapter endeavors to explore the continuum of developments in the intensive, 40+-year study of how cannabinoids regulate food intake, gastrointestinal motility and secretion, fat and carbohydrate disposition, mitochondrial respiration and core body temperature. It is anticipated that this work will offer new insight and provide a newfound appreciation of the pleiotropic mechanisms through which cannabinoids control energy homeostasis.

Keywords: Cannabinoids, appetite, metabolism, hypothalamus, brain stem, GI tract, body temperature, POMC neurons, contraction, secretion, transmitter release

HISTORICAL BACKGROUND/INTRODUCTORY REMARKS

Throughout history, marijuana (a.k.a., *Cannabis sativa*, *Cannabis indica*, *ta-ma*, bhang, Indian hemp) has been among the world's most widely cultivated plant. Its first recorded use dates back over 12,000 years [1]. It has been used extensively

*Address correspondence to Edward J. Wagner:Department of Basic Medical Sciences, College of Osteopathic Medicine, Western University of Health Sciences, 309 E. Second Street, Pomona, CA 91766, Tel: 909-469-5239, Fax: 909-469-5698, E-mail: ewagner@westernu.edu

Eric Murillo-Rodríguez, Emmanuel S. Onaivi, Nissar A. Darmani & Edward Wagner (Eds.)

for the strength of its stalk fibers by the ancient Chinese, Greek and Roman civilizations [2-7]. These cultures, along with the Egyptians, Indians and Assyrians from ancient and medieval periods, were also using cannabis to varying degrees for a number of different medicinal purposes (*e.g.*, constipation, malaria, pain relief, fever reduction, sleep induction, appetite stimulation); often times mixing it with other substances such as alcohol or opium [1-5,7]. In addition, they were aware of the intoxicant and aphrodisiac properties of cannabis, as well as its ability to cause impotence [2-5,7]. In America, cannabis was used for many of these same expressed purposes going back to colonial times, and this use continued right up until the passage of the Marijuana Tax Act in 1937 [2,3,5,6]. In fact, various preparations of cannabis extract were listed in the National Formulary and U.S. Pharmacopoeia up until 1941 [2, 6].

Fast forward to the 1960s, and it is here when we find that tetrahydrocannabinol (THC) was first identified as the primary bioactive constituent of marijuana [8]. This seminal discovery prompted structure-function analyses that ultimately revealed four classes of compounds with pharmacological and behavioral properties similar to THC: tricyclic molecules with an intact dibenzopyran ring system like THC, bicyclic molecules (*e.g.* CP-55,940), aminoalkylindoles (*e.g.*, WIN 55,212) and arachidonylethanolamides (*e.g.*, anandamide [1]). It was another, nearly 30 years before one of the receptors to which THC binds was discovered and cloned from the brain and testis of the rat and human – namely, the cannabinoid CB1 receptor [9,10]. These discoveries were followed shortly thereafter by the identification of anandamide as an endogenous agonist for the CB1 receptor [11]. In 1993, Munro and colleagues [12] identified the CB2 receptor as a second subtype of cannabinoid receptor located primarily in peripheral tissues.

It is now known that both CB1 and CB2 receptors are metabotropic, $G_{i/o}$-coupled receptors that negatively modulate adenylyl cyclase activity, cAMP production, protein kinase A (PKA) activation and Ca^{2+} influx through voltage-gated Ca^{2+} channels. They also enhance K^+ efflux through a variety of K^+ channels such as the Kv4.2 channel and the G protein-gated, inwardly-rectifying K^+ (GIRK)1 channel. In addition, they modulate the activity of AMP-dependent protein kinase (AMPK) in a site-specific manner, increase the activity of mitogen-activated protein kinase (MAPK) in microglia, and reduce nitric oxide production in macrophages (for review see [13]). Interestingly there is a metabotropic orphan receptor, termed GPR55, for which lysophosphatidylinositol is the endogenous agonist and CB1 receptor antagonists like SR141716A and AM251 appear to act as partial agonists. This receptor is expressed throughout the body, and has been implicated in the regulation of neurotransmitter release, vascular tone, bone remodeling, pain, cell proliferation and energy balance. In contrast to the effects seen following the activation of CB1 receptors, GPR55 stimulation leads to intracellular Ca^{2+} mobilization and increased transmitter release. This makes sense when one considers that SR141716A and AM251 are capable of activating this receptor. In peripheral tissues GPR55 stimulation has been reported to trigger the activation of phosphatidylinositol-3-kinase (PI3K), Bmx, phospholipase C, MAPK, and RhoA (for review see [14]).

In the time that has elapsed since its prohibition, the studies conducted have largely supported the idea that cannabinoids have widespread medicinal applications; with considerable efficacy in the treatments of chemotherapy-associated nausea, pain and glaucoma [1,15]. However, the mood-altering, euphoric properties invoked following their inhalation or ingestion still remain the primary reason behind their use [1,15,16]. In fact, there is an ongoing surge in the recreational use of synthetic aminoalkylindoles (*e.g.*, JWH018, WIN 55,212-2) and other CB1 receptor agonists such as HU-210 that have been impregnated in herbal blends and incense, and marketed under names like Spice, K2 and Banana Cream Nuke [17-20]. Although long considered benign compared with drugs of abuse such as heroin or cocaine, evidence gathered over the past 30 years suggests that CB1 receptor agonists activate a major brain reward pathway comprising the midbrain dopamine neurons [21-24]. This suggests a common denominator for the rewarding properties of heroin, cocaine, ethanol and marijuana [25]. Moreover, the abuse of the synthetic cannabinoids found in the aforementioned herbal mixtures has been associated with a disturbing number fatalities reported over the past several years [20].

This chapter will focus on the role of cannabinoids in the regulation of energy homeostasis. We will start with an overview of the biosynthesis, transport and metabolism of endogenous cannabinoids. Next we will discuss cannabinoid effects on food intake. Then we will talk about cannabinoid actions on energy expenditure. Finally, we will summarize the current state of what we know concerning the cannabinoid regulation of energy balance, and the direction that future research is likely to take us.

OVERVIEW OF ENDOGENOUS CANNABINOID BIOSYNTHESIS, TRANSPORT AND METABOLISM

Biosynthesis of Endogenous Cannabinoids

Endogenous cannabinoids are derivatives of unsaturated fatty acids, distributed in the central nervous system (CNS), peripheral nerves, uterus, leukocytes, spleen and testicles [26]. These lipid molecules serve as ligands for CB_1 and CB_2 receptors, as well as GPR55. The first endogenous cannabinoid discovered was anandamide (arachidonylethanolamide), which was isolated from porcine brain in 1992 [26]. The second endogenous cannabinoid uncovered was 2-AG, which was first identified in the intestine of canine gut [27]. Some additional endocannabinoids that have been identified include O-arachidonoylethanolamine, 2-arachidonyl glyceryl ether and docosatetraenoyl-ethanolamide [26,28,29]. Endogenous cannabinoids are not stored in cells like neurotransmitters; rather they are synthesized as needed [26].

The two best-described endogenous cannabinoids are anandamide and 2-AG, which as mentioned above are lipids that differ from amino acid, amine and peptide transmitters in more complex ways than merely their chemical makeup [30]. It is now widely accepted that phospholipids such as phosphatidylcholine or phosphatidylinositol are not only constituents of the cell membrane, but are also precursors for transmembrane signaling molecules and serve as important biologically active lipids in cell-to-cell communication [29]. The molecular structures that anandamide and 2-AG share are a polyunsaturated fatty acid tail and a polar head group consisting of ethanolamine and glycerol [29]. Even though endogenous cannabinoids bear a resemblance to eicosanoids, they are unique because of their alternate biosynthetic routes. Aside from eicosanoids and in contrast to classical and peptide transmitter synthesis anandamide and 2-AG are produced quickly by receptor-stimulated cleavage of membrane lipid precursors from mainly neurons and glia cells then released quickly from these cells after their assembly [29,30].

The first step in the biosynthesis of endogenous cannabinoids involves Ca^{2+} influx into the cell through voltage-dependent Ca^{2+} channels, and Ca^{2+} freed from intracellular stores upon excitement of inositol 1, 4, 5-trisphosphate (IP_3) receptors [26,29]. This increase in intracellular Ca^{2+} is critical for the activation of the biosynthetic enzymes [31]. Anandamide synthesis occurs primarily by a reaction involving precursors in the cell membrane such as phosphatidylethanolamine (PE) and phospholipids [26,29]. The reaction is carried out *via* N-acyltransferase (NAT, a.k.a. transacylase), which transfers the arachidonate group from the sn-1 glycerol ester position of phospholipids like phosphatidylcholine to the primary amino group of PE [26,29,31,32]. Once N-arachidonoyl-PE is generated phospholipase D (PLD) converts it to anandamide [26]. Yet another pathway of anandamide synthesis involves the condensation of arachidonic acid and ethanolamine by an enzyme originally termed anandamide synthase [26,29]. It is now known that this reaction is actually carried out by fatty acid amide hydrolase in the presence of high concentrations of the arachidonic acid and ethanolamine; performing a reaction opposite that of the normal hydrolysis reaction involved in anandamide degradation ([29]; see below).

There are two possible pathways through which 2-AG can be synthesized. The first method requires the activation of phospholipase C (PLC) through neurotransmitter receptors such as G_q-coupled metabotropic glutamate receptors or muscarinic cholinergic receptors, which produces IP_3 and 1,2-diacylglycerol, the latter of which can then be converted into 2-AG by the enzyme 1,2-diacylglycerol lipase (DGL [29]). Purification of rat brain DGL has been reported, and inhibitors of PLC and DGL prevent 2-AG synthesis in cell cultures of cortical neurons [29,33]. In addition, DGL is found in close synaptic apposition with presynaptically localized CB1 receptors [34]. Collectively, these findings signify that the PLC/DGL pathway plays an integral role in the formation of 2-AG. The second proposed route of 2-AG formation involves phospholipase A_1 (PLA$_1$), which is thought to generate a lysophospholipid that is subsequently hydrolyzed to 2-AG by lyso-PLC activation [29].

Transport and Metabolism of Endogenous Cannabinoids

Newly synthesized anandamide or 2-AG, released into the extracellular space, subsequently activates G-protein coupled cannabinoid receptors, predominantly in a retrograde synaptic signaling fashion [30]. Both anandamide and 2-AG are hydrophobic molecules and therefore are confined in their movements through their aqueous environments [29]. However, growing evidence suggests that carrier-mediated transport may represent a means through which these lipid molecules can be rapidly and selectively removed from the synaptic cleft [35]. Indeed, N-(4-hydroxyphenyl) arachidonylamide (AM404) blocks anandamide accumulation in rat cortical neurons and astrocytes *in vitro*, whereas prostaglandin E_2 (PGE_2) was ineffective [36]. It also enhances the suppression of inhibitory neurotransmission by 2-AG in hippocampal slices [37]. Anandamide also accumulates in cerebellar granule cells in a saturable, stereoselective and Na^+-independent fashion that is sensitive to noncompetitive inhibition by the fatty acid phloretin [38,39]. The structural determinants for substrate recognition and subsequent facilitated diffusion by the anandamide transporter include a polar, hydroxyl-containing head group and a carboxamide group [39]. Given the structural similarities between anandamide and 2-AG, this would help explain why 2-AG is cleared from the media of human astrocytoma cells just as rapidly and effectively as anandamide, and how 2-AG is able to compete with anandamide (and *vice versa*) to varying degrees for carrier-mediated translocation *via* the anandamide transporter in different cell types [28,29,39,40].

Once inside the cell, anandamide is broken down to arachidonic acid and ethanolamine by fatty acid amide hydrolase (FAAH) [26]. This enzyme is mostly found in liver and brain tissues and expressed less in the spleen, kidney, testis and lungs [26]. Within the brain FAAH is widely expressed, but most prominently in the cortex, hippocampus, amygdala and cerebellum [41]. Anandamide can also be metabolized into PGE_2-ethanolamide and 12(S)-hydroxy-arachidonylethanolamide *via* the cyclooxygenase-2 and lipooxygenase, respectively [26]. Hydrolysis of 2-AG is carried out by monoglyceride lipase (MGL), a serine hydrolase, which breaks down monoglycerides into fatty acid and glycerol [42]. As with FAAH, MDL has a widespread distribution throughout the brain, with appreciable expression being observed in areas rich with CB1 receptors such as the hippocampus, cortex, thalamus and cerebellum [43]. The hippocampal distribution of MGL is laminar in appearance, which is indicative of a presynaptic distribution in the termination zones

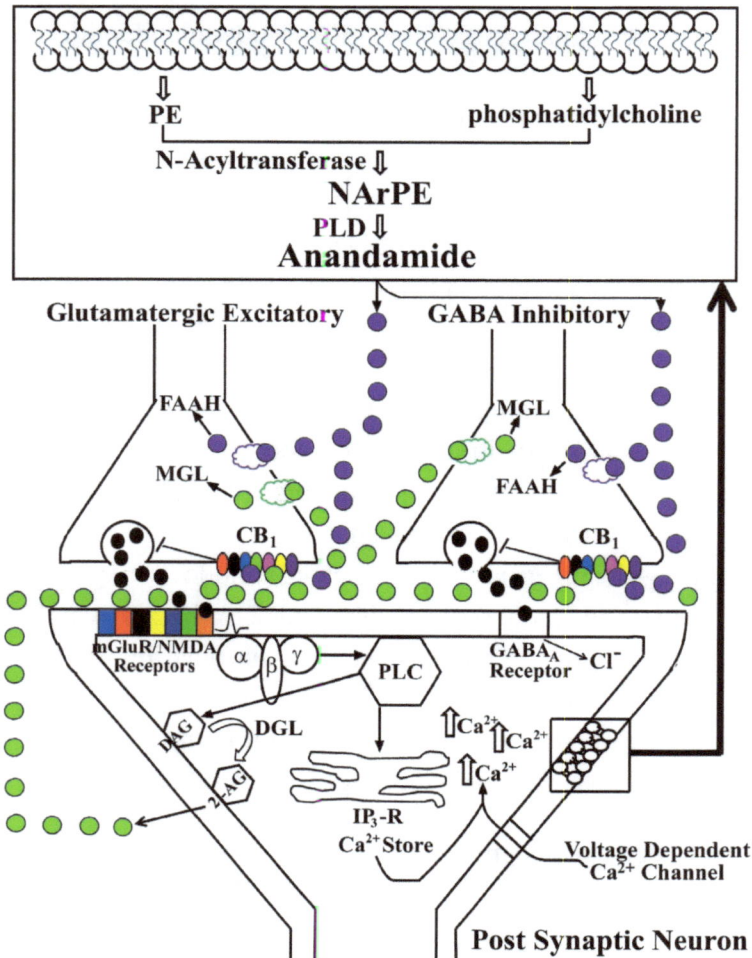

Figure 1: A summary of the mechanisms that are responsible for endogenous cannabinoid biosynthesis, release, transport and metabolism. Calcium mobilization through the release from intracellular stores triggered by inositol 1, 4, 5 triphosphate (IP$_3$), as well as influx through voltage-gated Ca2$^+$ channels, is necessary to activate the biosynthetic enzymes. The activation of phospholipase C (PLC) can be initiated through group I metabotropic glutamate receptors (mGluR)s or ionotropic *N*-methyl-D-aspartate glutamate (NMDA) receptors. Once PLC is activated it will produce IP$_3$ and 1,2-diacylglycerol (DAG), the latter of which is converted to 2-AG through the activity of the enzyme 1,2 diacylglycerol lipase (DGL). Anandamide is produced from the membrane precursors phosphatidylethanolamine (PE) and phospholipids like phosphatidylcholine, which are transformed into N-arachidonoyl-PE (NArPE) *via* N-acyltransferase. NArPE is then acted on by phospholipase D (PLD) to form anandamide. Once 2-AG and anandamide are released from the postsynaptic cell, they activate CB$_1$ receptors located primarily on presynaptic nerve terminals to inhibit both glutamate and GABA release. Carrier-mediated facilitated diffusion removes 2-AG and anandamide from the synaptic cleft. 2-AG is then broken down into arachidonic acid and glycerol by monoglyceride lipase (MGL) and anandamide is hydrolyzed into arachidonic acid and ethanolamine *via* fatty acid amide hydrolase (FAAH).

of glutamatergic Schaffer collaterals and mossy fibers, which renders it strategically localized to degrade 2-AG at CA3-CA1 pyramidal cell and dentate-CA3 pyramidal cell synapses [29,43]. This is substantiated by the fact that MGL inhibitors like arachidonoyl fluorophosphonate appreciably augment the presynaptic inhibitory effects of endogenously produced 2-AG on inhibitory and excitatory neurotransmission in the hippocampus [44]. The dynamics of the synthesis, signaling, transport and metabolism are graphically depicted in Fig. **1**.

CANNABINOID EFFECTS ON ENERGY INTAKE

As mentioned above it has long been known anecdotally that cannabinoids stimulate food intake, and this has since been proven experimentally in both humans and animal models [45-49]. Studies in rodents have revealed that CB1 receptor agonists increase the amount of time spent eating and decrease the time spent resting, whereas CB1 receptor antagonists decrease the amount of time spent eating and increase the time spent grooming and resting [50,51]. The hyperphagia elicited by CB1 receptor agonists exhibits an inverted U dose-response relationship, and this is due most likely to the cataleptic effect of cannabinoids observed at higher doses [47,51-53]. In addition, the hyperphagic and hypophagic effects of CB1 receptor agonists and antagonists, respectively, are greatly accentuated in subjects fed a palatable, carbohydrate-rich or high-fat diets [47,51,54-57].

In a seminal study conducted back in 1971, Abel [45] reported that marijuana smoking significantly increased marshmallow consumption in human subjects who were brought in for the expressed purpose of evaluating marijuana's effect on memory and intellectual performance. Collectively, these and other observations gradually led to the idea that various formulations of THC could be clinically applicable as therapeutic adjuncts in ameliorating the cachexia associated with various pathological states. Indeed, smoked marijuana or orally ingested dronabinol (Marinol) are both efficacious in lessening the pain severity, anorexia, weight loss, nausea and vomiting seen with chronic pain, HIV/AIDS and a number of different types of cancer (*e.g.*, lung, gastrointestinal, pancreatic, prostate, Hodgkin's disease [58-65]). By contrast, the CB1 receptor antagonist SR141716A (Rimonabant) significantly decreased body weight and waist circumference, as well as normalized the lipid profile, of obese patients taking part in the RIO-North America clinical trial [66]. Were it not for some untoward side effects (*e.g.*, respiratory tract infection, arthralgia, depressed mood) experienced by a small percentage of participants, this compound would have undoubtedly proved to be an effective therapeutic adjunct in the treatment of obesity.

In all of the many studies touting the therapeutic efficacy of cannabinoid receptor agonists, whether they be case reports, case series or randomized, double-blind studies with placebo-treated controls, the considerable majority of participants were male [62-65]. However, in the one study where the gender ratio was more evenly split, the ability of cannabis extract and THC to stimulate appetite and improve quality of life in cachexic cancer patients was rendered ineffective [67]. This suggests that there are gender differences in the cannabinoid-induced increase in energy intake, and this idea has been substantiated in rodent animal models. Indeed, a ~10X greater dose of the CB1 receptor agonist CP55940 is required to elicit increased consumption of sweetened condensed milk in female rats that is equivalent to that observed in males [68]. Male guinea pigs also are more sensitive to the appetite-stimulating properties of the cannabinoid agonist WIN 55,212-2, and microstructural analysis of meal pattern reveals that the more robust hyperphagia observed in males is associated with increases in meal size, frequency and duration, whereas in females it is associated only with an increase in meal frequency [69].

Regulation of Gastrointestinal Motility, Secretion, Inflammation and Brain-Gut Communication

It is clear that cannabinoids exert widespread actions in regulating gastrointestinal function, and serve as chemical messengers that help mediate communication between the gut and brain. For example, CB1 receptors are expressed in nerve fibers, as well as in virtually all cholinergic motor neurons and, to a lesser degree, in substance P-containing neurons within the myenteric plexus of the guinea pig and rat [70]. These receptors are poised to mediate the inhibition of electrically-evoked contractions in the small intestine and peristalsis in the ileum, the latter of which is due to presumptive increases in nitric oxide production and the opening of apamin-sensitive K^+ channels [71,72]. CB1 receptor activation can also indirectly inhibit cholinergic contractions of longitudinal muscle from the murine ileum by negatively modulating purinergic P2X receptor-mediated increases in acetylcholine release [73]. In the gastric fundus both anandamide and WIN 55,212-2 inhibit cholinergic twitch contractions as well as non-adrenergic, non-cholinergic mediated relaxations [74]. Collectively, these actions serve to suppress gastrointestinal motility [75-79], which would slow the transit of luminal contents and allow for increased absorption of digested nutrients [80-82]. This also makes sense when one considers that the cannabinoid-induced increase in caloric content requires additional time for the nutrient macromolecules to be hydrolyzed into their absorbable units. Some have proposed that this is due most likely to a reduction in propulsive activity, with decreases in the frequency of gastric and intestinal contractions occurring without any change in intraluminal pressure [75]. Still others have shown that the THC-induced decrease in pyloric contractility is associated with a reduction in intragastric pressure [83].

Cannabinoids also are involved in regulating gastrointestinal secretion. For example, CB1 receptors are expressed in vasoactive intestinal peptide and neuropeptide Y (NPY)/cholinergic neurons, as well as in paravascular nerves and fibers, within the submucosal plexus of the guinea pig ileum [84]. The CB1/CB2 receptor agonist WIN 55,212-2 decreases the electrogenic ion transport caused by electrical field stimulation and capsaicin that is precluded by extrinsic denervation of the ileum [84]. WIN 55,212-2 and HU-210 both decrease pentagastrin- and 2-deoxy-D-glucose-induced gastric acid secretion; effects that are attenuated by cervical vagotomy and ganglionic blockade [85]. In addition, inhibition of MGL mitigates against gastric damage induced by nonsteroidal anti-inflammatory drugs in mice [86]. Moreover, cholera toxin upregulates CB1 receptor expression and increases anandamide secretion in the small intestine; effects which appear to counter the increased fluid accumulation caused by the toxin [87]. Both methanandamide and CP 55,940 increase orexigenic ghrelin release from the gastric mucosa, and smoked medicinal cannabis elevates plasma levels of ghrelin in HIV-infected men [88,89]. By contrast, both SR141716A and the anorexigenic anandamide analog oleoylethanolamide decrease circulating ghrelin levels in fed rats [90].

THC and cannabidiol both exert anti-inflammatory actions that ameliorate the damage and disturbed colonic motility seen with 2,4,6-trinitrobenzene-induced acute colitis in the rat [91]. Moreover, WIN 55,212-2 inhibits cytokine and chemokine secretion from rat pancreatic acini, and pretreatment with the agonist significantly attenuates the increase in amylase release as well as the morphological damage caused by caerulin-induced pancreatitis [92]. Another cannabinoid receptor, GPR55, also exerts anti-inflammatory effects that can influence gastrointestinal motility under conditions such as lipopolysaccharide-induced septic ileus [93]. These anti-inflammatory actions may be due to the ability of cannabinoids to activate/desensitize transient receptor potential, vanilloid type (TRPV)1-4 channels that have been found in the jejunum and ileum [94].

CB1 receptors also are expressed in vagal afferents innervating the stomach and duodenum, the levels of which are increased by fasting and reduced by refeeding in a cholecystokinin (CCK)-dependent manner [95]. These afferents convey chemical information on the luminal contents, as well as mechanical information on the tension in the gut wall, and when activated they transmit a satiety signal to the nucleus of the tractus solitarius (NTS; [96]). CB1 receptor activation blocks the cytokine-induced increase in intracellular calcium within vagal nerve terminals in the NTS, and in doing so blocks the malaise and anorexia caused by pro-inflammatory mediators such as tumor necrosis factor [97]. THC can also inhibit $5HT_3$ receptor-mediated currents in rat nodose ganglion neurons [98], and alter the unit activity of over 50% of NTS neurons, the considerable majority of which were catecholaminergic, glucose-responsive and glucose-sensitive neurons [99]. In 2004, Debenev and co-workers [100] reported that the cannabinoid receptor agonists WIN 55,212-2 and anandamide suppress both excitatory and inhibitory synaptic inputs impinging upon efferent neurons the dorsal motor nucleus of the vagus (DMNV), some of which project to the stomach. It is now known that endogenous cannabinoids are synthesized and released on demand in DMNV neurons, where they activate CB1 receptors located on presynaptic GABAergic nerve terminals in retrograde fashion to inhibit $GABA_A$ receptor mediated synaptic currents *via* a process known as depolarization-induced suppression of inhibition (DSI; [101]). Endogenous cannabinoids also appear to stimulate GABA release in the DMNV by activating TRPV1 channels on the terminals of glutamatergic neurons emanating from the NTS [102]. Collectively, these effects culminate in increased consumption, as evidenced by the fact that CP55940 administered into the fourth ventricle stimulates the intake of sweetened condensed milk [68]. CB2 receptors also reside in the DMNV, where they appear to serve an anti-emetic function [103]. However, their exact role related to regulating energy balance remains to be elucidated. In addition, peripheral CB1 receptors mediate the analgesia that alleviates the visceral pain arising from colorectal distention [104].

Regulation of the Hypothalamic Feeding Circuitry

The neuroanatomical substrates of the hypothalamic feeding circuitry comprise both orexigenic and anorexigenic components. The orexigenic neuronal populations include the neuropeptide Y (NPY) and ghrelin neurons with cell bodies located in the arcuate nucleus (ARC) of the mediobasal hypothalamus [105-109]. In addition, there are orexin (hypocretin) and melanin concentrating hormone (MCH) neurons with cell bodies emanating from the lateral hypothalamus that serve to stimulate feeding [110-113]. Inhibitory inputs to the hypothalamic feeding circuitry arise predominantly from the hypothalamic ventromedial nucleus (VMN; [114-116]), and from proopiomelanocortin (POMC) neurons originating in the ARC [117,118]. Cocaine amphetamine related transcript (CART), a neuropeptide that is found in a large percentage POMC neurons, as well as in neurons in the dorsomedial nucleus (DMN), lateral hypothalamic area (LHA) and paraventricular nucleus (PVN), also suppresses feeding [119-122]. In addition, α-melanocyte stimulating hormone (α-MSH) derived from the POMC gene decreases food intake [118]. By contrast, opioids like the POMC derivative β-endorphin stimulate feeding [107,123]. On the other hand, male transgenic β-endorphin knockout mice exhibit hyperphagia associated with increased adiposity and other abnormalities such as hyperinsulinemia and glucose intolerance [124]. Agouti-related peptide (AgRP) colocalizes with NPY in a subpopulation of ARC neurons, and stimulates feeding by antagonizing the actions of α-MSH at melanocortin (MC)4 receptors [125-129]. This hypothalamic feeding circuit is modulated by peripheral hormones emanating from the gut (*e.g.*, peptide YY (PYY), ghrelin, glucagon-like peptide (GLP)-1) and by leptin emanating from adipose tissue [117,130-133]. In addition, leptin and PYY inhibit energy intake by increasing the firing rate of the inhibitory inputs (*e.g.*, POMC neurons) and decreasing that observed in excitatory inputs such as the NPY neurons, whereas ghrelin exerts the opposite effect on these neurons [117,134-137]. While there is considerable synaptic reciprocity and redundancy [113,128,138-140], all of the neural components comprising the hypothalamic feeding circuit project to the PVN [141,142] where they can synapse on corticotrophin-releasing hormone (CRH) neurons [108,142], alter the firing rate of parvocellular PVN neurons [143] and exert effects on feeding [113]. Given that CRH suppresses food intake [144], it is apparent that the PVN is an important locus for accommodating afferent signals concerning energy status and integrating them into an efferent feeding response.

CB1 receptors are expressed in the ARC, preoptic area, PVN, VMN, LHA and DMN [121,145]. Accordingly, it should not be surprising that both endogenous and exogenous CB1 receptor agonists can stimulate food intake when administered directly into nuclei comprising the hypothalamic feeding circuitry. For example, anandamide delivered directly into the VMN stimulates food consumption [146], as does THC when administered into the PVN [147]. 2-AG levels in the hypothalamus are increased by food deprivation, and reduced during refeeding [148]. Hypothalamic 2-AG concentrations also are elevated in obese Zucker (*fa/fa*) rats, as well as in obese *db/db* (leptin receptor deficient) and *ob/ob* (leptin deficient) mice [149]. In addition, orexigenic ghrelin increases hypothalamic 2-AG and, to a lesser extent, anandamide concentrations [150], whereas anorexigenic leptin decreases hypothalamic concentrations of both 2-AG and anandamide [149]. With regard to the former, both THC and 2-AG, as well as ghrelin, increase the activity of AMPK in the hypothalamus, and the ability of ghrelin to elevate hypothalamic AMPK activity is blocked by SR141716A [150,151].

Thus, both exogenous and endogenous cannabinoids are poised to regulate energy homeostasis, in part, *via* their actions on cellular substrates within the hypothalamic feeding circuitry. In the LHA, endogenous cannabinoids disinhibit MCH neurons by reducing $GABA_A$ receptor-mediated synaptic input impinging on these cells *via* DSI[152,153]. In addition, WIN 55,212-2 administered directly into the ventral tegmental area (VTA) increases c-fos expression in orexin (hypocretin) neurons [154]. On the other hand, WIN 55,212-2 has been shown to inhibit the activity of these neurons by reducing excitatory input onto these cells [153], which has ramifications concerning the mechanism(s) through which cannabinoids regulate arousal. Both anandamide and CP55, 940 were reported to increase KCl-evoked NPY release from hypothalamic explants [155]. This contrasts with the observation that SR141716A was able to decrease food intake in NPY-deficient mice just as efficaciously as it did in their wildtype controls [149]. In addition, WIN 55,212-2 did not affect the membrane potential or firing rate of NPY neurons, nor did it affect the synaptic input impinging upon these cells [156]. Collectively, this would indicate that NPY neurons are not critical to the ability of cannabinoids to regulate energy homeostasis. In 2008, Sinnayah and coworkers [154] reported that WIN 55,212-2 and the CB1 receptor antagonist AM251 respectively increase and decrease food intake in AgRP-overexpressing A^y mice. This would suggest that POMC neurons are not involved in the cannabinoid regulation of energy balance. On the other hand, WIN 55,212-2 presynaptically attenuates whereas AM251 accentuates convergent, excitatory glutamatergic and inhibitory GABAergic input onto both murine and guinea pig POMC neurons [53,157,158]. CB1 receptor activation can also augment an A-type K^+ current (I_A) through postsynaptic Kv4.2 channels that serves to directly inhibit these cells [53,159]. Moreover, transgenic FAAH-deficient mice exhibit reduced numbers of CART-immunoreactive fibers in the ARC, DMN and the periventricular nucleus, and week-long treatment with SR141716A restored the number of CART fibers to levels observed in their wildtype counterparts [160]. Furthermore, SR141716A was unable to decrease food intake CART-deficient mice [160].

These multifaceted actions of cannabinoids at POMC synapses are sexually differentiated. For example, the potency of WIN 55,212-2 to presynaptically inhibit GABA$_A$ receptor-mediated input is reduced ~6X in males as compared to females [69,161]. In addition, the cannabinoid-induced augmentation of the I_A is observed only in females, whereas in males CB1 receptor activation leads to the activation of GIRK1 channels [158,159]. Coupled with the fact that there is a greater CB1 receptor density in the hypothalamus of male rats as compared to females [162], these sexually differentiated actions of cannabinoids at POMC synapses help explain why males are more responsive to the hyperphagia caused by WIN 55,212-2 than are females [69].

This sexually discrepant, cannabinoid regulation of appetite can be further modified by gonadal steroid hormones. For example, estradiol markedly attenuates the ability of CB1 receptor agonists to presynaptically inhibit ionotropic glutamate receptor-mediated excitation of POMC neurons, and to augment the I_A in these cells [53,161]. This negative modulatory effect of the steroid is evident within minutes following bath application to hypothalamic slices, and lasts at least 24 hr following systemic administration [53,161]. The ability of estradiol to disrupt cannabinoid signaling is due to the activation of estrogen receptor (ER)α and the G_q-coupled membrane ER, which triggers a signal transduction cascade that involves the activation of PI3K, protein kinase C (PKC)δ and, to a lesser extent, PKA [163,164]. This is consistent with the estradiol-induced downregulation of CB1 receptors in the hypothalami of ovariectomized rats [162]. Collectively, this would render CB1 receptors less effective in decreasing glutamatergic neurotransmission; leading to increased excitation of POMC neurons and augmented anorexigenic tone within the hypothalamic feeding circuitry. This undoubtedly accounts, at least in part, for the ability of estradiol to dampen cannabinoid-induced hyperphagia in the female rodent [53,164].

In the PVN, corticosteroids rapidly decrease excitatory glutamatergic synaptic input onto both parvocellular and magnocellular neurons *via* a $G\alpha_s$-cAMP-PKA pathway that increases concentrations of anandamide and 2-AG to inhibit transmission [165,166]. Leptin antagonizes the corticosteroid-induced increases in endogenous cannabinoid levels, and thus the inhibitory effects on glutamate release, *via* a phosphodiesterase-3B-mediated decrease in intracellular cAMP production [166]. Given that CRH suppresses food intake [144], this corticosteroid effect may very well represent a fast negative feedback mechanism through which a critical anorexigenic component of the hypothalamic feeding circuitry is quieted during fasting by virtue of an increase in endogenous cannabinoid tone within the PVN. Ghrelin also reduces glutamatergic neurotransmission at synapses with parvocellular neurons in a manner that is sensitive to antagonism by AM251 or the DGL inhibitor tetrahydrolipstatin, thereby implicating the involvement of endogenous cannabinoids [150].

Regulation of the Hedonic Aspects of Food Intake

In addition to regulating gastrointestinal function and aspects of energy balance related to nutrient status and the like, compelling evidence indicates that cannabinoids influence the hedonic, rewarding components of appetitive behavior. Indeed, the nucleus accumbens (NAc) constitutes one of two brain sites for cannabinoid reward, as rats will readily self-administer THC into this region and establish conditioned place preference for the drug [25]. WIN 55,212-2 decreases GABAergic and glutamatergic input onto NAc neurons [167], and endogenous cannabinoids inhibit corticofugal glutamatergic input impinging on these cells *via* a process known as long-term depression [168-170]. These collective, cannabinoid-induced changes in synaptic transmission within the NAc ultimately increase dopamine release from mesolimbic terminals [23,171]. The cell bodies of these mesolimbic dopamine neurons emanate from the VTA, and the focal injection of WIN 55,212-2 or AM251 into this region respectively increases or decreases food intake [154]. Dopamine, in turn, decreases the content of anandamide and 2-AG in the limbic forebrain (of which the NAc is a part) *via* the activation of D1 and D2 receptors, respectively [172]. These latter findings contrast with a report from Sinnayah and co-workers [154], who observed that AM251 enhances electrically stimulated dopamine release from the NAc shell.

On the other hand, the concentrations of anandamide and 2-AG within the limbic forebrain are increased by fasting to an even greater extent than they are in the hypothalamus [148]. The NAc is an important neuroanatomical substrate for the μ-opioid receptor-mediated intake of high-fat food [173]. It also projects to the ventral palladium, which is an important integrative center for the hedonic liking and ingestion of palatable food [174]. It should not be a surprise, therefore, that anandamide or 2-AG administered into the shell of the NAc increase c-fos expression, food intake and sucrose-induced liking reactions [148,175], whereas SR141716A decreases dopamine release in the NAc shell that is caused by the ingestion of highly palatable food [176]. Thus, a fasting-induced increase in endogenous cannabinoid tone in the NAc will enhance motivation and incentive to procure palatable food, as well as the reward experienced upon its consumption (for review see [34]).

CANNABINOID EFFECTS ON ENERGY EXPENDITURE

Regulation of Lipogenesis and Glucose Homeostasis

Considerable evidence suggests that cannabinoids regulate the disposition of carbohydrates and fat. CB1 receptor activation is reported to attenuate glucose-stimulated insulin secretion and Ca^{2+} oscillations in pancreatic β islet cells [177], whereas the activation of GPR55 by O-1602 does just the opposite [178]. In 3T3-L1 cells THC stimulates adipogenesis (as measured by increased peroxisome proliferator-activated receptor γ expression) and lipid accumulation [179]. It also decreases both basal and isoproterenol-induced lipolysis, as well as NAPE-specific PLD expression, and increases adiponectin and transforming growth factor β expression [179]. THC increases glucose uptake in both normal 3T3-L1 cells and those made insulin resistant following exposure to tumor necrosis factor-α [180]. This latter finding is associated with an increase in the expression of glucose transporter-4, and while THC *per se* decreased the expression of insulin receptor substrate-1 (IRS-1) and IRS-2 in normal cells, it markedly increases IRS-1 and IRS-2 expression in insulin-resistant cells [180]. Moreover, HU210 increases the hepatic expression of lipogenic transcription factors such as SREBP-1c and enzymes like acetyl coenzyme-A carboxylase and fatty acid synthase, and consumption of a high-fat diet increases hepatic anandamide synthesis [181]. This explains how CB1 receptor agonists increase fatty acid synthesis in the liver, and why CB1 receptor knockout mice are resistant to increased adiposity, as well as to elevations in circulating insulin, triglycerides and leptin when fed a high-fat diet [181]. Furthermore, ethanol exposure enhances DGL-β expression and 2-AG production in hepatic stellate cells, and the resultant CB1 receptor activation leads to steatosis *via* increased lipogenesis and decreased fatty acid oxidation [182]. These lipogenic effects can be attributed to decreased AMPK activity in the liver and adipose tissue [151]. In the liver, the cannabinoid-induced decrease in AMPK activity can also accentuate hepatic gluconeogenesis *via* increased expression of phosphoenolpyruvate carboxykinase and glucose-6-phosphatase [151,183].

Interestingly, cannabinoid-induced lipogenesis may also be influenced by colonic bacteria and ambient levels of lipopolysaccharide (LPS), as evidenced in part by the fact that prebiotic treatment of mice with genetically- (*ob/ob*) or diet-induced obesity decreases colonic CB1 receptor expression and anandamide levels, as well as circulating LPS concentrations (an index of inflammation and gut permeability), and increases colonic FAAH expression [184]. Similar findings were observed with antibiotic treatment in lean mice, and in *Myd88$^{-/-}$* mice fed a high-fat diet [184]. In addition, SR141716A decreased plasma LPS levels, whereas HU210 increased them [184].

Regulation of Thermogenesis and Core Body Temperature

Cannabinoids elicit other metabolic effects as well. For example, WIN 55,212-2 dose dependently decreases uncoupling protein (UCP)1 expression in differentiated brown adipocytes, and this is associated with respective increases and decreases in visfatin and adiponectin expression in white adipocytes [185]. This is consistent with the observation that THC inhibits mitochondrial O_2 consumption in both human spermatozoa and oral cancer cells [186,187]. CB1 receptor activation also diminishes the Krebs'-Szentgyörgyi cycle's velocity, thereby decreasing the oxidative metabolism of glucose [188]. At the organismal level, WIN 55,212-2 decreases O_2 consumption and CO_2 production in the female guinea pig [164], and THC reduces both the basal and hypothermia-stimulated rates of O_2 consumption in the mouse [189]. The decrease in O_2 consumption caused by the intracerebroventricular or intrahypothalamic administration of THC is associated with a reduction in core body temperature [190], and the reduction in core body temperature caused by the systemic or intrahypothalamic administration of WIN 55,212-2 is blocked by pre-treatment with SR141716A [191]. This CB1 receptor-mediated hypothermia can be attributed in part to increased thermosensitivity and decreased firing of primary thermodetector units, increased thermosensitivity and firing of heat-sensitive interneurons, as well as decreased thermosensitivity and firing of cold-sensitive interneurons, in the preoptic area of the anterior hypothalamus [192]. Just like with energy intake, the cannabinoid-induced hypothermia is sexually differentiated, as evidenced by the fact that male guinea pigs exhibit a ~0.5°C greater reduction in core body temperature in response to 1 mg/kg WIN 55,212-2 than their female counterparts [69]. Interestingly, the magnitude and duration of the cannabinoid-induced hypothermia is appreciably dampened by estradiol in ovariectomized guinea pigs, which is consistent with the negative modulatory effect of the steroid on the cannabinoid-induced hyperphagia [53]. By contrast, SR141716A increases thermogenesis in brown adipose tissue of the rat, an effect that is associated with increased expression of UCP1 and attenuated following sympathetic denervation [193]. A similar thermogenic effect is observed with AM251 in the guinea pig [69].

SUMMARY, CONCLUSIONS AND FUTURE DIRECTIONS

The research conducted over the past half-century clearly and collectively points to a prominent and pervasive role for cannabinoids in regulating energy homeostasis. Exogenous and endogenous cannabinoids exert pleiotropic actions that occur *via* complex interactions between the gut, liver, pancreas, brainstem, hypothalamus and the limbic forebrain. The increased endogenous cannabinoid tone created by a negative energy balance signals *via* the ghrelin released from the oxyntic mucosa, the vagal afferents innervating the gastrointestinal tract, the NTS and DMNV neurons in the medulla, the POMC, parvocellular PVN, MCH and possibly orexin neurons in the hypothalamus, and the mesolimbic dopaminergic neurons that terminate in the NAc to convey information about nutrient bioavailability and to promote an increase in appetitive behavior. Exogenous cannabinoids can signal *via* these same neuroanatomical substrates to evoke the sensation of a negative energy balance and thereby stimulate food intake in an otherwise satiated individual. Cannabinoids also act *via* vagal efferents and those within the myenteric plexus to inhibit gastrointestinal motility, which increases the transit time of the luminal contents and increases their exposure to the mucosal surface, thereby augmenting the absorption of ingested nutrients. Once the nutrients are absorbed, cannabinoids then promote anabolic pathways (*e.g.*, gluconeogenesis, glycogenesis, lipogenesis, protein synthesis) due in large part to tissue-specific alterations in AMPK activity that facilitate macromolecular assembly and storage in the liver, adipose tissue and striated muscle. In addition, cannabinoids interact with the hypothalamic thermoregulatory center to bring about a reduction in core body temperature, and decrease mitochondrial respiration and metabolic heat production. Moreover, they can modulate the activity of vagal and submucosal efferents to inhibit hydrochloric acid secretion and electrolyte transport. Finally, cytokine release from secretory epithelia is reduced by cannabinoids, and this undoubtedly accounts in part for their ability to diminish gastrointestinal inflammation.

The question arises: where to go from here? While undoubtedly great strides have been made in advancing our understanding of how cannabinoids regulate energy homeostasis, the overall picture is far from complete and remains a work in progress. One aspect that certainly warrants further investigation is the role of GPR55 in regulating energy balance. Indeed, there is a loss-of-function mutation of GPR55, in which valine is substituted for glycine at the 195th position, that is comparatively more prevalent in a cohort of female Japanese individuals afflicted with anorexia nervosa [194]. Moreover, GPR55 expression is elevated in the visceral and subcutaneous fat of obese individuals [195]. Many cannabinoid effects pertaining to energy intake and/or expenditure are subject to modulation by a variety of different hormones (*e.g.*, CCK, leptin, ghrelin, estradiol, glucocorticoids). It will therefore be essential to ascertain the signal transduction mechanisms through which these hormones influence the coupling of CB1 receptors (and perhaps GPR55) to their effector systems in their target cells and tissues. In addition, several of the endpoints related to the cannabinoid regulation of energy homeostasis (*e.g.*, food intake, meal pattern, core body temperature) are sexually differentiated, with males responding more robustly than their female counterparts. Thus, clinicians and researchers alike will need to take this into consideration when developing rational strategies for utilizing cannabinoid-based, adjunct pharmacotherapies to ameliorate the cachexia associated with cancer and HIV/AIDS. Lastly, it is imperative that we continue to explore how cannabinoids interact with the immune system, mucosal epithelial cells and gut microbiota to modulate the gastrointestinal inflammation that is associated with obesity. The cannabinoid researchers of today stand on the shoulders of the pioneers that have led the way up to this point, and are poised to make the discoveries that will give us an even greater appreciation for the critical role that cannabinoids play in regulating energy homeostasis.

ACKNOWLEDGEMENTS

Declared none.

CONFLICT OF INTEREST

The authors confirm that this chapter content has no conflicts of interest.

REFERENCES

[1]   Adams IB, Martin BR. Cannabis: pharmacology and toxicology in animals and humans. Addiction 1996; 91:1585-1614.
[2]   Mikuriya TH. Marijuana in medicine: past, present and future. Calif Med 1969; 110:34-40.
[3]   Hindmarch I. A social history of the use of Cannabis Sativa. Contemp Rev 1972; 220:252-257.
[4]   Hamarneh S. Pharmacy in medieval Islam and the history of drug addiction. Med Hist 1972; 16:226-237.
[5]   Brunner TF. Marijuana in ancient Greece and Rome? The literary evidence. Bull Hist Med 1973; 47:344-355.
[6]   Winek CL. Some historical aspects of marijuana. Clin Toxicol 1977; 10:242-253.
[7]   Touw M. The religious and medical uses of Cannabis in China, India and Tibet. J Psychoactive Drugs 1981; 13:23-34.
[8]   Mechoulam R, Gaoni Y. A total synthesis of dl-Δ^1-tetrahydrocannabinol, the active constituent of hashish. J Am Chem Soc 1965; 87:3273-3275.
[9]   Matsuda LA, Lolait SJ, Brownstein MJ, Young AC, Bonner TI. Structure of a cannabinoid receptor and functional expression of the cloned cDNA. Nature 1990; 346:561-564.
[10]   Gérard CM, Mollereau C, Vassart G, Parmentier M. Molecular cloning of a human cannabinoid receptor which is also expressed in testis. Biochem J 1991; 279:129-134.
[11]   Devane WA, Hanus L, Breuer A, Pertwee RG, Stevenson LA, Griffin G *et al*. Isolation and structure of a brain constituent that binds to the cannabinoid receptor. Science 1992; 258:1946-1949.
[12]   Munro S, Thomas KL, Abu-Shaar M. Molecular characterization of a peripheral receptor for cannabinoids. Nature 1993; 365:61-65.
[13]   Viveros M-P, Bermúdez-Silva F-J, Lopez-Rodriguez A-B, Wagner EJ. The endocannabinoid system as a pharmacological target derived from its CNS role in energy homeostasis and reward: applications in eating disorders and addiction. Pharmaceuticals 2011; 4:1101-1136.
[14]   Henstridge CM. Off-target cannabinoid effects mediated by GPR55. Pharmacology 2012; 89:179-187.
[15]   Howlett AC. Reverse pharmacology applied to the cannabinoid receptor. Trends Pharmacol Sci 1990; 11:395-397.
[16]   Chait LD. Delta-9-tetrahydrocannabinol content and human marijuana self- administration. Psychopharmacology (Berl) 1989; 98:51-55.
[17]   Atwood BK, Huffman J, Straiker A, Mackie K. JWH018, a common constituent of 'Spice' herbal blends, is a potent and efficacious cannabinoid CB1 receptor agonist. Br J Pharmacol 2010; 160:585-593.
[18]   Järbe TUC, Deng H, Vadivel SK, Makriyannis A. Cannabinergic aminoalkylindoles, including AM678=JWH018 found in 'Spice', examined using drug (Δ^9-tetrahydrocannabinol) discrimination in rats. Behav Pharmacol 2011; 22:498-507.

[19]   Hu X, Primack BA, Barnett TE, Cook RL. College students and use of K2: an emerging drug of abuse in young persons. Subst Abuse Treat Prev Policy 2011; 6:16.

[20]   Fattore L, Fratta W. Beyond THC: the new generation of cannabinoid designer drugs. Front Behav Neurosci 2011; 5:doi:10.3389/fnbeh.2011.00060.

[21]   Wise RA. Addictive drugs and brain stimulation reward. Annu Rev Neurosci 1996; 19:319-340.

[22]   French ED. Delta^9-tetrahydrocannabinol excites rat VTA dopamine neurons through activation of cannabinoid CB1 but not opioid receptors. Neurosci Lett 1997; 226:159-162.

[23]   Tanda G, Pontieri FE, Di Chiara G. Cannabinoid and heroin activation of mesolimbic dopamine transmission by a α_1 opioid receptor mechanism. Science 1997; 276:2048-2050.

[24]   Wickelgren I. Marijuana: harder than thought? Science 1997; 276:1967-1968.

[25]   Zangen A, Solinas M, Ikemoto S, Goldberg SR, Wise RA. Two brain sites for cannabinoid reward. J Neurosci 2006; 26:4901-4907.

[26]   Habayeb OMH, Bell SC, Konje JC. Endogenous cannabinoids: Metabolism and their role in reproduction. Life Sci 2002; 70:1963-1977.

[27]   Mechoulam R, Ben Shabat S, Hanus L, Ligumsky M, Kaminski NE, Schatz AR *et al*. Identification of an endogenous 2-monoglyceride, present in canine gut, that binds to cannabinoid receptors. Biochem Pharmacol 1995; 50:83-90.

[28]   Jarrahian A, Manna S, Edgemond WS, Campbell WB, Hillard CJ. Structure-activity relationships among *N*-arachidonylethanolamine (anandamide) head group analogues for the anandamide transporter. J Neurochem 2000; 74:2597-2606.

[29]   Freund TF, Katona I, Piomelli D. Role of endogenous cannabinoids in synaptic signaling. Physiol Rev 2003; 83:1017-1066.

[30]   Piomelli D, Giuffrida A, Calignano A, Rodríguez de Fonseca F. The endocannabinoid system as a target for therapeutic drugs. Trends Pharmacol Sci 2000; 21:218-224.

[31]   Sugiura T, Kondo S, Sukagawa A, Tonegawa T, Nakane S, Yamashita A *et al*. Transacylase-mediated and phosphodiesterase-mediated synthesis of N-arachidonoylethanolamine, an endogenous cannabinoid-receptor ligand, in rat brain microsomes. Biochem Biophys Res Commun 1996; 218:113-117.

[32]   Sugiura T, Kondo S, Sukagawa A, Tonegawa T, Nakane S, Yamashita A *et al*. Transacylase-mediated and phosphodiesterase-mediated synthesis of N-arachidonoylethanolamine, an endogenous cannabinoid-receptor ligand, in rat brain microsomes - Comparison with synthesis from free arachidonic acid and ethanolamine. Eur J Biochem 1996; 240:53-62.

[33]   Farooqui AA, Rammohan KW, Horrocks LA. Isolation, characterization, and regulation of diacylglycerol lipases from the bovine brain. Ann NY Acad Sci 1989; 559:25-36.

[34]   Di Marzo V, Ligresti A, Cristino L. The endocannabinoid system as a link between homeostatic and hedonic pathways involved in energy balance regulation. Int J Obesity 2009; 33:S18-S24.

[35]   Hirsch D, Stahl A, Lodish HF. A family of fatty acid transporters conserved from mycobacterium to man. Proc Natl Acad Sci 1998; 95:8625-8629.

[36]   Beltramo M, Stella N, Calignano A, Lin SY, Makriyannis A, Piomelli D. Functional role of high-affinity anandamide transport, as revealed by selective inhibition. Science 2012; 277:1094-1097.

[37]   Hájos N, Kathuria S, Dinh T, Piomelli D, Freund TF. Endocannabinoid transport tightly controls 2-arachidonoyl glycerol actions in the hippocampus: effects of low temperature and the transport inhibitor AM404. Eur J Neurosci 2004; 19:2991-2996.

[38]   Hillard CJ, Edgemond WS, Jarrahian A, Campbell WB. Accumulation of N-arachidonoylethanolamine (anandamide) into cerebellar granule cells occurs *via* facilitated diffusion. J Neurochem 1997; 69:631-638.

[39]   Piomelli D, Beltramo M, Glasnapp S, Lin SY, Goutopoulos A, Xie X-Q *et al.* Structural determinants for recognition and translocation by the anandamide transporter. Proc Natl Acad Sci 1999; 96:5802-5807.

[40]   Bisogno T, Maccarrone M, De Petrocellis L, Jarrahian A, Finazzi-Agrò A, Hillard C *et al.* The uptake by cells of 2-arachidonylglycerol, an endogenous agonist of cannabinoid receptors. Eur J Biochem 2001; 268:1982-1989.

[41]   Thomas EA, Cravatt BF, Danielson PE, Gilula NB, Sutcliffe JG. Fatty acid amide hydrolase, the degradative enzyme for anandamide and oleamide, has selective distribution in neurons within the central nervous system. J Neurosci Res 1997; 50:1047-1052.

[42]   Karlsson M, Contreras JA, Hellman U, Tornqvist H, Holm C. cDNA cloning, tissue distribution, and identification of the catalytic triad of monoglyceride lipase: Evolutionary relationship to esterases, lysophospholipases, and haloperoxidases. J Biol Chem 1997; 272:27218-27223.

[43]   Dinh TP, Carpenter D, Leslie FM, Freund TF, Katona I, Sensi SL *et al.* Brain monoglyceride lipase participating in endocannabinoid inactivation. Proc Natl Acad Sci 2002; 99:10819-10824.

[44]   Hashimotodani Y, Ohno-Shosaku T, Kano M. Presynaptic monoacylglycerol lipase activity determines basal endocannabinoid tone and terminates retrograde endocannabinoid signaling in the hippocampus. J Neurosci 2007; 27:1211-1219.

[45]   Abel EL. Effects of marihuana on the solution of anagrams, memory and appetite. Nature 1971; 231:260-261.

[46]   Williams CM, Rogers PJ, Kirkham TC. Hyperphagia in pre-fed rats following oral Δ^9-THC. Physiol Behav 1998; 65:343-346.

[47]   Koch JE. Δ^9-THC stimulates food intake in Lewis rats: Effects on chow, high-fat and sweet high-fat diets. Pharmacol Biochem Behav 2001; 68:539-543.

[48]   Budney AJ, Hughes JR, Moore BA, Novy PL. Marijuana abstinence effects in marijuana smokers maintained in their home environment. Arch Gen Psychiatry 2001; 58:917-924.

[49]   Williams CM, Kirkham TC. Observational analysis of feeding induced by Δ^9-THC and anandamide. Physiol Behav 2002; 76:241-250.

[50]   Hodge J, Bow JP, Plyler KS, Vemuri K, Wisniecki A, Salamone JD *et al.* The cannabinoid CB1 receptor inverse agonist AM 251 and antagonist AM 4113 produce similar effects on the behavioral satiety sequence in rats. Behav Brain Res 2008; 193:298-305.

[51]   Escartín-Pérrez RE, Cendejas-Trejo NM, Cruz-Martínez AM, González-Hernández B, Mancilla-Díaz JM, Florán-Garduño B. Role of cannabinoid CB1 receptors on macronutrient selection and satiety in rats. Physiol Behav 2009; 96:646-650.

[52]   Tseng AH, Craft RM. Sex differences in antinociceptive and motoric effects of cannabinoids. Eur J Pharmacol 2001; 430:41-47.

[53]   Kellert BA, Nguyen MC, Nguyen C, Nguyen QH, Wagner EJ. Estrogen rapidly attenuates cannabinoid-induced changes in energy homeostasis. Eur J Pharmacol 2009; 622:15-24.

[54]   Rowland NE, Mukherjee M, Robertson K. Effects of the cannabinoid receptor antagonist SR 141716, alone and in combination with dexfenfluramine or naloxone, on food intake in rats. Psychopharmacology (Berl) 2001; 159:111-116.

[55]   Williams CM, Kirkham TC. Reversal of Δ^9-THC hyperphagia by SR141716 and naloxone but not dexfenfluramine. Pharmacol Biochem Behav 2002; 71:341-348.

[56]   Ravinet-Trillou C, Arnone M, Delgorge C, Gonalons N, Keane P, Maffrand J-P *et al*. Anti-obesity effect of SR141716, a CB1 receptor antagonist, in diet-induced obese mice. Am J Physiol Regul Integr Comp Physiol 2003; 284:R345-R353.

[57]   Hildebrandt AL, Kelly-Sullivan DM, Black SC. Antiobesity effects of chronic CB1 receptor antagonist treatment in diet-induced obese mice. Eur J Pharmacol 2003; 462:125-132.

[58]   Sacks N, Hutcheson JR, Watts JM, Webb RE. Case report: the effect of tetrahydrocannabinol on food intake during chemotherapy. J Am Coll Nutr 1990; 9:630-632.

[59]   Nelson K, Walsh D, Deeter P, Sheehan F. A phase II study of delta-9-tetrahydrocannabinol for appetite stimulation in cancer-associated anorexia. J Palliat Care 1994; 10:14-18.

[60]   Beal JE, Olson R, Laubenstein L, Morales JO, Bellman P, Yangco B *et al*. Dronabinol as a treatment for anorexia associated with weight loss in patients with AIDS. J Pain Symptom Manage 1995; 10:89-97.

[61]   Jatoi A, Windschitl HE, Loprinzi CL, Sloan JA, Dakhil SR, Mailliard JA *et al*. Dronabinol *versus* megestrol acetate *versus* combination therapy for cancer-associated anorexia: a north central cancer treatment group study. J Clin Oncol 2002; 20:567-573.

[62]   Woolridge E, Barton S, Samuel J, Osorio J, Dougherty A, Holdcroft A. Cannabis use in HIV for pain and other medical symptoms. J Pain Symptom Manage 2005; 29:358-367.

[63]   Haney M, Rabkin J, Gunderson E, Foltin RW. Dronabinol and marijuana in HIV+ marijuana smokers: acute effects on caloric intake and mood. Psychopharmacology (Berl) 2005; 181:170-178.

[64]   Walsh D, Kirkova J, Davis MP. The efficacy and tolerability of long-term use of dronabinol in cancer-related anorexia: A case series. J Pain Symptom Manage 2005; 30:493-495.

[65]   Lynch ME, Young J, Clark AJ. A case series of patients using medical marihuana for management of chronic pain under the Canadian Marihuana Medical Access Regulations. J Pain Symptom Manage 2006; 32:497-501.

[66]   Pi-Sunyer FX, Aronne LJ, Heshmati HM, Devin J, Rosenstock J. Effect of Rimonabant, a Cannabinoid-1 receptor blocker, on weight and cardiometabolic risk factors in overweight or obese patients. JAMA 2006; 295:761-775.

[67]   Strasser F, Luftner D, Possinger K, Ernst G, Ruhstaller T, Meissner W *et al*. Comparison of orally administered cannabis extract and delta-9-tetrahydrocannabinol in treating patients with cancer-related anorexia-cachexia syndrome: A multicenter, phase III, randomized, double-blind, placebo-controlled clinical trial from the cannabis-study-group. J Clin Oncol 2006; 24:3394-3400.

[68]   Miller CC, Murray TF, Freeman KG, Edwards GL. Cannabinoid agonist, CP 55,940, facilitates intake of palatable foods when injected into the hindbrain. Physiol Behav 2004; 80:611-616.

[69]   Diaz S, Farhang B, Hoien J, Stahlman M, Adatia N, Cox JM *et al*. Sex differences in the cannabinoid modulation of appetite, body temperature and neurotransmission at POMC synapses. Neuroendocrinology 2009; 89:424-440.

[70]   Coutts AA, Irving AJ, Mackie K, Pertwee RG, Anavi-Goffer S. Localisation of cannabinoid CB_1 receptor immunoreactivity in the guinea pig and rat myenteric plexus. J Comp Neurol 2002; 448:410-422.

[71]   Pertwee RG, Fernando SR, Griffin G, Ryan W, Razdan RK, Compton DR *et al.* Agonist-antagonist characterization of 6'-cyanohex-2'-yne-delta^8-tetrahydrocannabinol in two isolated tissue preparations. Eur J Pharmacol 1996; 315:195-201.

[72]   Heinemann Á, Shahbazian A, Holzer P. Cannabinoid inhibition of guinea-pig intestinal peristalsis *via* inhibition of excitatory and activation of inhibitory neural pathways. Neuropharmacology 1999; 38:1289-1297.

[73]   Baldassano S, Zizzo MG, Serio R, Mulè F. Interaction between cannabinoid CB1 receptors and endogenous ATP in the control of spontaneous mechanical activity in the mouse ileum. Br J Pharmacol 2009; 158:243-251.

[74]   Storr M, Gaffal E, Saur D, Schusdziarra V, Allescher HD. Effect of cannabinoids on neural transmission in rat gastric fundus. Can J Physiol Pharmacol 2002; 80:67-76.

[75]   Shook JE, Burks TF. Psychoactive cannabinoids reduce gastrointestinal propulsion and motility in rodents. J Pharmacol Exp Ther 1989; 249:444-449.

[76]   Izzo AA, Mascolo N, Capasso R, Germanò MP, De Pasquale R, Capasso F. Inhibitory effect of cannabinoid agonists on gastric emptying in the rat. Naunyn-Schmiedeberg's Arch Pharmacol 1999; 360:221-223.

[77]   McCallum RW, Soykan I, Sridhar KR, Ricci DA, Lange RC, Plankey MW. Delta-9-tetrahydrocannabinol delays the gastric emptying of solid food in humans: a double-blind, randomized study. Aliment Pharmacol Ther 1999; 13:77-80.

[78]   Landi M, Croci T, Rinaldi-Carmona M, Maffrand J-P, Le Fur G, Manara L. Modulation of gastric emptying and gastrointestinal transit in rats through intestinal cannabinoid CB$_1$ receptors. Eur J Pharmacol 2002; 450:77-83.

[79]   Esfandyari T, Camilleri M, Ferber I, Burton D, Baxter K, Zinsmeister AR. Effect of a cannabinoid agonist on gastrointestinal transit and postprandial satiation in healthy human subjects: a randomized, placebo-controlled study. Neurogastroenterol Motil 2006; 18:831-838.

[80]   Hunt JN, Stubbs DF. The volume and energy content of meals as determinants of gastric emptying. J Physiol (Lond) 1975; 245:209-225.

[81]   Männistö P. The effect of crystal size, gastric content and emptying rate on the absorption of nitrofurantoin in healthy human volunteers. Int J Clin Pharmacol 1978; 16:223-228.

[82]   Miller LJ, Malagelada J-R, Taylor WF, Go VLW. Intestinal control of human postprandial gastric function: the role of components of jejunoileal chyme in regulating gastric secretion and gastric emptying. Gastroenterology 1981; 80:763-769.

[83]   Krowicki ZK, Moerschbaecher JM, Winsauer PJ, Digavalli SV, Hornby PJ. Δ^9-Tetrahydrocannabinol inhibits gastric motility in the rat through cannabinoid CB1 receptors. Eur J Pharmacol 1999; 371:187-196.

[84]   MacNaughton WK, Van Sickle MD, Keenan CM, Cushing K, Mackie K, Sharkey KA. Distribution and function of the cannabinoid-1 receptor in the modulation of ion transport in the guinea pig ileum: relationship to capsaicin-sensitive nerves. Am J Physiol Gastrointest Liver Physiol 2004; 286:g863-g871.

[85]   Adami M, Frati P, Bertini S, Kulkarni-Narla A, Brown DR, de Caro G *et al.* Gastric antisecretory role and immunohistochemical localization of cannabinoid receptors in the rat stomach. Br J Pharmacol 2002; 135:1598-1606.

[86]   Kinsey SG, Nomura DK, O'Neal ST, Long JZ, Mahadevan A, Cravatt BF *et al.* Inhibition of monoacylglycerol lipase attenuates nonsteroidal anti-inflammatory drug-induced gastric hemorrhages in mice. J Pharmacol Exp Ther 2011; 338:795-802.

[87]   Izzo AA, Capasso F, Costagliola A, Bisogno T, Marsicano G, Ligresti A *et al*. An endogenous cannabinoid tone attenuates cholera toxin-induced fluid accumulation in mice. Gastroenterology 2003; 125:765-774.

[88]   Zbucki RL, Sawicki B, Hryniewicz A, Winnicka MM. Cannabinoids enhance gastric X/A - like cells activity. Folia Histochem Cytobiol 2008; 46:219-224.

[89]   Riggs PK, Vaida F, Rossi SS, Sorkin LS, Gouaux B, Grant I *et al*. A pilot study of the effects of cannabis on appetite hormones in HIV-infected adult men. Brain Res 2012; 1431:46-52.

[90]   Cani PD, Montoya ML, Neyrinck AM, Delzenne NM, Lambert DM. Potential modulation of plasma ghrelin and glucagon-like peptide-1 by anorexigenic cannabinoid compounds, SR141716A (rimonabant) and oleoylethanolamide. Br J Nutrition 2004; 92:757-761.

[91]   Jamontt JM, Molleman A, Pertwee RG, Parsons ME. The effects of Δ^9-tetrahydrocannabinol and cannabidiol alone and in combination on damage, inflammation and *in vitro* motility disturbances in rat colitis. Br J Pharmacol 2010; 160:712-723.

[92]   Petrella C, Agostini S, Alema GS, Casolini P, Carpino F, Giuli C *et al*. Cannabinoid agonist WIN55,212 *in vitro* inhibits interleukin-6 (IL-6) and monocyte chemo-attractant protein-1 (MCP-1) release by rat pancreatic acini and *in vivo* induces dual effects on the course of acute pancreatitis. Neurogastroenterol Motil 2010; 22:1248-e323.

[93]   Lin X-H, Yuece B, Li Y-Y, Feng Y-J, Feng J-Y, Yu L-Y *et al*. A novel CB receptor GPR55 and its ligands are involved in regulation of gut movement in rodents. Neurogastroenterol Motil 2011; 23:862-e342.

[94]   De Petrocellis L, Orlando P, Moriello AS, Aviello G, Stott C, Izzo AA *et al*. Cannabinoid actions at TRPV channels: effects on TRPV3 and TRPV4 and their potential relevance to gastrointestinal inflammation. Acta Physiol 2012; 204:255-266.

[95]   Burdyga G, Lal S, Varro A, Dimaline R, Thompson DG, Dockray GJ. Expression of cannabinoid CB1 receptors by vagal afferent neurons is inhibited by cholecystokinin. J Neurosci 2004; 24:2708-2715.

[96]   Gil K, Bugajski A, Thor P. Electrical vagus nerve stimulation decreases food consumption and weight gain in rats fed a high-fat diet. J Physiol Pharmacol 2011; 62:637-646.

[97]   Rogers RC, Hermann GE. Tumor necrosis factor activation of vagal afferent terminal calcium is blocked by cannabinoids. J Neurosci 2012; 32:5237-5241.

[98]   Yang KHS, Isaev D, Morales M, Petroianu G, Galadari S, Oz M. The effect of Δ^9-tetrahydrocannabinol on 5-HT$_3$ receptors depends on the current density. Neuroscience 2010; 171:40-49.

[99]   Himmi T, Dallaporta M, Perrin J, Orsini J-C. Neuronal responses to Δ^9-tetrahydrocannabinol in the solitary tract nucleus. Eur J Pharmacol 1996; 312:273-279.

[100].Derbenev AV, Stuart TC, Smith BN. Cannabinoids suppress synaptic input to neurones of the rat dorsal motor nucleus of the vagus nerve. J Physiol (Lond) 2004; 559:923-938.

[101]   Roux J, Wanaverbecq N, Jean A, Lebrun B, Trouslard J. Depolarization-induced release of endocannabinoids by murine dorsal motor nucleus of the vagus nerve neurons differentially regulates inhibitory and excitatory neurotransmission. Neuropharmacology 2009; 56:1106-1115.

[102]   Derbenev AV, Monroe MJ, Glatzer NR, Smith BN. Vanilloid-mediated heterosynaptic facilitation of inhibitory synaptic input to neurons of the rat dorsal motor nucleus of the vagus. J Neurosci 2006; 26:9666-9672.

[103]   Van Sickle MD, Duncan M, Kingsley PJ, Mouihate A, Urbani P, Mackie K *et al*. Identification and functional characterization of brainstem cannabinoid CB$_2$ receptors. Science 2005; 310:329-332.

[104] Brusberg M, Arvidsson S, Kang D, Larsson H, Lindström E, Martinez V. CB1 receptors mediate the analgesic effects of cannabinoids on colorectal distention-induced visceral pain in rodents. J Neurosci 2009; 1554:1564.

[105] Kotz CM, Grace MK, Briggs JE, Billington CJ, Levine AS. Naltrexone induces arcuate nucleus neuropeptide Y gene expression in the rat. Am J Physiol Regul Integr Comp Physiol 1996; 271:R289-R294.

[106] Glaum SR, Hara M, Bindokas VP, Lee CC, Polonsky KS, Bell GI *et al*. Leptin, the *obese* gene product, rapidly modulates synaptic transmission in the hypothalamus. Mol Pharmacol 1996; 50:230-235.

[107] Kalra SP, Horvath TL. Neuroendocrine interactions between galanin, opioids and neuropeptide Y in the control of reproduction and appetite. Ann NY Acad Sci 1998; 863:236-240.

[108] Smith MS, Grove KL. Integration of the regulation of reproductive function and energy balance: lactation as a model. Frontiers Neuroendocrinol 2002; 23:225-256.

[109] Toshinai K, Date Y, Murakami N, Shimada M, Mondal MS, Shimbara T *et al*. Ghrelin-induced food intake is mediated *via* the orexin pathway. Endocrinology 2003; 144:1506-1512.

[110] Edwards CMB, Abusnana S, Sunter D, Murphy KG, Ghatei MA, Bloom SR. The effect of the orexins on food intake: comparison with neuropeptide Y, melanin-concentrating hormone and galanin. J Endocrinol 1999; 160:R7-R12.

[111] Ballinger AB, Williams G, Corder R, El-Haj T, Farthing MJG. Role of hypothalamic neuropeptide Y and orexigenic peptides in anorexia associated with experimental colitis in the rat. Clin Sci 2001; 100:221-229.

[112] Della-Zuana O, Presse F, Ortola C, Duhault J, Nahon JL, Levens N. Acute and chronic administration of melanin-concentrating hormone enhances food intake and body weight in Wistar and Sprague-Dawley rats. Int J Obesity 2002; 26:1289-1295.

[113] Abbott CR, Kennedy AR, Wren AM, Rossi M, Murphy KG, Seal LJ *et al*. Identification of hypothalamic nuclei involved in the orexigenic effect of melanin-concentrating hormone. Endocrinology 2003; 144:3943-3949.

[114] Stricker EM. Hyperphagia. New England J Med 1978; 298:1010-1013.

[115] Beverly JL, Martin RJ. Increased GABA shunt activity in VMN of three hyperphagic rat models. Am J Physiol Regul Integr Comp Physiol 1989; 25:R1225-R1231.

[116] Varma M, Laviano A, Meguid MM, Gleason JR, Yang Z-J, Oler A. Comparison of early feeding pattern dynamics in female and male rats after reversible ventromedial nucleus of hypothalamus block. J Investig Med 2000; 48:417-4262.

[117] Cowley MA, Cone RD, Enriori P, Louiselle I, Williams SM, Evans AE. Electrophysiological actions of peripheral hormones on melanocortin neurons. Ann NY Acad Sci 2003; 994:175-186.

[118] Marks DL, Cone RD. The role of the melanocortin-3 receptor in cachexia. Ann NY Acad Sci 2003; 994:258-266.

[119] Lambert PD, Couceyro PR, McGirr KM, Dall Vechia SE, Smith Y, Kuhar MJ. CART peptides in the central control of feeding and interactions with neuropeptide Y. Synapse 1998; 29:293-298.

[120] Vrang N, Tang-Christensen M, Larsen PJ, Kristensen P. Recombinant CART peptide induces c-Fos expression in central areas involved in central control of feeding behavior. Brain Res 1999; 818:499-509.

[121] Cota D, Marsicano G, Tschöp M, Grübler Y, Flachskamm C, Schubert M *et al.* The endogenous cannabinoid system affects energy balance *via* central orexigenic drive and peripheral lipogenesis. J Clin Invest 2003; 112:423-431.

[122] Horvath TL. The hardship of obesity: a soft-wired hypothalamus. nature neuroscience 2005; 8:561-565.

[123] Gulati K. Differential effects of intrahypothalamic administration of opioids on food intake in naive and tolerant rats. Pharmacol Biochem Behav 1995; 52:689-694.

[124] Appleyard SM, Hayward M, Young JI, Butler AA, Cone RD, Rubinstein M *et al.* A role for endogenous β-endorphin in energy homeostasis. Endocrinology 2003; 144:1753-1760.

[125] Huszar D, Lynch CA, Fairchild-Huntress V, Dunmore JH, Fang Q, Berkemeier LR *et al.* Targeted disruption of the melanocortin-4 receptor results in obesity in mice. Cell 1997; 88:131-141.

[126] Fong TM, Mao C, MacNeil T, Kalyani R, Smith T, Weinberg D *et al.* ART (protein product of agouti-related transcript) as an antagonist of MC-3 and MC-4 receptors. Biochem Biophys Res Commun 1997; 237:629-631.

[127] Hanada R, Nakazato M, Matsukura S, Murakami N, Yoshimatsu H, Sakata T. Differential regulation of melanin-concentrating hormone and orexin genes in the agouti-related protein/melanocortin-4 receptor system. Biochem Biophys Res Commun 2000; 268:88-91.

[128] Zheng H, Corkern MM, Crousillac SM, Patterson LM, Phifer CB, Berthoud H-R. Neurochemical phenotype of hypothalamic neurons showing Fos expression 23 h after intracranial AgRP. Am J Physiol Regul Integr Comp Physiol 2002; 282:R1773-R1781.

[129] Olszewski PK, Wickwire K, Wirth MM, Levine AS, Giraudo SQ. Agouti-related protein: appetite or reward? Ann NY Acad Sci 2003; 994:187-191.

[130] Batterham RL, Bloom SR. The gut hormone peptide YY regulates appetite. Ann NY Acad Sci 2003; 994:162-168.

[131] Seo S, Ju S, Chung H, Lee D, Park S. Acute effects of glucagon-like peptide-1 on hypothalamic neuropeptide and AMP activated kinase expression in fasted rats. Endocrine Journal 2008; 55:867-874.

[132] Chen W, Yan Z, Liu S, Zhang G, Sun D, Hu S. The changes of pro-opiomelanocortin neurons in type 2 diabetes mellitus rats after ileal transposition: the role of POMC neurons. J Gastrointest Surg 2011; 15:1618-1624.

[133] Baraboi E-D, St Pierre DH, Shooner J, Timofeeva E, Richard D. Brain activation following peripheral administration of the GLP-1 receptor agonist exendin-4. Am J Physiol Regul Integr Comp Physiol 2011; 301:R1011-R1024.

[134] Takahashi KA, Cone RD. Fasting induces a large, leptin-dependent increase in the intrinsic action potential frequency of orexigenic arcuate nucleus neuropeptide Y/agouti-related protein neurons. Endocrinology 2005; 146:1043-1047.

[135] Ghamari-Langroudi M, Colmers WF, Cone RD. PYY$_{3-36}$ inhibits the action potential firing activity of POMC neurons of arcuate nucleus through postsynaptic Y2 receptors. Cell Metabolism 2005; 2:191-199.

[136] Hill JW, Williams KW, Ye C, Luo J, Balthasar N, Coppari R *et al.* Acute effects of leptin require PI3K signaling in hypothalamic proopiomelanocortin neurons in mice. J Clin Invest 2008; 118:1796-1805.

[137] Andrews ZB, Liu Z-W, Walllingford N, Erion DM, Borok E, Friedman JM *et al.* UCP2 mediates ghrelin's action on NPY/AgRP neurons by lowering free radicals. Nature 2008; 454:846-851.

[138] Broberger C. Hypothalamic cocaine- and amphetamine-regulated transcript (CART) neurons: histochemical relationship to thyrotropin-releasing hormone, melanin-concentrating hormone, orexin/hypocretin and neuropeptide Y. Brain Res 1999; 848:101-113.

[139] Bäckberg M, Hervieu G, Wilson S, Meister B. Orexin receptor-1 (OX-R1) immunoreactivity in chemically identified neurons of the hypothalamus: focus on orexin targets involved in control of food and water intake. Eur J Neurosci 2002; 15:315-328.

[140] Guan J-L, Uehara K, Lu S, Wang Q-P, Funahashi H, Sakurai T *et al*. Reciprocal synaptic relationships between orexin- and melanin-concentrating hormone-containing neurons in the rat lateral hypothalamus: a novel circuit implicated in feeding regulation. Int J Obesity 2002; 26:1523-1532.

[141] Goldsmith PC, Boggan JE, Thind KK. Opioid synapses on vasopressin neurons in the paraventricular and supraoptic nuclei of juvenile monkeys. Neuroscience 1991; 45:709-719.

[142] Horvath TL. Endocannabinoids and the regulation of body fat: the smoke is clearing. J Clin Invest 2003; 113:323-326.

[143] Davidowa H, Li Y, Plagemann A. Altered responses to orexigenic (AGRP, MCH) and anorexigenic (α-MSH, CART) neuropeptides of paraventricular hypothalamic neurons in early postnatally overfed rats. Eur J Neurosci 2003; 18:613-621.

[144] Zorilla EP, Taché Y, Koob GF. Nibbling at the CRF receptor control of feeding and gastrointestinal motility. Trends Pharmacol Sci 2003; 24:421-427.

[145] Romero J, Wenger T, De Miguel R, Ramos JA, Fernández-Ruiz JJ. Cannabinoid receptor binding did not vary in several hypothalamic nuclei after hypothalamic deafferentation. Life Sci 1998; 63:351-356.

[146] Jamshidi N, Taylor DA. Anandamide administration into the ventromedial hypothalamus stimulates appetite in rats. Br J Pharmacol 2001; 134:1151-1154.

[147] Verty ANA, McGregor IS, Mallet PE. Paraventricular hypothalamic CB1 cannabinoid receptors are involved in the feeding stimulatory effects of Δ^9-tetrahydrocannabinol. Neuropharmacology 2005; 49:1101-1109.

[148] Kirkham TC, Williams CM, Fezza F, Di Marzo V. Endocannabinoid levels in rat limbic forebrain and hypothalamus in relation to fasting, feeding and satiation: stimulation of eating by 2-arachidonyl glycerol. Br J Pharmacol 2002; 136:550-557.

[149] Di Marzo V, Goparahu SK, Wang L, Liu J, Bátkai S, Járai Z *et al*. Leptin-regulated endocannabinoids are involved in maintaining food intake. Nature 2001; 410:822-825.

[150] Kola B, Farkas I, Christ-Crain M, Wittmann G, Lolli F, Amin F *et al*. The orexigenic effect of ghrelin is mediated through central activation of the endogenous cannabinoid system. PLoS ONE 2008; 3:e1797. doi:10.1371/journal.pone.0001797.

[151] Kola B, Hubina E, Tucci SA, Kirkham TC, Garcia EA, Mitchell SE *et al*. Cannabinoids and ghrelin have both central and peripheral metabolic and cardiac effects *via* AMP-activated protein kinase. J Biol Chem 2005; 280:25196-25201.

[152] Jo Y-H, Chen Y-JL, Chua SC, Talmage DA, Role LW. Integration of endocannabinoid and leptin signaling in an appetite-related neural circuit. Neuron 2005; 48:1055-1066.

[153] Huang H, Acuna-Goycolea C, Li Y, Cheng HM, Obrietan K, van den Pol AN. Cannabinoids excite hypothalamic melanin-concentrating hormone but inhibit hypocretin/orexin neurons: implications for cannabinoid actions on food intake and cognitive arousal. J Neurosci 2007; 27:4870-4881.

[154] Sinnayah P, Jobst EE, Rathner JA, Caldera-Siu AD, Tonelli-Lemos L, Eusterbrock AJ *et al.* Feeding induced by cannabinoids is mediated independently of the melanocortin system. PLoS ONE 2008; 3:e2202.

[155] Gamber KM, Macarthur H, Westfall TC. Cannabinoids augment the release of neuropeptide Y in the rat hypothalamus. Neuropharmacology 2005; 49:646-652.

[156] van den Pol AN, Yao Y, Fu L-Y, Foo K, Huang H, Coppari R *et al.* Neuromedin B and gastrin-releasing peptide excite arcuate nucleus neuropeptide Y neurons in a novel transgenic mouse expressing strong *Renilla* green fluorescent protein in NPY neurons. J Neurosci 2009; 29:4622-4639.

[157] Hentges ST, Low MJ, Williams JT. Differential regulation of synaptic inputs by constitutively released endocannabinoids and exogenous cannabinoids. J Neurosci 2005; 25:9746-9751.

[158] Ho J, Cox JM, Wagner EJ. Cannabinoid-induced hyperphagia: Correlation with inhibition of proopiomelanocortin neurons? Physiol Behav 2007; 92:507-519.

[159] Tang SL, Tran V, Wagner EJ. Sex differences in the cannabinoid modulation of an A-type K^+ current in neurons of the mammalian hypothalamus. J Neurophysiol 2005; 94:2983-2986.

[160] Osei-Hyiaman D, Depetrillo M, Harvey-White J, Bannon AW, Cravatt BF, Kuhar MJ *et al.* Cocaine- and amphetamine-related transcript is involved in the orexigenic effect of endogenous anandamide. Neuroendocrinology 2005; 81:273-282.

[161] Nguyen QH, Wagner EJ. Estrogen differentially modulates the cannabinoid-induced presynaptic inhibition of amino acid neurotransmission in proopiomelanocortin neurons of the arcuate nucleus. Neuroendocrinology 2006; 84:123-137.

[162] Riebe CJN, Hill MN, Lee TTY, Hillard CJ, Gorzalka BB. Estrogenic regulation of limbic cannabinoid receptor binding. Psychoneuroendocrinology 2010; 35:1265-1269.

[163] Jeffery GS, Peng KC, Wagner EJ. The role of phosphatidylinositol-3-kinase and AMP-activated kinase in the rapid estrogenic attenuation of cannabinoid-induced changes in energy homeostasis. Pharmaceuticals 2011; 4:630-651.

[164] Washburn N, Borgquist A, Wang K, Jeffery GS, Kelly MJ, Wagner EJ. Receptor subtypes and signal transduction mechanisms contributing to the estrogenic attenuation of cannabinoid-induced changes in energy homeostasis. Neuroendocrinology 2013; 97:160-175.

[165] Di S, Malcher-Lopes R, Halmos KC, Tasker JG. Nongenomic glucocorticoid inhibition *via* endocannabinoid release in the hypothalamus: a fast feedback mechanism. J Neurosci 2003; 23:4850-4857.

[166] Malcher-Lopes R, Di S, Marcheselli VS, Weng F-J, Stuart CT, Bazan NG *et al.* Opposing crosstalk between leptin and glucocorticoids rapidly modulates synaptic excitation *via* endocannabinoid release. J Neurosci 2006; 26:6643-6650.

[167] Hoffman AF, Lupica CR. Direct actions of cannabinoids on synaptic transmission in the nucleus accumbens: a comparison with opioids. J Neurophysiol 2001; 85:72-83.

[168] Hoffman AF, Oz M, Caulder T, Lupica CR. Functional tolerance and blockade of long-term depression at synapses in the nucleus accumbens after chronic cannabinoid exposure. J Neurosci 2003; 23:4815-4820.

[169] Fourgeaud L, Mato S, Bouchet D, Hémar A, Worley PF, Manzoni OJ. A single *in vivo* exposure to cocaine abolishes endocannabinoid-mediated long-term depression in the nucleus accumbens. J Neurosci 2004; 24:6939-6945.

[170] Mato S, Robbe D, Puente N, Grandes P, Manzoni OJ. Presynaptic homeostatic plasticity rescues long-term depression after chronic Δ^9-tetrahydrocannabinol exposure. J Neurosci 2005; 25:11619-11627.

[171] Cheer JF, Wassum KM, Heien MLAV, Phillips PEM, Wightman RM. Cannabinoids enhance subsecond dopamine release in the nucleus accumbens of awake rats. J Neurosci 2004; 24:4393-4400.

[172] Patel S, Rademacher DJ, Hillard CJ. Differential regulation of the endocannabinoids anandamide and 2-arachidonylglycerol within the limbic forebrain by dopamine receptor activity. J Pharmacol Exp Ther 2003; 306:880-888.

[173] Will MJ, Franzblau EB, Kelley AE. Nucleus accumbens μ-opioids regulate intake of a high-fat diet *via* activation of a distributed brain network. J Neurosci 2003; 23:2882-2888.

[174] Smith KS, Berridge KC. The ventral pallidum and hedonic reward: neurochemical maps of sucrose "liking" and food intake. J Neurosci 2005; 25:8637-8649.

[175] Mahler SV, Smith KS, Berridge KC. Endocannabinoid hedonic hotspot for sensory pleasure: anandamide in nucleus accumbens shell enhances 'liking' of a sweet reward. Neuropsychopharmacol 2007; 32:2267-2278.

[176] Melis T, Succu S, Sanna F, Boi A, Argiolas A, Melis MR. The cannabinoid antagonist SR 141716A (Rimonabant) reduces the increase of extra-cellular dopamine release in the rat nucleus accumbens induced by a novel high palatable food. Neurosci Lett 2007; 419:231-235.

[177] Nakata M, Yada T. Cannabinoids inhibit insulin secretion and cytosolic Ca^{2+} oscillation in islet β-cells *via* CB1 receptors. Regul Pept 2008; 145:49-53.

[178] Romero-Zerbo SY, Rafacho A, Díaz-Arteaga A, Suárez J, Quesada I, Imbernon M *et al*. A role for putative cannabinoid receptor GPR55 in the islets of Langerhans. J Endocrinol 2011; 211:177-185.

[179] Teixeira D, Pestana D, Faria A, Calhau C, Azevedo I, Monteiro R. Modulation of adipocyte biology by Δ^9-tetrahydrocannabinol. Obesity 2010; 18:2077-2085.

[180] Gallant M, Odei-Addo F, Frost CL, Levendal R-A. Biological effects of THC and a lipophilic cannabis extract on normal and insulin resistant 3T3-L1 adipocytes. Phytomedicine 2009; 16:942-949.

[181] Osei-Hyiaman D, Depetrillo M, Pacher P, Liu J, Radaeva S, Bátkai S *et al*. Endocannabinoid activation at hepatic CB1 receptors stimulates fatty synthesis and contributes to diet-induced obesity. J Clin Invest 2005; 115:1298-1305.

[182] Jeong W, Osei-Hyiaman D, Park O, Liu J, Bátkai S, Mukhopadhyay P *et al*. Paracrine activation of hepatic CB1 receptors by stellate cell-derived endocannabinoids mediates alcoholic fatty liver. Cell Metabolism 2008; 7:227-235.

[183] Lim CT, Kola B, Korbonits M. AMPK as a mediator of hormonal signaling. J Mol Endocrinol 2010; 44:87-97.

[184] Muccioli GG, Naslain D, Bäckhed F, Reigstad CS, Lambert DM, Delzenne NM *et al*. The endocannabinoid system links gut microbiota to adipogenesis. Mol Syst Biol 2010; 6:392.

[185] Perwitz N, Fasshauer M, Klein J. Cannabinoid receptor signaling directly inhibits thermogenesis and alters expression of adiponectin and visfatin. Horm Metab Res 2006; 38:356-358.

[186] Badawy ZS, Chohan KR, Whyte DA, Penefsky HS, Brown OM, Souid A-K. Cannabinoids inhibit the respiration of human sperm. Fertil Steril 2009; 91:2471-2476.

[187]   Whyte DA, Al-Hammadi S, Balhaj G, Brown OM, Penefsky HS, Souid A-K. Cannabinoids inhibit cellular respiration of human oral cancer cells. Pharmacology 2010; 85:328-335.

[188]   Duarte JMN, Ferreira SG, Carvalho RA, Cunha RA, Köfalvi A. CB_1 receptor activation inhibits neuronal and astrocytic intermediary metabolism in the rat hippocampus. Neurochem Int 2012; 60:1-8.

[189]   Pertwee RG, Tavendale R. Effects of Δ^9-tetrahydrocannabinol on the rates of oxygen consumption of mice. Br J Pharmacol 1977; 60:559-568.

[190]   Fitton AG, Pertwee RG. Changes in body temperature and oxygen consumption rate of conscious mice produced by intrahypothalamic and intracerebroventricular injections of Δ^9-tetrahydrocannabinol. Br J Pharmacol 1982; 75:409-414.

[191]   Rawls SM, Cabassa J, Geller EB, Adler MW. CB_1 receptors in the preoptic anterior hypothalamus regulate WIN 55212-2 [(4,5-dihydro-2-methyl-4(4-morpholinylmethyl)-1-(1-naphthalenyl-carbonyl)-6H-pyrrolo[3,2,1ij]quinolin-6-one]-induced hypothermia. J Pharmacol Exp Ther 2002; 301:963-968.

[192]   Schmeling WT, Hosko MJ. Effect of Δ^9-tetrahydrocannabinol on hypothalamic thermosensitive units. Brain Res 1980; 187:431-443.

[193]   Verty ANA, Allen AM, Oldfield BJ. The effects of Rimonabant on brown adipose tissue in rat: implications for energy expenditure. Obesity 2008; 17:254-261.

[194]   Ishiguro H, Onaivi ES, Horiuchi Y, Imai K, Komaki G, Ishikawa T *et al*. Functional polymorphism in the GPR55 gene is associated with anorexia nervosa. Synapse 2011; 65:103-108.

[195]   Moreno-Navarrete JM, Catalán V, Whyte L, Díaz-Arteaga A, Vázquez-Martínez R, Rotellar R *et al*. The L-α-lysophosphatidylinositol/GPR55 system and its potential role in human obesity. Diabetes 2012; 61:281-291.

Send Orders for Reprints at reprints@benthamscience.net

CHAPTER 4

Structural Biology of Endocannabinoid Targets and Enzymes: Components Tuned to the Flexibility of Endogenous Ligands

Dow P. Hurst, Jagjeet Singh and Patricia H. Reggio*

Center for Drug Discovery, Department of Chemistry and Biochemistry, University of North Carolina at Greensboro, Greensboro, NC 27402, USA

Abstract: The lipid bilayer plays a major role in the "life-cycle" of the endocannabinoids, anandamide and 2-AG. These ligands are synthesized on demand in the lipid bilayer; act at membrane embedded cannabinoid receptors that may be accessed *via* the lipid bilayer; and, are degraded by membrane associated enzymes that have lipid entry portals for their respective endocannabinoids (2-AG-Monoacylglycerol lipase (MGL); AEA-Fatty acid amide hydrolase (FAAH)). Transport for degradation (especially for AEA) remains a hot research topic, as AEA must leave the plasma membrane and travel inside the cell to FAAH which is associated with the membrane of the endoplasmic reticulum. This review focuses on structural features of each of the components of the endocannabinoid signaling system, including the enodogenous ligands themselves. For the homo-allylic double bond pattern in their arachidonyl acyl chains confers the "dynamic plasticity" that these ligands require to navigate the bilayer, thread through entry portals of the receptors, and enter lipid entry portals of the enzymes that comprise the endocannabinoid signaling system.

Keywords: Cannabinoid, CB1, CB2, GPCR, endocannabinoid, anandamide, 2-AG, FAAH, MGL, FABP, FLAT, EMT, S1P1, lpid entry portal, delta-9-THC,virodhamine, NADA, arachidonic acid, retrograde signaling, GPR18, GPR55.

INTRODUCTION

When first isolated, the cannabinoid receptor [1] was named for the natural compounds in *Cannabis sativa L.* that produce effects at this receptor such as delta-9-tetrahydrocannabinol (**1, Chart 1**) [2]. Early work indicated that the cannabinoid CB1 receptor, for example, was a G protein coupled receptor (GPCR) (1) with very high density in the brain [3]. Why would a drug of abuse receptor have such high density in the brain? It would be nearly ten years before

---

*Address correspondence to Patricia H. Reggio:** Department of Chemistry and Biochemistry, UNC Greensboro, Greensboro, NC 27402 USA; Tel: 336 334 5333; Fax: 336 334 5402; Email: phreggio@uncg.edu

Eric Murillo-Rodríguez, Emmanuel S. Onaivi, Nissar A. Darmani & Edward Wagner (Eds.)

this question was resolved by the discovery that the CB1 receptor was the mediator of retrograde signaling at synapses in the brain [4, 5]. Additional surprises were in store for the field. When the endogenous ligands for the CB1 and CB2 receptors, anandamide [6] and 2-arachidonylglcerol [7], were identified, these compounds belonged to an entirely different chemical class than any other Class A GPCR endogenous ligand isolated to date. The endocannabinoids were not peptides such as those that activated GPCRs like the opioid receptors (met-enkephalin or leu-enkephalin) nor were they small amines such as those that activate many Class A GPCRs such as the dopamine, serotonin and β-2 adrenergic receptors. Instead, the cannabinoid endogenous ligands were lipid-derived arachidonic acid derivatives [6,7]. Today, the endogenous cannabinoid system has been nearly fully characterized to include the endogenous cannabinoids, the cannabinoid receptors, synthetic enzymes, degradative enzymes and possibly, transporters. This review will focus on the structures of every component of the endocannabinoid system, beginning with the endocannabinoids themselves. For it is the structures of the endocannabinoids to which the proteins in the endocannabinoid system have clearly been tuned.

Endocannabinoid Ligands: Structure and Conformation

The endogenous cannabinoids are unsaturated fatty acid derivatives with ethanolamide, glycerol or glycerol ether headgroups. The first enodogenous cannabinoid to be identified was N-arachidonylethanolamine (AEA, also called anandamide, **2, Chart 1**). This compound was isolated by Mechoulam and co-workers from porcine brain [6]. While AEA is an arachidonic acid derivative, ethanolamines of other unsaturated fatty acids have been identified to have high cannabinoid receptor affinity, including N-homo-γ-linolenoylethanolamine (**3, Chart 1**) and N-docosatetraenoylethanolamine (**4, Chart 1**) [8]. sn-2-arachidonylglycerol (2-AG; **5, Chart 1**) was originally reported to be the endogenous ligand for the CB2 receptor [9]. 2-AG is a full agonist that binds to both CB1 and CB2 and is found in the brain in much higher concentrations than AEA (170-fold) [10]. A related compound, 2-eicosa-5',8',11',14'-tetraenylglycerol (2-AG ether, noladin ether, **6, Chart 1**), has been identified to be another endogenous cannabinoid [11], although it is uncertain that this compound exists in mammals [12]. Additional endogenous cannabinoids have been found in nervous tissue from mammals. These include the "capsaicin-like" agonist, *N*-arachidonoyl dopamine (NADA, **7, Chart 1**) [13, 14] and the endogenous antagonist, virodhamine (**8, Chart 1**) [15].

CHART 1

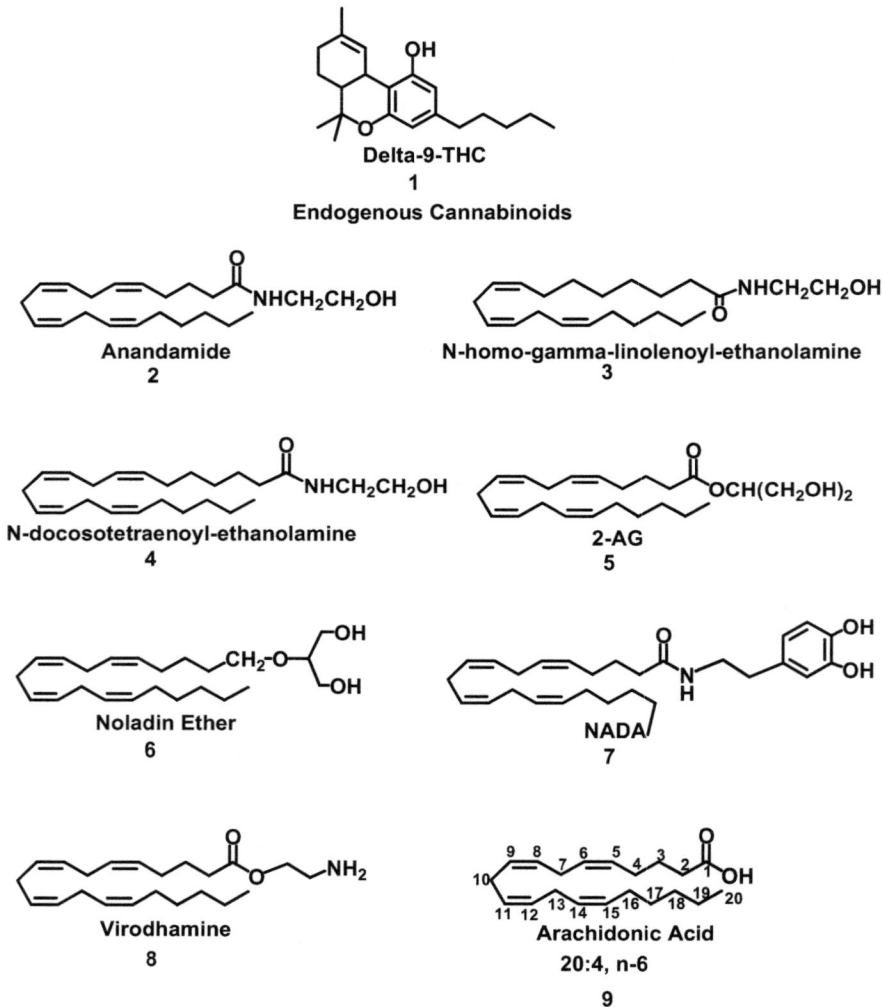

Delta-9-THC
1

Endogenous Cannabinoids

Anandamide
2

N-homo-gamma-linolenoyl-ethanolamine
3

N-docosotetraenoyl-ethanolamine
4

2-AG
5

Noladin Ether
6

NADA
7

Virodhamine
8

Arachidonic Acid
20:4, n-6
9

Chart 1: The structures of classical cannabinoids and endogenous cannabinoids are illustrated here.

Endocannabinoid SAR for CB1 and CB2 reveals many more possible substitutions in the head group than in the fatty acid portions of these molecules

[16]. All of the active endogenous cannabinoids contain a fatty acid chain with multiple homoallylic double bonds. These are fatty acid chains with *cis* double bonds separated by one methylene carbon. The most common enodcannabinoid fatty acid, arachidonic acid, contains 20 carbons and four homoallylic double bonds with the first double bond beginning at the C6 carbon on the fatty acid chain (20:4, n-6). The conformations accessible for this type of fatty acid chain have been studied extensively and they have been characterized as being extremely flexible [17] due to the existence of low free energy regions that are quite broad [18]. The barrier to rotation about Csp2-Csp3 bonds in these chains has been reported to be less than 1 kcal/mol [18]. Monte Carlo/simulated annealing calculations identified a broad distribution of torsion angles about the skew torsion angles 119°(s) and -119°(s') for the C5-C6-C7-C8 torsion angle in AEA, for example (see **Chart 1, 9** for numbering system). The effect of these low energy rotational barriers is that methylene carbons in fatty acid chains like arachidonic acid can act as pivot points, allowing these fatty acid chains to assume very diverse shapes, from extended to U-, L- or C-shapes. The resultant molecules have very striking "maneuverability". This is in contrast to saturated fatty acid chains which have higher energy barriers (3.0 kcal/mol) for rotation about their Csp3-Csp3 bonds and tend to assume straighter conformations. In fatty acid chains where the number of homoallylic double bonds has been reduced, there is a decreasing tendency to form folded conformations, but the chain will still have curvature associated with the unsaturated regions [19]. The SAR of the AEA acyl chain has been shown to correlate with such changes in the fatty acid chain [20].

Early pharmacophore models for AEA binding at CB1 focused on specific shapes such as the J-shape [21] or the helical shape [22]. Focusing upon a hairpin-like conformation, Di Marzo and co-workers developed lipopeptides with conformational restrictions. None of these compounds had high CB1 affinity, but some showed 30-50-fold less affinity than AEA (**2**) [23]. In Monte Carlo/simulated annealing studies, Barnett-Norris and co-workers studied the low free energy conformations of high CB1 affinity ligands AEA (**2**), 2-AG (**3**), and a dimethylheptyl analog of AEA (16,16-dimethyldocosa-*cis*-5,8,11,14-tetraenoyle-thanolamine) and compared these to the conformationally restricted prostanoid ligand, N-(2-hydroxyethyl)prostaglandin-B_2-ethanolamide (PGB$_2$-EA), which has no affinity for CB1 [24]. The highest populated conformations for AEA (**2**) and 2-AG (**3**) were the angle-iron and U-shaped conformations. The relative population of these two conformations was influenced by the environment (water *vs.* CHCl$_3$). Results were similar for a dimethylheptyl AEA derivative, however, PGB$_2$-EA did not form angle-iron (extended) conformers. Instead, it existed primarily in an L-shape. The authors suggested that the low probability for PGB$_2$-EA to form extended conformations may be the reason for its poor CB1 affinity.

To further explore the relationship between molecular conformations and CB1 affinity, Barnett-Norris and co-workers extended their Monte Carlo/simulated annealing conformational studies to a series of ethanolamide-fatty acid congeners of AEA in which the homoallylic double bond pattern was varied [20]. These included AEA (20:4, n-6 (Ki =39.2 ± 5.7 nM) and its 22:4, n-6 (Ki = 34.4 ± 3.2 nM); 20:3, n-6 (Ki = 53.4± 5.5 nM); and 20:2, n-6 (Ki > 1500 nM) congeners [25]. All congeners had a family of conformers that were in extended conformations, as well as one of U/J shaped conformers. However, the relative populations of these two families depended on the homoallylic double bond pattern. While the analogs with at least three homoallylic double bonds had the U/J-shaped family predominating, for the low affinity 20:2, n-6 ethanolamide, the extended conformer family predominated. There also was a difference in curvature of the U/J-shaped conformers in the entire series. Considering the C-3 to C-17 region of each analog (for numbering system, see AA (**9**), **Chart 1**), the average radii of curvature (with their 95% confidence intervals) were the following: for the 20:2,n-6 analog- 5.8 Å (5.3-6.2); for the 20:3, n-6 analog- 4.4 Å (4.1-4.7); for the 20:4, n-6 analog- 4.0 Å (3.7-4.2); and for the 22:4, n-6 analog- 4.0 Å (3.6-4.5). These results suggest that the ability to form tightly curved structures leads to higher CB1 affinity for this series of compounds [20].

In summary, SAR studies of AEA and 2-AG and their analogs suggest that high CB1 affinity ligands must be able to move between two conformational extremes: they must be able to adopt extended conformations [19], but they also must be able to adopt tightly curved conformations [21-23]. One possible explanation for this is that one set of conformations is needed for approaching and entering the receptor, while the other set is important once inside the receptor.

Endocannabinoid Mediated Retrograde Signaling

Endocannabinoids have been shown to act as retrograde messengers throughout the brain [26]. They can be involved both in short- and long-term forms of synaptic plasticity [27, 28] (for a recent review, see [29]). A role for endocannabinoids in short-term synaptic plasticity was demonstrated initially. This form of plasticity includes depolarization-induced suppression of inhibition (DSI) [5,30] and depolarization-induced suppression of excitation (DSE) [31]. A role for endocannabinoids in the mediation of presynaptic long-term depression (eCB-LTD) at both excitatory [32, 33] and inhibitory [34, 35] synapses was demonstrated subsequently. Both AEA and 2-AG have been identified as endocannabinoid regulators of synaptic function [29]. However, 2-AG appears to be the primary endocannabinoid involved in activity-dependent retrograde signaling, while the role of AEA in synaptic transmission is still debated. There is evidence of functional cross-talk between 2-AG and AEA [36] and depending on the type of presynaptic activity, 2-AG and AEA have been shown to be recruited differentially from the same post-synaptic neuron [37, 38].

To understand the short- and long-term impacts of 2-AG and AEA on synaptic signaling, it is important to examine the biosynthetic and degradative pathways for each. The biosynthetic enzymes for 2-AG are localized in dendritic spines and somatodendritic compartments on post-synaptic neurons [29,36]. Cannabinoid CB1 receptors are often expressed pre-synaptically, however. Thus, 2-AG, once synthesized, must diffuse "backwards" across the synapse to the pre-synaptic location of the cannabinoid receptor. It is still unclear how 2-AG accomplishes this movement from the post-synaptic cell plasma membrane. It is possible that the movement is *via* simple diffusion or energy-independent carrier proteins may facilitate 2-AG's movement. Once 2-AG reaches CB1, it will bind in the binding site cavity of the receptor, activating the receptor. CB1 activation results in multiple effects. Most important for retrograde signaling, however, is the inhibition of neurotransmitter release from the pre-synaptic cell that is mediated by voltage-activated Ca^{2+} channel inhibition and inwardly rectifying K^+ channel enhancement in the nerve terminal membrane [5, 30, 31, 37-40].

Synthesis of 2-AG and Anandamide Occurs in the Lipid Bilayer

At synapses, membrane vesicles are used to store neurotransmitters, however, endocannabinoids cannot be "stored" because of their lipid-derived nature. These ligands can readilty partition into membrane and diffuse through membrane and therefore cannot be contained. For this reason, endocannabinoids are synthesized on demand. 2-AG is synthesized in two steps. First diacylglycerol is generated by phospholipase C-β hydrolysis of phosphatidylinositol-4,5-bisphosphate. Then, diacylglycerol is hydrolyzed by diacylglycerol lipase (DAGL-α) to produce 2-AG [41, 42]. In an alternate first step, phosphatidic acid can produce diacylglycerol in a phospholipase-A2 or –D catalyzed reaction [43].

Anandamide is generated from a phosopholipid precursor, N-arachidonoyl phosphatidylethanolamine (NAPE) in two-steps [44]. First NAPE synthesis is catalyzed in a calcium dependent manner by a yet to be identified transacylase that catalyzes the transfer of sn-1 located arachidonic acid (AA) on phosphatidyl choline to the nitrogen atom of phosphatidylethanolamine (PE). Then, NAPE is hydrolyzed to anandamide (AEA) by a NAPE-specific phospholipase-D (PLD) which has been cloned [49], purified and characterized [50]. NAPE-PLD has been shown to selectively reduce NAPE and increase AEA levels when overexpressed in cells [45]. The discovery that AEA levels are not reduced in NAPE-PLD knock-out mice [53] or by siRNA knockdown of NAPE-PLD in macrophages [54], suggests that other biosynthetic pathways exist for AEA. In support of this, tissues from NAPE-PLD knock-out mice have been found to have enzymatic activity for the conversion of NAPE to AEA in a calcium dependent manner [53].

AEA can be synthesized by a calcium-independent mechanism that is sensitive to methyl arachidonoyl fluorophosphate (MAFP). Here NAPE is first converted to 2-lyso-NAPE by the group IB secretory phospholipase A2 (PLA2); then, 2-lyso-NAPE is metabolized to yield AEA [55]. However, additional enzymes must be involved in 2-lyso-NAPE production because PLA2 has a very restricted tissue expression. In the RAW264.7 mouse macrophage cell line, NAPE can be hydrolyzed by phospholipase C to produce phosphoanandamide (pAEA). Phosphatases (including the putative tyrosine phosphatase PTPN22 [46]) then can dephosphorylate pAEA to yield AEA. In macrophages, this pathway is responsible for the endotoxin (LPS)-induced increase in AEA biosynthesis [46, 47]. Another alternative pathway for AEA synthesis involves αβ-hydrolase 4 (Abhd4). This enzyme can act on either NAPE or lyso-NAPE to produce the glycerophospho-arachidonoyl ethanolamide (GpAEA). GpAEA is then acted upon by a metal-dependent, phosphodiesterase to produce AEA [56].

Does the Lipid Bilayer Orient Endocannabinoids for Productive Interaction with Endocannabinoid System Components?

The lipid bilayer plays a central role in the life-cycle of endocannabinoids. To understand the mechanism of endocannabinoid action, it becomes important to know where endocannabinoids may be located in a lipid bilayer and what conformations they may adopt in this environment. Both molecular dynamics and NMR spectrosciopy can be used to provide this information.

Molecular Dynamics Simulations in Lipid. Molecular dynamics simulations of AEA in a 1,2-dioleoyl-*sn*-glycero-3-phosphocholine (DOPC) phospholipid bilayer have shown that the AEA polar headgroup resides in the polar phospholipid headgroup region of the bilayer at the lipid-water interface, while the AEA nonpolar acyl chain extends into the hydrocarbon core of the membrane. These simulations also revealed that (i) in the DOPC bilayer environment, an AEA elongated conformation is preferred, yet many AEA conformations are sampled. Other conformations observed include angle-iron/extended/helical conformers, as well as more compact conformations such as J and U shaped conformations; (ii) the AEA headgroup has extensive hydrogen bonding interactions with DOPC which are short-lived; and (iii) C-H bond order parameters decrease as one moves towards the center of the bilayer and these order parameters are low compared to those seen for fatty acid saturated acyl chains [48]. The orientation of AEA in DOPC is illustrated in Fig. (**1**).

NMR Spectroscopic Studies in Lipid. An NMR study of AEA in a dipalmitoylphosphatidylcholine multilamellar model membrane bilayer system has revealed information about AEA conformation, location, and dynamic properties [49]. These studies revealed that AEA adopts an extended conformation with the headgroup residing at the phospholipid polar group level and its terminal methyl group extending to the bilayer center. ^{2}H NMR experiments showed that AEA exhibits dynamic properties similar to membrane phospholipids, producing no bilayer perturbations. *Thus, both experimental and MD studies reveal that AEA tends to favor an extended conformation in the bilayer, but AEA also dynamically samples many other conformations.*

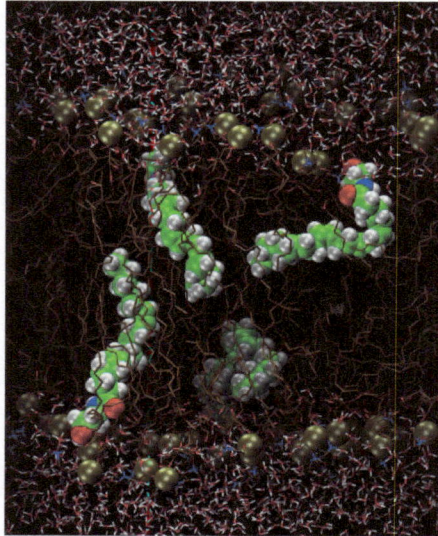

Figure 1: This is a frame from a multinanosecond simulation of AEA in a DOPC bilayer (48). Four AEA molecules are shown here, contoured at their Van der Waals radii. Two AEAs are in the upper leaflet of the membrane and two are in the lower leaflet. The phosphorus atoms of DOPC are shown as gold balls, while the remainder of the phospholipid head group atoms (nitrogens, blue; oxygens, red) and the fatty acid chains (orange) are shown in tube display. Water molecules are also shown in tube display. Here it is clear that AEA can adopt very different conformations in the lipid bilayer. These include extended, L-shaped and U-shaped conofrmations.

CANNABINOID RECEPTORS

The endocannabinoids have been shown to mediate retrograde signaling in the CNS. This signaling occurs when a calcium signal in a post-synaptic cell triggers the synthesis of 2-AG in the plasma membrane. 2-AG then diffuses (backwards) across the synapse to activate CB1 receptors located pre-synaptically. Receptor interaction, therefore, is the next major step for endocannabinoid signaling.

CB$_1$ Receptor. The Class A (rhodopsin family) of G-protein coupled receptors (GPCRs) includes the cannabinoid CB$_1$ and CB$_2$ receptors (see Fig. **(2)**). CB$_1$ was initially cloned from a rat cerebral cortex cDNA library [50]. Early sequence analyses revealed that CB_1 had highest homology with the endothelial differentiation gene (EDG) receptor family (now split into the lysophosphatidic acid (LPA) receptors and the spinghosine-1-phosphate (S1P) receptors) [51]. CB_1 receptors are expressed in the central nervous system (CNS) [52,53]. Such brain regions as the basal ganglia, cerebellum, and hippocampus are particularly rich in CB_1 receptors [54]. Outside the CNS, CB_1 receptors are found in human testis [55], retina [56], sperm cells [57], colonic tissues [58], peripheral neurons [59], adipocytes [60], and other organs including human adrenal gland, heart, lung, prostate, uterus, and ovary [61-63].

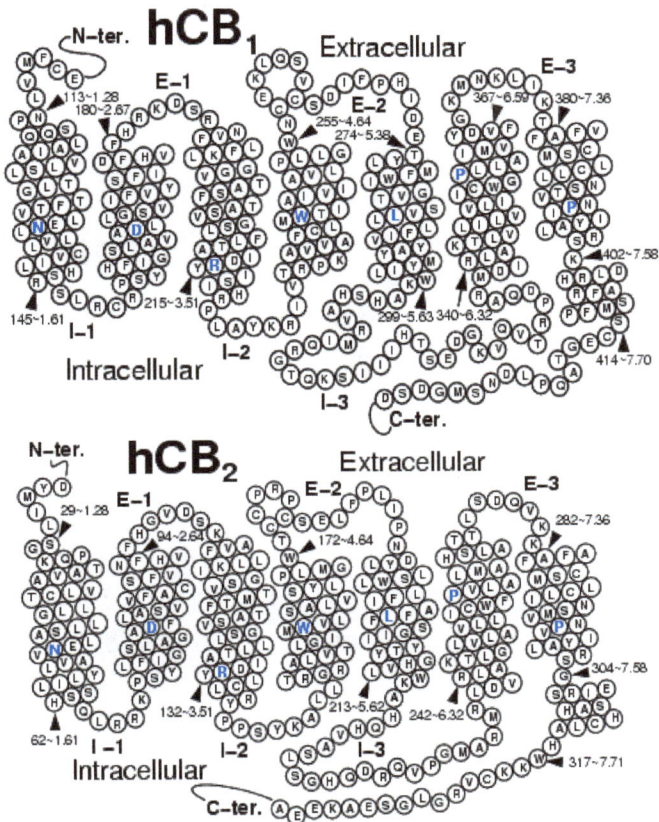

Figure 2: Helix net representations of the human CB_1 and CB_2 receptor sequences.

CB_1 receptors signal *via* multiple second effector systems (for a review see [64]). Agonists inhibit forskolin-stimulated adenylyl cyclase *via* a pertussis toxin-sensitive G-protein [65, 66]. CB_1 receptors inhibit N-, P-, and Q-type calcium channels and activate inwardly rectifying potassium channels In heterologous cells [65, 67,68]. In neuronal cells, CB_1 inhibits PKA-dependent voltage-gated N-type Ca^{2+} channels (N-type VGCCs) [69]. Calcium channel inhibition and activation of inwardly rectifying potassium currents is pertussis toxin-sensitive and independent of cAMP inhibition. This suggests a direct G protein mechanism [67]. In certain circumstances, CB_1 can couple to Gs proteins to activate adenylyl cyclase [70-72]. CB_1 also mediates Ca^{2+} fluxes that are Gq/PLC-dependent in rat insulinoma beta-cells [73]. β-arrestins have been reported to play a role in CB_1 desensitization [74,75] and CB_1 stimulation *in vitro* and *in vivo* results in activation of ERK1/2 kinases in a variety of cell types [76].

CB_2 Receptor. The cannabinoid CB_2 receptor was cloned from a human promyelocytic leukemia cell HL60 cDNA library [77]. Within the transmembrane regions, human CB_2 receptor has 78% homology to human CB_1 receptor and 64% homology throughout the whole protein [77]. The CB_1 receptor is highly conserved across human, rat and mouse. In contrast, the CB_2 receptor has 93% amino acid identity between rat and mouse and 81% amino acid identity between rat and human. CB_2 signals *via* Gi/o-proteins to inhibit adenylyl cyclase, stimulate both the mitogen-activated protein kinase [78,79], and phosphoinositide 3-kinase pathways [80]. CB_2 also produces activation of *de novo* ceramide production or cyclooxygenase-2 (COX-2) induction [81].

The CB_2 receptor is highly expressed throughout the immune system [62,82]. In the CNS, CB_2 is expressed in the CNS under both pathological [83] and physiological conditions [84]. Brain CB_2 receptors have been shown to modulate cocaine's rewarding and locomoter-stimulating effects [85]. The high expression of CB_2 in the immune system combined with the fact that CB_2 knock-out mice fail to respond to the immunomodulatory effects of classical cannabinoids [86], suggests that CB_2 receptor ligands may have potential therapeutic applications as immunomodulators for the treatment of inflammation and allergy. The CB_2 receptor also has been shown to modulate leukocyte migration [87-90], activation [91], and antigen processing [92]. In ovariectomized mice [93], the CB_2 receptor has been reported to protect from bone loss. However, CB_2 activation has also been reported to protect from bone loss [94].

Putative Cannabinoid Receptors

The endogenous cannabinoids control a large number of physiological processes [95]. While most of these effects have been attributed to action at either the cannabinoid CB_1 or CB_2 receptors, some effects are clearly not CB_1- or CB_2-mediated. It is possible that some of these cannabinoid effects may not be receptor mediated at all. However, several orphan receptors, including GPR55, GPR18, GPR35 and GPR119 have been proposed to be putative cannabinoid receptors [96]. Recent studies have confirmed that among these, GPR18 and GPR55 recognize a range of cannabinoid ligands. Cannabinoid effects have also been attributed to the TRPV1 channel (for a review see [97]) and the peroxisome proliferator-activated receptors (PPARs) (for a review see [96]).

GPR18. Samuelson and co-workers first isolated GPR18 from mouse in 1996 [98]. Gantz and colleagues subsequently isolated GPR18 from human and dog [99]. As indicated by northern blot analysis of several human tissues, GPR18 is highly expressed in human spleen and testis [99]. GPR18 has also been found in the thymus, peripheral blood leukocytes and small intestine, all associated with the immune system. This suggests that GPR18 may play an immunomodulatory role [99]. In 2006, eicosa-5,8,11,14-tetraenoylamino-acetic acid (N-arachidonoylglycine; NAGly (**10**); **Chart 2**) was identified as the endogenous ligand for GPR18 [100]. Since NAGly (**10**) is an arachidonic acid derivative, it bears structural similarity to AEA (**2**). Because GPR18 is activated by the atypical cannabinoid, abnormal-cannabidiol (Abn-CBD) and several endogenous and synthetic cannabinoids, GPR18 has been proposed to be the long-sought abn-CBD receptor [101] and therefore another cannabinoid receptor.

GPR55 is a rhodopsin-like (Class A) GPCR, that was de-orphanized as a cannabinoid receptor [102,103]. GPR55 is highly expressed in human striatum [104] (Genbank accession # NM-005683) and couples to Gα13 [105,106], Gα12 or Gαq [107] proteins. In the human CNS, GPR55 is found predominantly in the caudate, putamen, and striatum [104]. In models of inflammatory and neuropathic pain, GPR55$^{-/-}$ mice have been shown to be protected. This suggests that GPR55 antagonists may have therapeutic potential as analgesics for both these pain

CHART 2

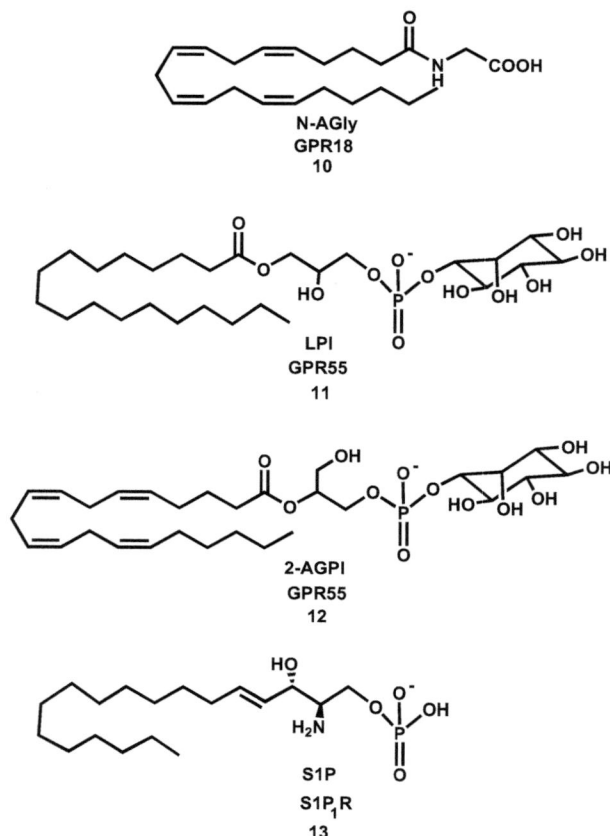

Chart 2: The structures of endogenous ligands of the GPR18, GPR55 and S1P$_1$ Receptors are illustrated here.

types [108]. A possible therapeutic use for GPR55 antagonists is in the treatment of osteoporosis, due to the physiological evidence that GPR55 is associated with bone resorption [109]. Other studies indicate that GPR55 activation is pro-carcinogenic [110-112]. Lysophosphatidylinositol (LPI, **11**) has been identified as an endogenous GPR55 agonist [113], with 2-arachidonoyl-sn-glycero-3-phosphoinositol (2-AGPI; **12**) possessing the best LPI activity observed to date [114]. Neither LPI nor 2-AGPI, however, bind to CB1 or CB2 receptors. Several labs have confirmed that GPR55 is a cannabinoid receptor [106, 107, 115] activated by various cannabinoid and atypical cannabinoid compounds. Using a β-arrestin green fluorescent protein biosensor to assess a cohort of CB$_1$/ CB$_2$ ligands for GPR55 activity, Kapur *et al.* [116] confirmed LPI (**11**) as a GPR55 agonist, while observing that the cannabinoid antagonists AM251 and SR141716A were also GPR55 agonists. These GPR55 ligands activated the G-protein dependent signaling of PKCβII and had comparable efficacy in inducing β-arrestin trafficking. The potent synthetic cannabinoid agonist CP55940 acted as a GPR55 antagonist/partial agonist, inhibiting GPR55 internalization, the formation of β-arrestin GPR55 complexes, and the phosphorylation of ERK1/2 [116].

While the rest of this review will focus solely on the CB_1 and CB_2 receptors, it is interesting to note that both of the putative cannabinoid receptors, GPR18 and GPR55 recognize arachidonic acid-derived endogenous ligands (N-AGly (GPR18) and 2-AGPI (GPR55)).

Cannabinoid Receptor Structure. The Ballesteros-Weinstein numbering system for GPCRs will be used here in all discussions of receptor residues [117]. In this numbering system, the most highly conserved Class A residue in each transmembrane helix (TMH) is labeled 50. This is preceded by the TMH number. In this system, for example, the most highly conserved residue in TMH3 is R3.50. The residue immediately before this would be labeled 3.49 and the residue immediately after this would be labeled 3.51. Loop residues are labelled by their absolute sequence numbers.

The cannabinoid CB_1 and CB_2 receptors (see Fig. (**2**)) belong to the Class A (rhodopsin (Rho) family) of GPCRs. Today, the GPCR field is benefiting from the increasing number of Class-A GPCR x-ray crystal structures that have been solved. These include rhodopsin (Rho) [118-120], meta-rhodopsin II [121], the β_2-adrenergic receptor (β_2-AR) [122-125], the β_1-adrenergic receptor (β_1-AR) [126,127], the adenosine A_{2A} receptor [128,129], the CXCR4 receptor [130], the dopamine D_3 receptor [131], the histamine H_1 receptor [132], the nociceptin/orphanin FQ receptor [133], the mu [134], delta [135] and kappa [136] opioid receptors and the $S1P_1$ receptor [137]. These crystal structures reveal a common topology that includes: (1) an extracellular N terminus; (2) seven transmembrane alpha helices (TMHs) arranged to form a closed bundle; (3) loops connecting TMHs that extend intra- and extracellularly; and, except for the CXCR4 receptor [130], (4) an intracellular C terminus that begins with a short helical segment (Helix 8) oriented parallel to the membrane surface. Ligand binding occurs within the TMH bundle, with additional ligand interactions occurring with extracellular (EC) loop residues in some structures.

In the binding pocket of each Class A GPCR, there is a set of residues that change conformation upon agonist binding. These "toggle switch" residues typically include a residue on TMH6 close to the TMH6 CWXP motif and a residue that interacts with this TMH6 residue. In CB_1R, the "toggle switch" pair has been shown by mutation to be between W6.48 and F3.36 [138]. In the crystal structure of the agonist bound beta-2-adrenergic receptor, the residues that comprise the "toggle switch" are F6.44, P5.50 and I3.40 [139]. When the toggle switch within the binding pocket is tripped by agonist binding, TMH6 straightens and moves away from the TMH bundle using the CWXP hinge motif. This movement of TMH6 breaks the "ionic lock" between R3.50 and E/D6.30 at the intracellular end of the receptor. What results is an intracellular opening in the TMH3/4/5/6 region large enough to allow the G-alpha protein to insert its alpha-5 helix C-terminal region into the activated GPCR [140]. This sequence of events is consistent with the recent x-ray crystal structure of the β2-adrenergic receptor in complex with Gs protein [141]. Fig. **(3)** illustrates the CB2 receptor (TMHs and loops, orange) in a POPC bilayer that has been activated by 2-AG (in VdW, yellow) [142] interacting with a Gαi1β1γ2 protein [143]. The alpha subunit of the G protein is colored green here, while the beta subunit is colored cyan and the gamma subunit is colored magenta. The insertion of the C-terminal Gαi1 alpha helix into CB2 is modeled after the recent β-2-adrenergic receptor in complex with Gs [141]. The GDP that is held by the Gα protein between its ras and helical domains is contoured at its Van der Waals radius.

The x-ray crystal structure of the $S1P_1$ receptor fused to T4-lysozyme (T4L) [137] affords us for the first time a comparison of Class A GPCRs triggered by lipid-derived ligands (such as $S1P_1$ and CB receptors) *versus* those triggered by small aminergic endogenous ligands (such as the beta-adrenergic or serotonin receptors) or peptide endogenous ligands (such as the mu-, delta- and kappa-opioid receptors). In the $S1P_1$ receptor crystal structure, the receptor is in complex with the selective antagonist sphingolipidmimic (R)-3-amino-(3 hexylphenyl-amino)-4-oxobutylphosphonic acid (ML056) [144]. The resolution in the $S1P_1$/T4L

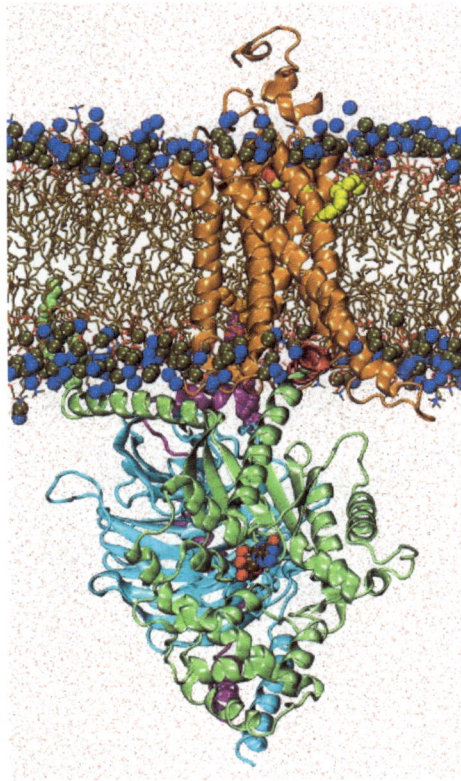

Figure 3: (A) This figure illustrates the CB_2 receptor (orange) in a POPC bilayer that has been activated by 2-AG (in VdW, yellow) [142]. The receptor is interacting with a G-protein, $G\alpha i1\beta 1\gamma 2$ [143]. The alpha subunit of the G protein is colored green here. The G protein beta subunit is colored cyan, while the gamma subunit is colored magenta. The insertion of the C-terminal alpha helix of the alpha subunit into CB_2 is modeled after the recent β-2-adrenergic receptor in complex with Gs [141].

crystal structure is 3.35 Å using traditional x-ray diffraction data processing methods. This resolution is reduced to 2.8 Å with an experimental microdiffraction data assembly method that can process data of rapidly decaying microcrystals [137]. The human $S1P_{1-5}$ receptors have very high (62-64%) sequence homology with the human cannabinoid CB_1 receptor in their transmembrane helix (TMH) regions. This high homology is interesting given that both the $S1P_{1-5}$ family of receptors and the cannabinoid CB_1/CB_2 receptors bind endogenous lipid-derived ligands. Because of this sequence homology, it is likely that structural motifs seen in the recent $S1P_1$ receptor x-ray crystal structure will have implications for the structures of the cannabinoid CB_1 and CB_2 receptors.

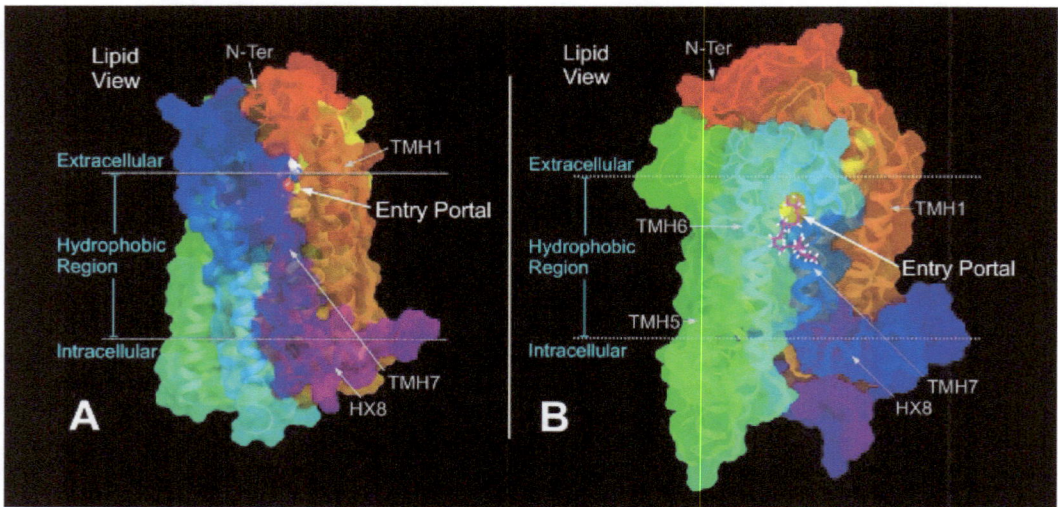

Figure 4: (A) The recent x-ray crystal structure of the $S1P_1$ receptor [137] shows that the N-terminus closes the receptor off to the extracellular milleu. The structure also shows a gap between TMH7 and TMH1 through which ligands may gain access to the binding pocket [137]. (B) This figure illustrates the result of molecular dynamics simulations of endogenous cannabinoid, 2-AG (5) binding to the membrane embedded CB_2 receptor. Here an opening forms between TMH6 and TMH7 in the CB_2 receptor as 2-AG (magenta) is poised to enter the receptor from the lipid bilayer [142].

The N-terminus in the $S1P_1$ crystal structure is one of its striking features. This terminus contains a helical segment that is packed across the TMH bundle (from TMH3 to TMH6) with the EC-1 and EC-2 loops packing against the N-terminal helix (see Fig. **(4A)**). **This arrangement occludes ligand access to the receptor from the extracellular milieu [137].** It is likely that this is similar in the CB receptors, particularly in CB_1 since the N-terminus of CB_1 is quite long (112 residues) (see Fig. **(4B)**). The primary function of this long N-terminus in CB_1 appears to be to retain the receptor in the endoplasmic reticulum (ER), diminishing cell surface expression [145].

Lipid Portal for Ligand Entry. The limited access to the ligand binding pocket from the extracellular milieu in the $S1P_1$ receptor suggests that this receptor may have been designed for ligand approach *via* the membrane bilayer. The spinghosine-1-phosphate receptors ($S1P_{1-5}$) are Class A GPCRs that bind the endogenous lipid, Sphingosine 1-phosphate (S1P) (**13; Chart 2**)). The lipid signaling molecule, S1P, regulates the cardiovascular and immune systems and functions in numerous physiological and pathophysiological conditions (for reviews, see Refs [146-148]). The $S1P_1$ crystal structure shows a gap between TMH7 and TMH1 through which ligands may gain access to the binding pocket (see Fig. **(4A)**) [137,149]. This gap originates from TMH1 leaning away from the TMH bundle, TMH1 also leans away from the TMH bundle in the β_2-adrenergic receptor structure (β_2-AR) [122,123], however, in the β_2-AR, this opening is filled by W7.40 and M1.39 and by the top of TMH2. Together these TMH1, TMH2 and TMH7 residues shield the bundle from the lipid bilayer. In $S1P_1$, TMH2 is straight and does help fill the TMH1/TMH7 opening and residues 7.40 and 1.39 are much smaller (V7.40 and F1.39), resulting is an opening to the lipid bilayer between TMH1 and TMH7 (see Fig. **(4A)**). The limited access to the ligand binding pocket from the extracellular milieu may explain why, in the presence of excess ligand, $S1P_1$ ligands, including S1P, show slow saturation of receptor binding [150].

A lipid portal for ligand entry has also been suggested by experimental and computational studies of the CB receptors. The isothiocyanate derivatized classical cannabinoid, (-)-7'-isothiocyanato-11-hydroxy-1',1'dimethylheptyl-hexahydro-cannabinol (AM841), enters the cannabinoid CB_1 receptor *via* the lipid bilayer at the level of C6.47 [151] (a CWXP motif residue that faces lipid), forming a covalent bond with this residue. Similar results were found for the CB_2 receptor [152]. Molecular dynamics simulations of 2-AG (**5**) with the CB_2 receptor in a palmitoyl-oleoyl-phosphatidylcholine (POPC) lipid bilayer have suggested that (1) the lipid face of TMH6/7 acts as a vestibule for 2-AG when it first partitions out of bulk lipid; (2) from the vestibule, 2-AG enters the CB_2 receptor binding pocket by passing between TMH6/7; (3) receptor activation is triggered by the passage of the 2-AG headgroup between TMH6/7 and into the TMH bundle [142]. Fig. **(4B)** illustrates the opening that forms between TMH6 and TMH7 in CB_2 as 2-AG is poised to enter the receptor from lipid. **These MD simulations suggest that the fatty acid portion of 2-AG (arachidonic acid) is key for getting the ligand to the receptor at the correct height in the bilayer so that the headgroup can enter the lipid portal [142]. The process of insertion into the portal requires that 2-AG first "dive" for the opening, leading with its headgroup and then progress inside the receptor by flexing its arachidonic acid chain as it threads through the portal. Such a process is facilitated by the homo-allylic double bond pattern of the arachidonic acid** chain which gives 2-AG tremendous flexibility While 2-AG does eventually pull completely inside the receptor (Fig. (5)) (assuming a folded conformation, with its head group interacting with EC-3 loop residue, D(275)), complete insertion of the acyl chain does not appear to be a requirement for receptor activation.

Degradative Enzymes: Lipid Portals for Endocannabinoid Entry

The endocannabinoids AEA and 2-AG are not stored in vesicles, they are synthesized upon demand in neurons and then efficiently metabolized to ensure rapid signal inactivation [10, 44]. Degradative enzymes for the endocannabinoids are integral membrane proteins accessed by the endocannabinoids *via* the lipid bilayer.

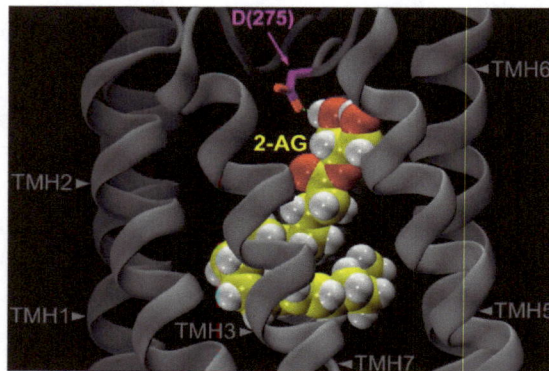

Figure 5: This figure illustrates the result of a continued molecular dynamics trajectory after the 2-AG headgroup has entered CB_2 *via* the TMH6/TMH7 portal and activated CB_2 [142]. 2-AG (VdW, yellow) does completely enter the CB_2 receptor (gray helices) and assumes a folded conformation within the ligand binding pocket, while continuing its interaction with D(275) in the EC-3 loop of CB2.

2-AG Degradation. The membrane-associated enzyme, monoacylglycerol lipase (MAGL) hydrolyzes 2-AG to glycerol and arachidonic acid after 2-AG interacts with the membrane-embedded CB receptor [153]. MAGL functions as a serine hydrolase [154]. In the mouse brain proteome, the majority of the 2-AG hydrolysis activity (~85%) is due to MGL, with the remaining hydrolysis activity attributed to ABHD6 and ABHD12, as well as a soluble fraction of MAGL [155]. MAGL is found mainly pre-synaptic and co-localized with the CB1 receptor in axon terminals [28]. This localization is ideal to terminate 2-AG/CB_1 signaling regardless of the source of the 2-AG [156]. Although ABHD6 represents only 4%

of brain 2-AG hydrolase activity, in neurons it rivals MAGL in efficacy. ABHD6 possesses typical α/β-hydrolase family fingerprints such as the lipase motif (GHSLG) and a fully conserved catalytic triad (postulated amino acid residues S246-D333-H372) [155]. ABHD6 appears to be an integral membrane protein whose active site is predicted to face the cell interior. Such an orientation suggests that ABHD6 is well suited to guard the intracellular pool of 2-AG at the site of generation (for an excellent review, see [156]).

Bertrand and co-workers reported the first crystal structure of human MAGL in its apo form and holo form with the covalent inhibitor SAR629 [157] (see Fig. **(6A)**). These structures are available in the Protein Data Bank (accession codes 3JW8 and 3JWE). MAGL is monomeric and shares the classic fold of the α/β hydrolase family which consists of an eight-stranded β-sheet composed of seven parallel strands and one antiparallel strand surrounded by α-helices. The fold provides a stable scaffold for the active sites of a wide variety of enzymes including proteases, lipases, esterases, dehalogenases, peroxidases, and epoxide hydrolases. The α/β hydrolase family possesses a highly conserved catalytic triad (Ser132-His279-Asp249 in MAGL) in the core domain and a 100% conserved histidine residue located after the last β-strand [158-160]. Newer members of α/β hydrolase family display additional structural features, mainly α helices. These features form "lid" or "capping" domains protecting access to the catalytic triad, which is buried in the canonical core domain of the enzyme [161]. Other smaller hydrolases such as Bacillus subtilis lipase do not share this lid, and the catalytic triad residues are solvent-exposed [162]. The structure of rat integral membrane FAAH also shows this lid feature, where the lid is presumed to be responsible for the interaction of FAAH with the lipid membrane [163]. In MAGL, the lid domain is formed from two large loops surrounding an amphipathic helix A4 (residues 156–190) (see Fig. **(6A)**, orange helix). An equivalent helix is found in rat FAAH. This helix has been described as the putative membrane-interacting region of the protein—or anchor helix [164]. It is likely the case also with MAGL, since the amphipathic helix A4 has its hydrophobic side exposed. The lid of MAGL is located at the entrance of a large elongated hydrophobic tunnel about 25 Å in length and 8 Å in width that has a polar bottom and terminates near the catalytic Ser132 (see Fig. **(6B)**). The topology of this tunnel is consistent with the topology of 2-AG which contains the highly flexible arachidonyl fatty acid chain that can maneuver easily in the tunnel, together with a polar glycerol head that is cleaved by the catalytic triad. Additional crystal structures of MAGL have been published [165,166] which differ mainly in the subset of the lid-domain (151–225) residues in the range of 151–173 that display large variations. A comparison to the apo structure (PDB ID 3HJU) [157] suggests that the lid-domain undergoes a substantial rearrangement upon ligand binding.

In α/β hydrolases, the oxyanion hole contains two nitrogen atoms stabilizing the negatively charged oxygen of the substrate during the transition state of the catalytic reaction [167, 168]. Based upon structural alignment of MAGL with other α/β hydrolase sequences, the water molecule linking catalytic Ser132 to Ala61 and Met133 is probably located in the oxyanion hole [157]. The catalytic triad provides activation of the nucleophilic serine, which cleaves the ester bond of 2-AG when stabilized *via* its carbonyl group to the oxyanion hole formed by main-chain nitrogen atoms of Ala61 and Met133. Bertrand suggests that the released glycerol molecule may diffuse toward a narrow "exit hole" (cytosolic port, Fig. **(6B)**) located at the same level as the catalytic triad, while arachidonic acid could diffuse back to the top of the tunnel and exit the protein [157]. Fig. **(6C)** shows the MGL protein associated with a POPC membrane containing multiple 2-AGs (VdW, gray). The amphipathic A4 helix (shown in orange) is inserted into the lower leaflet of the membrane. One 2-AG molecule (VdW, yellow) is poised to enter the lipid entry portal.

AEA Degradation. Studies have shown that fatty acid amide hydrolase (FAAH), an integral membrane-bound enzyme, is responsible for AEA metabolism into arachidonic acid and ethanolamine [163,169,170]. FAAH has been shown by immunohistochemistry to not be localized to the plasma membrane, but rather localized to the endoplasmic reticulum [171,172]. This means that AEA must diffuse or be carried to FAAH inside the cell (see Intracellular Trafficking of Anandamide and 2-AG section below). In the brain, FAAH can act as a general hydrolase metabolizing other fatty ethanolamides or fatty esters such as 2-AG [173-175]. It has been shown, however, that inactivation of 2-AG is mainly due to monoacylglycerol lipase (MAGL) in rat brain, while only traces of FAAH activity on 2-AG were detected [153,176-178]. The Cravatt group determined the three-dimensional structure of FAAH to 2.8 Å resolution by x-ray crystallography [163]. Coordinates and structure factors have been deposited in the Protein Data Bank (accession code 1MT5). The protein was crystallized from recombinantly expressed rat FAAH with the first 29 amino acids deleted at the NH$_2$-terminus. While this deleted region may participate in membrane binding [164], the truncated FAAH variant (residues 30 to 579) does associate with membranes and is able to degrade fatty acid amides in mammalian cells [179].

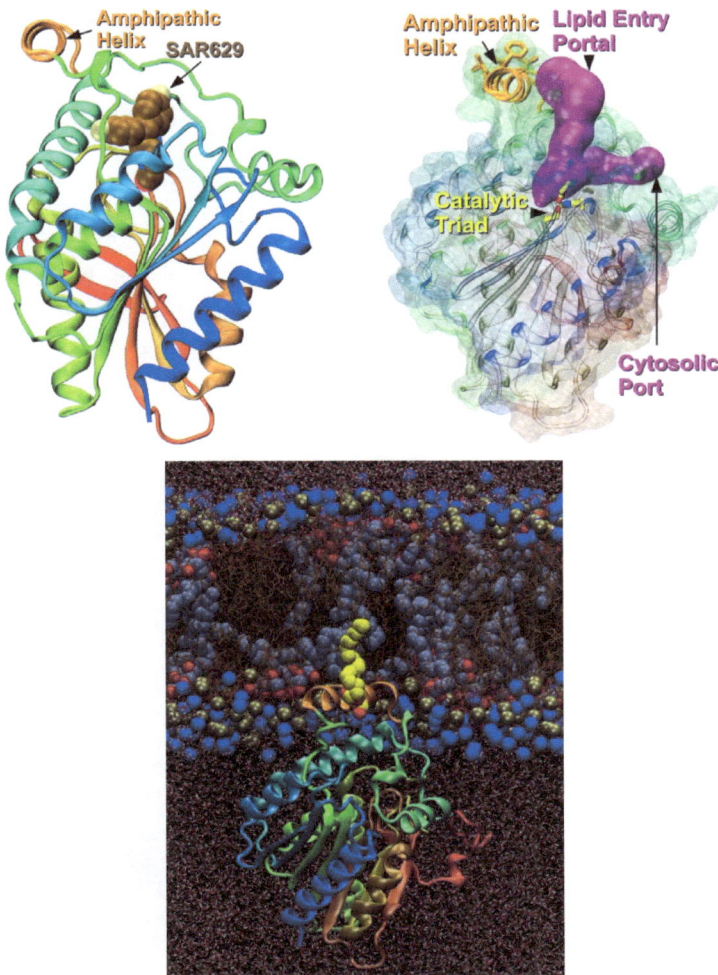

Figure 6: (A) The first crystal structure of human MGL in complex with the covalent inhibitor SAR629 is illustrated here [157]. SAR629 is contoured at its Van der Waals radii and colored gold. The amphipathic helix that allows association of MGL with the lipid bilayer is colored orange here. (B) The program Caver [197] was used here to outline the tunnels in MGL (magenta).

The lipid entry portal is adjacent to the amphipathic A4 helix (orange) that inserts into membrane. A second tunnel corresponds to the cytosolic port in MAGL. (C) This figure shows the MGL protein associated with a POPC membrane containing multiple 2-AGs (VdW, gray). The amphipathic A4 helix (orange) is inserted into the inner leaflet of the membrane. One 2-AG molecule (VdW, yellow) is poised to enter the lipid entry portal.

The crystal structure of FAAH shows that it is a dimeric enzyme (Fig. **(7A)**) with methoxy arachidonyl phosphonate (MAP) forming an adduct. This is consistent with chemical cross-linking studies that suggested the enzyme is dimeric in solution [179]. The core of FAAH is characterized by a twisted β sheet of 11 mixed strands surrounded by 24 α helices of various lengths. The active site of FAAH was initially identified based upon the location of core catalytic residues revealed by mutagenesis [180,181] and from the density of the inhibitor adduct methoxy arachidonyl phosphonate (MAP). The catalytic nucleophile Ser241 is covalently bound to the phosphorous of MAP, and the adjacent density can be modeled to accommodate the arachidonyl chain. The serine nucleophile in FAAH forms part of an unusual Ser-Ser-Lys catalytic triad with Ser217 and Lys142. The substrate binding pocket of FAAH includes a tunnel that leads from the surface and is occupied by the arachidonic acid acyl chain (see Fig. **(7B)**). This tunnel is lined with many aromatic and aliphatic amino acids. These residues include Ile491, a residue identified by ultraviolet crosslinking and mutagenesis studies to be important for substrate recognition [182].

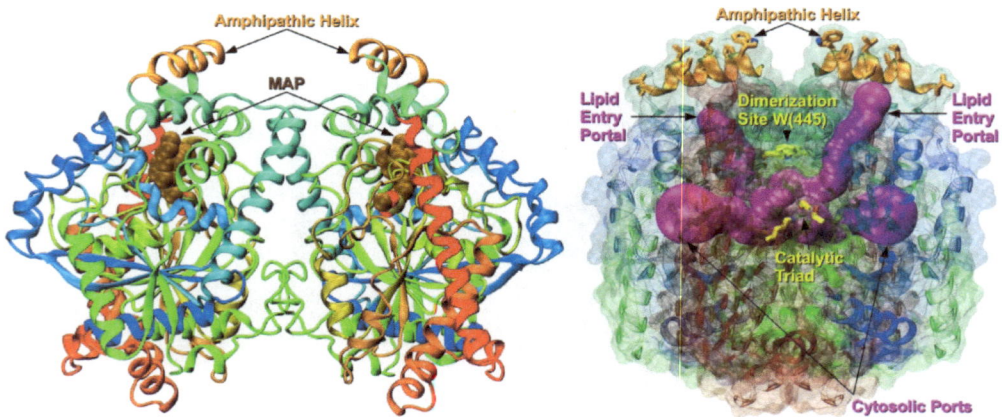

Figure 7: (A) The crystal structure of the dimeric enzyme, FAAH, in complex with the inhibitor adduct methoxy arachidonyl phosphonate (MAP) is illustrated here. (B) The substrate binding pocket of FAAH includes a tunnel leading from the surface of FAAH in which the arachidonoyl chain of MAP is inserted. This tunnel is lined with a preponderance of aromatic and aliphatic

amino acids. The two amphipathic helices α18 and α19 (orange) cap the active site and present several hydrophobic residues that likely constitute FAAH's membrane binding face. The program Caver [197] was used here to outline the tunnels in FAAH (magenta). A potential substrate entry tunnel is adjacent to α18 and α19 that may serve as a lipid entry portal. This tunnel terminates at the catalytic triad.

In FAAH, amino acids 410 to 438 form a helix-turn-helix motif that interrupts the AS fold. The two amphipathic helices α18 and α19 cap the active site and expose several hydrophobic residues that likely form FAAH's membrane binding face (see amphipathic helices in Fig. **(7B)**). A possible substrate entrance is adjacent to α18 and α19, and the arachidonic acid acyl chain of MAP contacts Phe432 of α18, which may indicate direct access between the FAAH active site and the hydrophobic membrane bilayer (see lipid entry portals in Fig. **(7B)**). The substrate entry is amphipathic, with hydrophobic residues on three sides of the rim and charged residues Arg486 and Asp403 on the remaining side. This amphipathic arrangement of residues may select for polar fatty acid amide head groups and their movement toward the active site. Overall, the close relationship between the membrane binding surface and the FAAH active site is similar to that of squalene cyclase [183] and prostaglandin H2 synthase [184], which also recognize lipid-soluble substrates and contain hydrophobic caps surrounding the entrances to their respective active sites. In all three enzymes, the hydrophobic cap is surrounded by positively charged amino acids that may interact with negatively charged phospholipids.

In FAAH, there is a second tunnel. This emerges from the active site at about an 80° angle from the arachidonyl-filled cavity. This tunnel splits into two tunnels to create a solvent-exposed cytosolic port and a route blocked by Trp445, a residue that forms a lock-and-key intersubunit contact (see Fig. **(7B)**). Thus, the FAAH active site appears to access both the cytoplasmic aqueous environment and the lipid bilayer. This arrangement may provide a cytosolic exit route for the polar amine substituents cleaved from the fatty acid amide substrates and could also provide entry for a waters required for deacylation of the FAAH–fatty acyl intermediate [181].

Intracellular Trafficking of AEA and 2-AG

AEA. Cellular uptake and intracellular trafficking of AEA is a crucial step in the "lifecycle" of this endocannabinoid as this transport delivers AEA to FAAH for degradation. The identity of a specific AEA transporter remains a hot topic for research in the endocannabinoid field as different research groups have identified different AEA intracellular binding proteins (AIBPs). These include fatty acid binding proteins 5 and 7 (FABP5 and FABP7) [185,186], the FAAH-like cytoplasmic AEA transporter (FLAT) [187], as well as heat shock protein 70 (HSP70) and albumin [188]. FABPs are a family of small, cytoplasmic proteins that bind and transport long chain fatty acids and other hydrophobic ligands. The overall structural motif of the family is a 10-strand β-barrel, with the first and second β strands connected by a helix-turn-helix motif (colored magenta in Fig. **(8)**) that acts as a portal through which fatty acids enter the protein [189]. It has been reported that FABP7 has the highest affinity for docosahexaenoic acid (DHA) [190]. This is consistent with FABP7 also binding AEA, since DHA is a highly unsaturated fatty acid with homo-allylic double bonds as is the arachidonyl chain of AEA. Fig. **(8)** shows AEA (orange) carried in the interior of FABP7 [191]. The FABP helix-turn-helix segment is highlighted here in magenta, while the rest of the β barrel is colored yellow. When AEA enters FABP7, the AEA carboxamide oxygen can interact with interior residues R126 and Y128, while the AEA hydroxyl group can interact with FABP7 interior residues, T53 and R106.

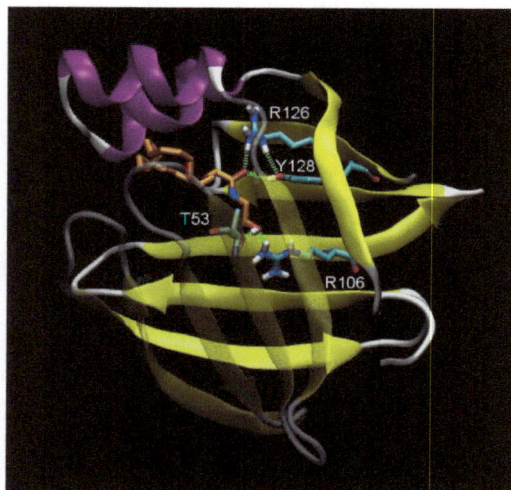

Figure 8: AEA is modeled here docked in FABP7. The overall structural motif of the FABP family is represented by a 10-strand β-barrel, with the first and second β strands connected by a helix-turn-helix motif (magenta) that acts as a dynamic portal through which fatty acids enter the protein [189]. When AEA enters FABP7, the carboxamide oxygen of AEA can interact with interior residues R126 and Y128, while the hydroxyl group of AEA can interact with FABP7 interior residues, T53 and R106.

2-AG. Only a few papers address the issue of 2-AG transport. Varying hypotheses have been proposed concerning 2-AG transport, from simple diffusion to carrier-mediated transport by the same endocannabinoid membrane transporter (EMT) proposed for AEA or *via* a different transporter [176, 192-195]. Recently, Chicca and co-workers have reported evidence for an endocannabinoid membrane transporter (EMT) that controls endocannabinoid extracellular and intracellular levels in an orchestrated manner together with cytoplasmic carrier proteins and degrading enzymes. This EMT is specific for arachidonic acid containing ligands: AEA, 2-AG, NADA, Noladin ether and virodhamine [196]. The structure of this EMT has yet to be solved.

CONCLUSIONS

This review has shown that the lipid bilayer plays a major role in the "life-cycle" of the endocannabinoids. AEA and 2-AG, are synthesized on demand in the lipid bilayer; act at membrane embedded cannabinoid receptors that may be accessed *via* the lipid bilayer; and, are degraded by membrane associated enzymes that have lipid entry portals for their respective endocannabinoids (2-AG-MAGL; AEA-FAAH). Transport for degradation (especially for AEA) remains a hot research topic, as AEA must leave the plasma membrane and travel inside the cell to FAAH which is associated with the membrane of the endoplasmic reticulum. The homo-allylic double bond pattern in the arachidonyl acyl chain of both endocannabinoids confers "dynamic plasticity" to their acyl chains that allows them to navigate through these entry portals and tunnels of various sizes and shapes. The field of endocannabinoids is expanding with the identification of two new putative cannabinoid receptors (GPR18 and GPR55). It is striking that both have endogenous ligands containing arachidonyl acyl chains as well. It is therefore very likely that "dynamic plasticity" will be important for these new ligands as well.

ACKNOWLEDGEMENTS

This work was supported by an NIH KO5 DA021358 grant to PHR.

CONFLICT OF INTEREST

The authors confirm that this chapter content has no conflicts of interest.

ABBREVIATIONS

2-AG	=	sn-2-arachidonylglycerol
2-AGPI	=	2-arachidonoyl-sn-glycero-3-phosphoinositol
Abhd4	=	αβ-hydrolase 4
AEA	=	N-arachidonylethanolamine
AM841	=	(-)-7'-isothiocyanato-11-hydroxy-1',1'dimethylheptyl-hexahydro-cannabinol
CB	=	cannabinoid
DAG	=	diacylglycerol
DAGL-α	=	diacylglycerol lipase
DOPC,1	=	2-dioleoyl-*sn*-glycero-3-phosphocholine
EMT	=	endocannabinoid membrane transporter
FAAH	=	fatty acid amide hydrolase
FABP	=	fatty acid binding protein
FLAT	=	FAAH-like cytoplasmic AEA transporter
GDP	=	Guanosine Diphosphate
GpAEA	=	glycerophospho-arachidonoyl ethanolamide
GPCR	=	G protein-coupled receptor
LPI	=	lysophosphatidylinositol
MAFP	=	methyl arachidonoyl fluorophosphate

MGL	=	monoacylglycerol lipase

MGL   =   monoacylglycerol lipase

ML056   =   (R)-3-amino-(3   hexylphenyl-amino)-4-
                                oxobutylphosphonic acid

NAGly, eicosa-5,8,11=   14-tetraenoylamino-acetic acid (N-arachidonoylglycine)

NAPE   =   N-arachidonoyl phosphatidylethanolamine

pAEA   =   phosphoanandamide

PLA2   =   phospholipase A2

PLD   =   phospholipase-D

POPC   =   palmitoyl-oleoyl-phosphatidylcholine

VdW   =   Van der Waals

β_1-AR   = β_1-adrenergic receptor

β_2-AR   = β_2-adrenergic receptor

REFERENCES

[1]   Devane WA, Dysarz FA, 3rd, Johnson MR, Melvin LS, Howlett AC. Determination and characterization of a cannabinoid receptor in rat brain. Mol Pharmacol 1988 Nov;34(5):605-13.

[2]   Gaoni Y, Mechoulam R. The isolation and structure of delta-1-tetrahydrocannabinol and other neutral cannabinoids from hashish. J Am Chem Soc 1971 Jan 13;93(1):217-24.

[3]   Herkenham M, Lynn AB, Little MD, Johnson MR, Melvin LS, de Costa BR, *et al.* Cannabinoid receptor localization in brain. Proc Natl Acad Sci U S A 1990 Mar;87(5):1932-6.

[4]   Katona I, Sperlagh B, Sik A, Kafalvi A, Vizi ES, Mackie K, *et al.* Presynaptically located CB1 cannabinoid receptors regulate GABA release from axon terminals of specific hippocampal interneurons. J Neurosci 1999 Jun 1;19(11):4544-58.

[5]   Wilson RI, Nicoll RA. Endogenous cannabinoids mediate retrograde signaling at hippocampal synapses. Nature 2001 Mar 29;410(6828):588-92.

[6]   Devane WA, Hanus L, Breuer A, Pertwee RG, Stevenson LA, Griffin G, *et al.* Isolation and structure of a brain constituent that binds to the cannabinoid receptor. Science 1992 Dec 18;258(5090):1946-9.

[7]   Mechoulam R, Ben-Shabat S, Hanus L, Ligumsky M, Kaminski NE, Schatz AR, *et al.* Identification of an endogenous 2-monoglyceride, present in canine gut, that binds to cannabinoid receptors. Biochem Pharmacol 1995 Jun 29;50(1):83-90.

[8]   Hanus L, Gopher A, Almog S, Mechoulam R. Two new unsaturated fatty acid ethanolamides in brain that bind to the cannabinoid receptor. J Med Chem 1993 Oct 1;36(20):3032-4.

[9]   Mechoulam R, Ben-Shabat S, Hanus L, Ligumsky M, Kaminski NE, Schatz AR, *et al.* Identification of an endogenous 2-monoglyceride, present in canine gut, that binds to cannabinoid receptors. Biochem Pharmacol 1995 Jun 29;50(1):83-90.

[10]   Stella N, Schweitzer P, Piomelli D. A second endogenous cannabinoid that modulates long-term potentiation. Nature 1997 Aug 21;388(6644):773-8.

[11]   Hanus L, Abu-Lafi S, Fride E, Breuer A, Vogel Z, Shalev DE, *et al.* 2-arachidonyl glyceryl ether, an endogenous agonist of the cannabinoid CB1 receptor. Proc Natl Acad Sci U S A 2001 Mar 27;98(7):3662-5.

[12]   Oka S, Tsuchie A, Tokumura A, Muramatsu M, Suhara Y, Takayama H, *et al.* Ether-linked analogue of 2-arachidonoylglycerol (noladin ether) was not detected in the brains of various mammalian species. J Neurochem 2003 Jun;85(6):1374-81.

[13]   Bezuglov V, Bobrov M, Gretskaya N, Gonchar A, Zinchenko G, Melck D, *et al.* Synthesis and biological evaluation of novel amides of polyunsaturated fatty acids with dopamine. Bioorg Med Chem Lett 2001 Feb 26;11(4):447-9.

[14]   Bisogno T, Melck D, Bobrov M, Gretskaya NM, Bezuglov VV, De Petrocellis L, *et al.* N-acyl-dopamines: novel synthetic CB(1) cannabinoid-receptor ligands and inhibitors of anandamide inactivation with cannabimimetic activity *in vitro* and *in vivo*. Biochem J 2000 Nov 1;351 Pt 3:817-24.

[15]   Porter AC, Sauer JM, Knierman MD, Becker GW, Berna MJ, Bao J, *et al.* Characterization of a novel endocannabinoid, virodhamine, with antagonist activity at the CB1 receptor. J Pharmacol Exp Ther 2002 Jun;301(3):1020-4.

[16]   Reggio PH. Endocannabinoid binding to the cannabinoid receptors: what is known and what remains unknown. Curr Med Chem 2010;17(14):1468-86.

[17]   Rabinovich AL, Ripatti PO. On the Conformational, Physical Properties and Function of Polyunsaturated AcylChains. Biochim Biophys Acta 1991;1085:53-6.

[18]   Rich MR. Conformational Analysis of Arachidonic and Related Fatty Acids Using Molecular Dynamics Simulations. Biochim Biophys Acta 1993;1178:87-96.

[19]   Reggio PH, Traore H. Conformational requirements for endocannabinoid interaction with the cannabinoid receptors, the anandamide transporter and fatty acid amidohydrolase. Chem Phys Lipids 2000 Nov;108(1-2):15-35.

[20]   Barnett-Norris J, Hurst DP, Lynch DL, Guarnieri F, Makriyannis A, Reggio PH. Conformational memories and the endocannabinoid binding site at the cannabinoid CB1 receptor. J Med Chem 2002 Aug 15;45(17):3649-59.

[21]   Thomas BF, Adams IB, Mascarella SW, Martin BR, Razdan RK. Structure-activity analysis of anandamide analogs: relationship to a cannabinoid pharmacophore. J Med Chem 1996 Jan 19;39(2):471-9.

[22]   Tong W, Collantes ER, Welsh WJ, Berglund BA, Howlett AC. Derivation of a pharmacophore model for anandamide using constrained conformational searching and comparative molecular field analysis. J Med Chem 1998 Oct 22;41(22):4207-15.

[23]   Di Marzo M, Casapullo A, Bifulco G, Cimino P, Ligresti A, Di Marzo V, *et al.* Synthesis, conformational analysis and CB1 binding affinity of hairpin-like anandamide pseudopeptide mimetics. J Pept Sci 2006 Sep;12(9):575-91.

[24]   Barnett-Norris J, Guarnieri F, Hurst DP, Reggio PH. Exploration of biologically relevant conformations of anandamide, 2-arachidonylglycerol, and their analogues using conformational memories. J Med Chem 1998 Nov 19;41(24):4861-72.

[25]   Sheskin T, Hanus L, Slager J, Vogel Z, Mechoulam R. Structural requirements for binding of anandamide-type compounds to the brain cannabinoid receptor. J Med Chem 1997 Feb 28;40(5):659-67.

[26]   Regehr WG, Carey MR, Best AR. Activity-dependent regulation of synapses by retrograde messengers. Neuron 2009 Jul 30;63(2):154-70.

[27]   Heifets BD, Castillo PE. Endocannabinoid signaling and long-term synaptic plasticity. Annu Rev Physiol 2009;71:283-306.

[28]   Kano M, Ohno-Shosaku T, Hashimotodani Y, Uchigashima M, Watanabe M. Endocannabinoid-mediated control of synaptic transmission. Physiol Rev 2009 Jan;89(1):309-80.

[29]   Castillo PE, Younts TJ, Chavez AE, Hashimotodani Y. Endocannabinoid signaling and synaptic function. Neuron 2012 Oct 4;76(1):70-81.

[30]   Ohno-Shosaku T, Maejima T, Kano M. Endogenous cannabinoids mediate retrograde signals from depolarized postsynaptic neurons to presynaptic terminals. Neuron 2001 Mar;29(3):729-38.

[31]   Kreitzer AC, Regehr WG. Retrograde inhibition of presynaptic calcium influx by endogenous cannabinoids at excitatory synapses onto Purkinje cells. Neuron 2001 Mar;29(3):717-27.

[32]   Gerdeman GL, Ronesi J, Lovinger DM. Postsynaptic endocannabinoid release is critical to long-term depression in the striatum. Nat Neurosci 2002 May;5(5):446-51.

[33]   Robbe D, Kopf M, Remaury A, Bockaert J, Manzoni OJ. Endogenous cannabinoids mediate long-term synaptic depression in the nucleus accumbens. Proc Natl Acad Sci U S A 2002 Jun 11;99(12):8384-8.

[34]   Chevaleyre V, Castillo PE. Heterosynaptic LTD of hippocampal GABAergic synapses: a novel role of endocannabinoids in regulating excitability. Neuron 2003 May 8;38(3):461-72.

[35]   Marsicano G, Wotjak CT, Azad SC, Bisogno T, Rammes G, Cascio MG, *et al.* The endogenous cannabinoid system controls extinction of aversive memories. Nature 2002 Aug 1;418(6897):530-4.

[36]   Di Marzo V. The endocannabinoid system: its general strategy of action, tools for its pharmacological manipulation and potential therapeutic exploitation. Pharmacol Res 2009 Aug;60(2):77-84.

[37]   Levenes C, Daniel H, Soubrie P, Crepel F. Cannabinoids decrease excitatory synaptic transmission and impair long-term depression in rat cerebellar Purkinje cells. J Physiol 1998 Aug 1;510 (Pt 3):867-79.

[38]   Hoffman AF, Lupica CR. Mechanisms of cannabinoid inhibition of GABA(A) synaptic transmission in the hippocampus. J Neurosci 2000 Apr 1;20(7):2470-9.

[39]   Takahashi KA, Linden DJ. Cannabinoid receptor modulation of synapses received by cerebellar Purkinje cells. J Neurophysiol 2000 Mar;83(3):1167-80.

[40]   Mackie K. Signaling *via* CNS cannabinoid receptors. Mol Cell Endocrinol 2008 Apr 16;286(1-2 Suppl 1):S60-5.

[41]   Piomelli D. The molecular logic of endocannabinoid signaling. Nat Rev Neurosci 2003 Nov;4(11):873-84.

[42]   Di Marzo V. Targeting the endocannabinoid system: to enhance or reduce? Nat Rev Drug Discov 2008 May;7(5):438-55.

[43]   Bisogno T, Melck D, De Petrocellis L, Di Marzo V. Phosphatidic acid as the biosynthetic precursor of the endocannabinoid 2-arachidonoylglycerol in intact mouse neuroblastoma cells stimulated with ionomycin. J Neurochem 1999 May;72(5):2113-9.

[44]   Di Marzo V, Fontana A, Cadas H, Schinelli S, Cimino G, Schwartz JC, *et al.* Formation and inactivation of endogenous cannabinoid anandamide in central neurons. Nature 1994 Dec 15;372(6507):686-91.

[45]   Okamoto Y, Morishita J, Wang J, Schmid PC, Krebsbach RJ, Schmid HH, *et al.* Mammalian cells stably overexpressing N-acylphosphatidylethanolamine-hydrolysing phospholipase D exhibit significantly decreased levels of N-acylphosphatidylethanolamines. Biochem J 2005 Jul 1;389(Pt 1):241-7.

[46]   Liu J, Wang L, Harvey-White J, Osei-Hyiaman D, Razdan R, Gong Q, *et al.* A biosynthetic pathway for anandamide. Proc Natl Acad Sci U S A 2006 Sep 5;103(36):13345-50.

[47]   Liu J, Batkai S, Pacher P, Harvey-White J, Wagner JA, Cravatt BF, *et al.* Lipopolysaccharide induces anandamide synthesis in macrophages *via* CD14/MAPK/phosphoinositide 3-kinase/NF-kappaB independently of platelet-activating factor. J Biol Chem 2003 Nov 7;278(45):45034-9.

[48]   Lynch DL, Reggio PH. Molecular Dynamics Simulations of the Endocannabinoid, N-Arachidonoylethanolamine (Anandamide) in a Phospholipid Bilayer: Probing Structure and Dynamics. J Med Chem 2005 2005;48:4824-33.

[49]   Tian X, Guo J, Yao F, Yang DP, Makriyannis A. The conformation, location, and dynamic properties of the endocannabinoid ligand anandamide in a membrane bilayer. J Biol Chem 2005 Aug 19;280(33):29788-95.

[50]   Matsuda LA, Lolait SJ, Brownstein MJ, Young AC, Bonner TI. Structure of a cannabinoid receptor and functional expression of the cloned cDNA. Nature 1990 Aug 9;346(6284):561-4.

[51]   Bramblett RD, Panu AM, Ballesteros JA, Reggio PH. Construction of a 3D model of the cannabinoid CB1 receptor: determination of helix ends and helix orientation. Life Sci 1995;56(23-24):1971-82.

[52]   Glass M, Dragunow M, Faull RL. Cannabinoid receptors in the human brain: a detailed anatomical and quantitative autoradiographic study in the fetal, neonatal and adult human brain. Neuroscience 1997 Mar;77(2):299-318.

[53]   Westlake TM, Howlett AC, Bonner TI, Matsuda LA, Herkenham M. Cannabinoid receptor binding and messenger RNA expression in human brain: an *in vitro* receptor autoradiography and *in situ* hybridization histochemistry study of normal aged and Alzheimer's brains. Neuroscience 1994 Dec;63(3):637-52.

[54]   Pertwee RG. Pharmacology of cannabinoid CB1 and CB2 receptors. Pharmacol Ther 1997;74(2):129-80.

[55]   Gerard CM, Mollereau C, Vassart G, Parmentier M. Molecular cloning of a human cannabinoid receptor which is also expressed in testis. Biochem J 1991 Oct 1;279 (Pt 1):129-34.

[56]   Straiker AJ, Maguire G, Mackie K, Lindsey J. Localization of cannabinoid CB1 receptors in the human anterior eye and retina. Invest Ophthalmol Vis Sci 1999 Sep;40(10):2442-8.

[57]   Schuel H, Chang MC, Burkman LJ, Picone RP, Makriyannis A, Zimmerman AM, *et al.* Cannabinoid Receptors in Sperm. Marijuana and Medicine. Totowa: Humana Press; 1999. p. 335-45.

[58]   Wright K, Rooney N, Feeney M, Tate J, Robertson D, Welham M, *et al.* Differential expression of cannabinoid receptors in the human colon: cannabinoids promote epithelial wound healing. Gastroenterology 2005 Aug;129(2):437-53.

[59] Ishac EJ, Jiang L, Lake KD, Varga K, Abood ME, Kunos G. Inhibition of exocytotic noradrenaline release by presynaptic cannabinoid CB1 receptors on peripheral sympathetic nerves. Br J Pharmacol 1996 Aug;118(8):2023-8.

[60] Roche R, Hoareau L, Bes-Houtmann S, Gonthier MP, Laborde C, Baron JF, *et al.* Presence of the cannabinoid receptors, CB1 and CB2, in human omental and subcutaneous adipocytes. Histochemistry and Cell Biology 2006 Aug;126(2):177-87.

[61] Bouaboula M, Rinaldi M, Carayon P, Carillon C, Delpech B, Shire D, *et al.* Cannabinoid-receptor expression in human leukocytes. Eur J Biochem 1993 May 15;214(1):173-80.

[62] Galiegue S, Mary S, Marchand J, Dussossoy D, Carriere D, Carayon P, *et al.* Expression of central and peripheral cannabinoid receptors in human immune tissues and leukocyte subpopulations. Eur J Biochem 1995 Aug 15;232(1):54-61.

[63] Rice W, Shannon JM, Burton F, Fiedeldey D. Expression of a brain-type cannabinoid receptor (CB1) in alveolar Type II cells in the lung: regulation by hydrocortisone. Eur J Pharmacol 1997 May 30;327(2-3):227-32.

[64] Turu G, Hunyady L. Signal transduction of the CB1 cannabinoid receptor. Journal of Molecular Endocrinology 2009 Feb;44(2):75-85.

[65] Felder CC, Joyce KE, Briley EM, Mansouri J, Mackie K, Blond O, *et al.* Comparison of the pharmacology and signal transduction of the human cannabinoid CB1 and CB2 receptors. Mol Pharmacol 1995 Sep;48(3):443-50.

[66] Howlett AC, Qualy JM, Khachatrian LL. Involvement of Gi in the inhibition of adenylate cyclase by cannabimimetic drugs. Mol Pharmacol 1986 Mar;29(3):307-13.

[67] Mackie K, Lai Y, Westenbroek R, Mitchell R. Cannabinoids activate an inwardly rectifying potassium conductance and inhibit Q-type calcium currents in AtT20 cells transfected with rat brain cannabinoid receptor. J Neurosci 1995 Oct;15(10):6552-61.

[68] Pan X, Ikeda SR, Lewis DL. Rat brain cannabinoid receptor modulates N-type Ca2+ channels in a neuronal expression system. Mol Pharmacol 1996 Apr;49(4):707-14.

[69] Azad SC, Kurz J, Marsicano G, Lutz B, Zieglgansberger W, Rammes G. Activation of CB1 specifically located on GABAergic interneurons inhibits LTD in the lateral amygdala. Learning & Memory (Cold Spring Harbor, NY. 2008 Mar;15(3):143-52.

[70] Glass M, Felder CC. Concurrent stimulation of cannabinoid CB1 and dopamine D2 receptors augments cAMP accumulation in striatal neurons: evidence for a Gs linkage to the CB1 receptor. J Neurosci 1997 Jul 15;17(14):5327-33.

[71] Abadji V, Lucas-Lenard JM, Chin C, Kendall DA. Involvement of the Carboxyl Terminus of the Third Intracellular Loop of the Cannabinoid CB1 Receptor in Constitutive Activation of G_s. J Neurochem 1999;72:2032-8.

[72] Kearn CS, Blake-Palmer K, Daniel E, Mackie K, Glass M. Concurrent stimulation of cannabinoid CB1 and dopamine D2 receptors enhances heterodimer formation: a mechanism for receptor cross-talk? Mol Pharmacol 2005 May;67(5):1697-704.

[73] De Petrocellis L, Marini P, Matias I, Moriello AS, Starowicz K, Cristino L, *et al.* Mechanisms for the coupling of cannabinoid receptors to intracellular calcium mobilization in rat insulinoma beta-cells. Exp Cell Res 2007 Aug 15;313(14):2993-3004.

[74] Breivogel CS, Lambert JM, Gerfin S, Huffman JW, Razdan RK. Sensitivity to delta9-tetrahydrocannabinol is selectively enhanced in beta-arrestin2 -/- mice. Behav Pharmacol 2008 Jul;19(4):298-307.

[75] Kouznetsova M, Kelley B, Shen M, Thayer SA. Desensitization of cannabinoid-mediated presynaptic inhibition of neurotransmission between rat hippocampal neurons in culture. Mol Pharmacol 2002 Mar;61(3):477-85.

[76] Howlett AC. Cannabinoid receptor signaling. Handb Exp Pharmacol 2005(168):53-79.

[77] Munro S, Thomas KL, Abu-Shaar M. Molecular characterization of a peripheral receptor for cannabinoids. Nature 1993 Sep 2;365(6441):61-5.

[78]   Bouaboula M, Poinot-Chazel C, Marchand J, Canat X, Bourrie B, Rinaldi-Carmona M, *et al.* Signaling pathway associated with stimulation of CB2 peripheral cannabinoid receptor. Involvement of both mitogen-activated protein kinase and induction of Krox-24 expression. Eur J Biochem 1996 May 1;237(3):704-11.

[79]   Bouaboula M, Desnoyer N, Carayon P, Combes T, Casellas P. Gi protein modulation induced by a selective inverse agonist for the peripheral cannabinoid receptor CB2: implication for intracellular signalization cross-regulation. Mol Pharmacol 1999 Mar;55(3):473-80.

[80]   Sanchez MG, Ruiz-Llorente L, Sanchez AM, Diaz-Laviada I. Activation of phosphoinositide 3-kinase/PKB pathway by CB(1) and CB(2) cannabinoid receptors expressed in prostate PC-3 cells. Involvement in Raf-1 stimulation and NGF induction. Cell Signal 2003 Sep;15(9):851-9.

[81]   Guzman M, Galve-Roperh I, Sanchez C. Ceramide: a new second messenger of cannabinoid action. Trends Pharmacol Sci 2001 Jan;22(1):19-22.

[82]   Howlett AC, Barth F, Bonner TI, Cabral G, Casellas P, Devane WA, *et al.* International Union of Pharmacology. XXVII. Classification of cannabinoid receptors. Pharmacol Rev 2002 Jun;54(2):161-202.

[83]   Benito C, Nunez E, Tolon RM, Carrier EJ, Rabano A, Hillard CJ, *et al.* Cannabinoid CB2 receptors and fatty acid amide hydrolase are selectively overexpressed in neuritic plaque-associated glia in Alzheimer's disease brains. J Neurosci 2003 Dec 3;23(35):11136-41.

[84]   Van Sickle MD, Duncan M, Kingsley PJ, Mouihate A, Urbani P, Mackie K, *et al.* Identification and functional characterization of brainstem cannabinoid CB2 receptors. Science 2005 Oct 14;310(5746):329-32.

[85]   Maurer SE, DeClue MS, Albertsen AN, Dorr M, Kuiper DS, Ziock H, *et al.* Interactions between catalysts and amphiphilic structures and their implications for a protocell model. Chemphyschem 2011 Mar 14;12(4):828-35.

[86]   Buckley NE, McCoy KL, Mezey E, Bonner T, Zimmer A, Felder CC, *et al.* Immunomodulation by cannabinoids is absent in mice deficient for the cannabinoid CB(2) receptor. Eur J Pharmacol 2000 May 19;396(2-3):141-9.

[87]   Massi P, Fuzio D, Vigano D, Sacerdote P, Parolaro D. Relative involvement of cannabinoid CB(1) and CB(2) receptors in the Delta(9)-tetrahydrocannabinol-induced inhibition of natural killer activity. Eur J Pharmacol 2000 Jan 17;387(3):343-7.

[88]   Jorda MA, Verbakel SE, Valk PJ, Vankan-Berkhoudt YV, Maccarrone M, Finazzi-Agro A, *et al.* Hematopoietic cells expressing the peripheral cannabinoid receptor migrate in response to the endocannabinoid 2-arachidonoylglycerol. Blood 2002 Apr 15;99(8):2786-93.

[89]   Kishimoto S, Gokoh M, Oka S, Muramatsu M, Kajiwara T, Waku K, *et al.* 2-arachidonoylglycerol induces the migration of HL-60 cells differentiated into macrophage-like cells and human peripheral blood monocytes through the cannabinoid CB2 receptor-dependent mechanism. J Biol Chem 2003 Jul 4;278(27):24469-75.

[90]   Franklin A, Stella N. Arachidonylcyclopropylamide increases microglial cell migration through cannabinoid CB2 and abnormal-cannabidiol-sensitive receptors. Eur J Pharmacol 2003 Aug 8;474(2-3):195-8.

[91]   Kishimoto S, Kobayashi Y, Oka S, Gokoh M, Waku K, Sugiura T. 2-Arachidonoylglycerol, an endogenous cannabinoid receptor ligand, induces accelerated production of chemokines in HL-60 cells. J Biochem (Tokyo) 2004 Apr;135(4):517-24.

[92]   McCoy KL, Matveyeva M, Carlisle SJ, Cabral GA. Cannabinoid inhibition of the processing of intact lysozyme by macrophages: evidence for CB2 receptor participation. J Pharmacol Exp Ther 1999 Jun;289(3):1620-5.

[93]   Idris AI, van 't Hof RJ, Greig IR, Ridge SA, Baker D, Ross RA, *et al*. Regulation of bone mass, bone loss and osteoclast activity by cannabinoid receptors. Nat Med 2005 Jul;11(7):774-9.

[94]   Ofek O, Karsak M, Leclerc N, Fogel M, Frenkel B, Wright K, *et al*. Peripheral cannabinoid receptor, CB2, regulates bone mass. Proc Natl Acad Sci U S A 2006 Jan 17;103(3):696-701.

[95]   Pertwee RG. Pharmacological actions of cannabinoids. In: Pertwee R, editor. Cannabinoids. Berlin, Heidelberg, New York: Springer; 2005. p. 1-51.

[96]   Hanson ML. Research and clinical findings--a wholistic view. Int J Orofacial Myology (Editorial). 2012 Nov;38:4-7.

[97]   Hanson Misialek L, Fazio RL, Denney RL, Myers WG. Limited predictive accuracy of the booklet category test in a criminal forensic sample. Appl Neuropsychol Adult 2013;20(2):77-82.

[98]   Samuelson LC, Swanberg LJ, Gantz I. Mapping of the novel G protein-coupled receptor Gpr18 to distal mouse chromosome 14. Mamm Genome 1996 Dec;7(12):920-1.

[99]   Gantz I, Muraoka A, Yang YK, Samuelson LC, Zimmerman EM, Cook H, *et al*. Cloning and chromosomal localization of a gene (GPR18) encoding a novel seven transmembrane receptor highly expressed in spleen and testis. Genomics 1997 Jun 15;42(3):462-6.

[100] Kohno M, Hasegawa H, Inoue A, Muraoka M, Miyazaki T, Oka K, *et al*. Identification of N-arachidonylglycine as the endogenous ligand for orphan G-protein-coupled receptor GPR18. Biochemical and Biophysical Research Communications 2006 Sep 1;347(3):827-32.

[101] Hanson MA, Gluckman PD, Ma RC, Matzen P, Biesma RG. Early life opportunities for prevention of diabetes in low and middle income countries. BMC Public Health 2012;12:1025.

[102] Brown AJ, Wise A, inventors; GlaxoSmithKline, assignee. Identification of modulators of GPR55 activity patent WO0186305. 2001.

[103] Drmota T, Greasley P, Groblewski T, inventors; Astrazeneca, assignee. Screening assays for cannabinoid-ligand type modulators of GPR55. USA patent WO2004074844. 2004.

[104] Sawzdargo M, Nguyen T, Lee DK, Lynch KR, Cheng R, Heng HH, *et al*. Identification and cloning of three novel human G protein-coupled receptor genes GPR52, PsiGPR53 and GPR55: GPR55 is extensively expressed in human brain. Brain Res Mol Brain Res 1999 Feb 5;64(2):193-8.

[105] Henstridge CM, Balenga NA, Ford LA, Ross RA, Waldhoer M, Irving AJ. The GPR55 ligand L-alpha-lysophosphatidylinositol promotes RhoA-dependent Ca2+ signaling and NFAT activation. Faseb J 2009 Jan;23(1):183-93.

[106] Ryberg E, Larsson N, Sjogren S, Hjorth S, Hermansson NO, Leonova J, *et al*. The orphan receptor GPR55 is a novel cannabinoid receptor. Br J Pharmacol 2007 Dec;152(7):1092-101.

[107] Lauckner JE, Jensen JB, Chen HY, Lu HC, Hille B, Mackie K. GPR55 is a cannabinoid receptor that increases intracellular calcium and inhibits M current. Proc Natl Acad Sci U S A 2008 Feb 19;105(7):2699-704.

[108] Staton PC, Hatcher JP, Walker DJ, Morrison AD, Shapland EM, Hughes JP, *et al*. The putative cannabinoid receptor GPR55 plays a role in mechanical hyperalgesia associated with inflammatory and neuropathic pain. Pain 2008 Sep 30;139(1):225-36.

[109] Whyte LS, Ryberg E, Sims NA, Ridge SA, Mackie K, Greasley PJ, *et al*. The putative cannabinoid receptor GPR55 affects osteoclast function *in vitro* and bone mass *in vivo*. Proc Natl Acad Sci U S A 2009 Sep 22;106(38):16511-6.

[110] Andradas C, Caffarel MM, Perez-Gomez E, Salazar M, Lorente M, Velasco G, *et al*. The orphan G protein-coupled receptor GPR55 promotes cancer cell proliferation *via* ERK. Oncogene 2010 Sep 6;30:245-52.

[111] Ford LA, Roelofs AJ, Anavi-Goffer S, Mowat L, Simpson DG, Irving AJ, *et al*. A role for L-alpha-lysophosphatidylinositol and GPR55 in the modulation of migration, orientation and polarization of human breast cancer cells. Br J Pharmacol 2010 Jun;160(3):762-71.

[112] Pineiro R, Maffucci T, Falasca M. The putative cannabinoid receptor GPR55 defines a novel autocrine loop in cancer cell proliferation. Oncogene 2010 Sep 13;30:142-52.

[113] Oka S, Nakajima K, Yamashita A, Kishimoto S, Sugiura T. Identification of GPR55 as a lysophosphatidylinositol receptor. Biochemical and Biophysical Research Communications 2007 Nov 3;362(4):928-34.

[114] Oka S, Toshida T, Maruyama K, Nakajima K, Yamashita A, Sugiura T. 2-Arachidonoyl-sn-glycero-3-phosphoinositol: A Possible Natural Ligand for GPR55. Journal of Biochemistry 2009 Jan;145(1):13-20.

[115] Johns DG, Behm DJ, Walker DJ, Ao Z, Shapland EM, Daniels DA, *et al*. The novel endocannabinoid receptor GPR55 is activated by atypical cannabinoids but does not mediate their vasodilator effects. Br J Pharmacol 2007 Nov;152(5):825-31.

[116] Kapur A, Zhao P, Sharir H, Bai Y, Caron MG, Barak LS, *et al*. Atypical responsiveness of the orphan receptor GPR55 to cannabinoid ligands. J Biol Chem 2009 Oct 23;284(43):29817-27.

[117] Carlson JC, Challis JK, Hanson ML, Wong CS. Stability of pharmaceuticals and other polar organic compounds stored on polar organic chemical integrative samplers and solid-phase extraction cartridges. Environ Toxicol Chem 2013 Feb;32(2):337-44.

[118] Palczewski K, Kumasaka T, Hori T, Behnke CA, Motoshima H, Fox BA, *et al*. Crystal structure of rhodopsin: A G protein-coupled receptor. Science 2000 Aug 4;289(5480):739-45.

[119] Okada T, Fujiyoshi Y, Silow M, Navarro J, Landau EM, Shichida Y. Functional role of internal water molecules in rhodopsin revealed by X-ray crystallography. Proc Natl Acad Sci U S A 2002 Apr 30;99(9):5982-7.

[120] Li J, Edwards PC, Burghammer M, Villa C, Schertler GF. Structure of bovine rhodopsin in a trigonal crystal form. J Mol Biol 2004 Nov 5;343(5):1409-38.

[121] Choe HW, Kim YJ, Park JH, Morizumi T, Pai EF, Krauss N, *et al*. Crystal structure of metarhodopsin II. Nature 2011 Mar 31;471(7340):651-5.

[122] Cherezov V, Rosenbaum DM, Hanson MA, Rasmussen SG, Thian FS, Kobilka TS, *et al*. High-resolution crystal structure of an engineered human beta2-adrenergic G protein-coupled receptor. Science 2007 Nov 23;318(5854):1258-65.

[123] Rasmussen SG, Choi HJ, Rosenbaum DM, Kobilka TS, Thian FS, Edwards PC, *et al*. Crystal structure of the human beta2 adrenergic G-protein-coupled receptor. Nature 2007 Nov 15;450(7168):383-7.

[124] Rosenbaum DM, Cherezov V, Hanson MA, Rasmussen SG, Thian FS, Kobilka TS, *et al*. GPCR engineering yields high-resolution structural insights into beta2-adrenergic receptor function. Science 2007 Nov 23;318(5854):1266-73.

[125] Rasmussen SGF, Choi H-J, Fung JJ, Pardon E, Casarosa P, Chae PS, *et al*. Structure of a Nanobody-Stabilized Active State of the Beta-2-Adrenoreceptor. Nature 2011;469:175-80.

[126] Warne T, Serrano-Vega MJ, Baker JG, Moukhametzianov R, Edwards PC, Henderson R, *et al*. Structure of a beta1-adrenergic G-protein-coupled receptor. Nature 2008 Jul 24;454(7203):486-91.

[127] Moukhametzianov R, Warne T, Edwards PC, Serrano-Vega MJ, Leslie AG, Tate CG, *et al.* Two distinct conformations of helix 6 observed in antagonist-bound structures of a {beta}1-adrenergic receptor. Proc Natl Acad Sci U S A 2011 May 17;108(20):8228-32.

[128] Jaakola VP, Griffith MT, Hanson MA, Cherezov V, Chien EY, Lane JR, *et al.* The 2.6 angstrom crystal structure of a human A2A adenosine receptor bound to an antagonist. Science 2008 Nov 21;322(5905):1211-7.

[129] Lebon G, Warne T, Edwards PC, Bennett K, Langmead CJ, Leslie AG, *et al.* Agonist-bound adenosine A2A receptor structures reveal common features of GPCR activation. Nature 2011 Jun 23;474(7352):521-5.

[130] Bokoch MP, Zou Y, Rasmussen SG, Liu CW, Nygaard R, Rosenbaum DM, *et al.* Ligand-specific regulation of the extracellular surface of a G-protein-coupled receptor. Nature 2010 Jan 7;463(7277):108-12.

[131] Chien EY, Liu W, Zhao Q, Katritch V, Han GW, Hanson MA, *et al.* Structure of the human dopamine d3 receptor in complex with a d2/d3 selective antagonist. Science 2010 Nov 19;330(6007):1091-5.

[132] Ovesen P, Rasmussen S, Kesmodel U. Effect of prepregnancy maternal overweight and obesity on pregnancy outcome. Obstet Gynecol 2011 Aug;118(2 Pt 1):305-12.

[133] Louie JK, Jamieson DJ, Rasmussen SA. 2009 pandemic influenza A (H1N1) virus infection in postpartum women in California. Am J Obstet Gynecol 2011 Feb;204(2):144 e1-6.

[134] Reefhuis J, Rasmussen SA, Honein MA. Prenatal *versus* postnatal repair of myelomeningocele. The New England journal of medicine (Comment (Letter). 2011 Jun 30;364(26):2555; author reply 6.

[135] Reefhuis J, Honein MA, Schieve LA, Rasmussen SA. Use of clomiphene citrate and birth defects, National Birth Defects Prevention Study, 1997-2005. Hum Reprod 2011 Feb;26(2):451-7.

[136] Markhus VH, Rasmussen S, Lie SA, Irgens LM. Placental abruption and premature rupture of membranes. Acta Obstet Gynecol Scand 2011 Sep;90(9):1024-9.

[137] Hartnack Tharin JE, Rasmussen S, Krebs L. Consequences of the Term Breech Trial in Denmark. Acta Obstet Gynecol Scand (Comparative Study). 2011 Jul;90(7):767-71.

[138] McAllister SD, Hurst DP, Barnett-Norris J, Lynch D, Reggio PH, Abood ME. Structural mimicry in class A G protein-coupled receptor rotamer toggle switches: the importance of the F3.36(201)/W6.48(357) interaction in cannabinoid CB1 receptor activation. J Biol Chem 2004 Nov 12;279(46):48024-37.

[139] Rosenbaum DM, Zhang C, Lyons JA, Holl R, Aragao D, Arlow DH, *et al.* Structure and function of an irreversible agonist-beta(2) adrenoceptor complex. Nature 2011 Jan 13;469(7329):236-40.

[140] Hamm HE, Deretic D, Arendt A, Hargrave PA, Koenig B, Hofmann KP. Site of G protein binding to rhodopsin mapped with synthetic peptides from the alpha subunit. Science 1988 Aug 12;241(4867):832-5.

[141] Rasmussen SG, DeVree BT, Zou Y, Kruse AC, Chung KY, Kobilka TS, *et al.* Crystal structure of the beta2 adrenergic receptor-Gs protein complex. Nature 2011 Sep 29;477(7366):549-55.

[142] Hurst DP, Grossfield A, Lynch DL, Feller S, Romo TD, Gawrisch K, *et al.* A lipid pathway for ligand binding is necessary for a cannabinoid G protein-coupled receptor. J Biol Chem 2010 Jun 4;285(23):17954-64.

[143] Wall MA, Coleman DE, Lee E, Iniguez-Lluhi JA, Posner BA, Gilman AG, *et al.* The structure of the G protein heterotrimer Gi alpha 1 beta 1 gamma 2. Cell 1995 Dec 15;83(6):1047-58.

[144] Kessler J, Rasmussen S, Godfrey K, Hanson M, Kiserud T. Venous liver blood flow and regulation of human fetal growth: evidence from macrosomic fetuses. Am J Obstet Gynecol 2011 May;204(5):429 e1-7.

[145] Andersson H, D'Antona AM, Kendall DA, Von Heijne G, Chin CN. Membrane assembly of the cannabinoid receptor 1: impact of a long N-terminal tail. Mol Pharmacol 2003 Sep;64(3):570-7.

[146] Ahluwalia IB, Singleton JA, Jamieson DJ, Rasmussen SA, Harrison L. Seasonal influenza vaccine coverage among pregnant women: pregnancy risk assessment monitoring system. J Womens Health (Larchmt) 2011 May;20(5):649-51.

[147] Nyberg MK, Johnsen SL, Rasmussen S, Kiserud T. Hemodynamics of fetal breathing movements: the inferior vena cava. Ultrasound Obstet Gynecol 2011 Dec;38(6):658-64.

[148] Hellebust H, Johnsen SL, Rasmussen S, Kiserud T. Maternal weight gain: a determinant for fetal abdominal circumference in the second trimester. Acta Obstet Gynecol Scand 2011 Jun;90(6):666-70.

[149] Hanson MA, Roth CB, Jo E, Griffith MT, Scott FL, Reinhart G, *et al*. Crystal structure of a lipid G protein-coupled receptor. Science 2012 Feb 17;335(6070):851-5.

[150] Simonsen AB, Jorgensen A, Laursen MB, Jorgensen MB, Rasmussen S, Simonsen O. Clinical, radiological and arthroscopic graduation of knee osteoarthritis. Ugeskr Laeger 2011 Mar 28;173(13):956-8.

[151] Picone RP, Khanolkar AD, Xu W, Ayotte LA, Thakur GA, Hurst DP, *et al*. (-)-7'-Isothiocyanato-11-hydroxy-1',1'-dimethylheptylhexahydrocannabinol (AM841), a high-affinity electrophilic ligand, interacts covalently with a cysteine in helix six and activates the CB1 cannabinoid receptor. Mol Pharmacol 2005 Dec;68(6):1623-35.

[152] Pei Y, Mercier RW, Anday JK, Thakur GA, Zvonok AM, Hurst D, *et al*. Ligand-binding architecture of human CB2 cannabinoid receptor: evidence for receptor subtype-specific binding motif and modeling GPCR activation. Chem Biol 2008 Nov 24;15(11):1207-19.

[153] Dinh TP, Carpenter D, Leslie FM, Freund TF, Katona I, Sensi SL, *et al*. Brain monoglyceride lipase participating in endocannabinoid inactivation. Proc Natl Acad Sci U S A 2002 Aug 6;99(16):10819-24.

[154] Fredrikson G, Tornqvist H, Belfrage P. Hormone-sensitive lipase and monoacylglycerol lipase are both required for complete degradation of adipocyte triacylglycerol. Biochim Biophys Acta 1986 Apr 15;876(2):288-93.

[155] Blankman JL, Simon GM, Cravatt BF. A comprehensive profile of brain enzymes that hydrolyze the endocannabinoid 2-arachidonoylglycerol. Chem Biol 2007 Dec;14(12):1347-56.

[156] Savinainen JR, Saario SM, Laitinen JT. The serine hydrolases MAGL, ABHD6 and ABHD12 as guardians of 2-arachidonoylglycerol signaling through cannabinoid receptors. Acta physiologica (Oxford, England) 2012 Feb;204(2):267-76.

[157] Bertrand T, Auge F, Houtmann J, Rak A, Vallee F, Mikol V, *et al*. Structural basis for human monoglyceride lipase inhibition. J Mol Biol 2010 Feb 26;396(3):663-73.

[158] Nardini M, Dijkstra BW. Alpha/beta hydrolase fold enzymes: the family keeps growing. Curr Opin Struct Biol 1999 Dec;9(6):732-7.

[159] Ollis DL, Cheah E, Cygler M, Dijkstra B, Frolow F, Franken SM, *et al*. The alpha/beta hydrolase fold. Protein Eng 1992 Apr;5(3):197-211.

[160] Schrag JD, Cygler M. Lipases and alpha/beta hydrolase fold. Methods Enzymol 1997;284:85-107.

[161] Brzozowski AM, Derewenda U, Derewenda ZS, Dodson GG, Lawson DM, Turkenburg JP, *et al*. A model for interfacial activation in lipases from the structure of a fungal lipase-inhibitor complex. Nature 1991 Jun 6;351(6326):491-4.

[162] van Pouderoyen G, Eggert T, Jaeger KE, Dijkstra BW. The crystal structure of Bacillus subtilis lipase: a minimal alpha/beta hydrolase fold enzyme. J Mol Biol 2001 May 25;309(1):215-26.

[163] Bracey MH, Hanson MA, Masuda KR, Stevens RC, Cravatt BF. Structural adaptations in a membrane enzyme that terminates endocannabinoid signaling. Science 2002 Nov 29;298(5599):1793-6.

[164] Cravatt BF, Giang DK, Mayfield SP, Boger DL, Lerner RA, Gilula NB. Molecular characterization of an enzyme that degrades neuromodulatory fatty-acid amides. Nature 1996 Nov 7;384(6604):83-7.

[165] Schalk-Hihi C, Schubert C, Alexander R, Bayoumy S, Clemente JC, Deckman I, *et al*. Crystal structure of a soluble form of human monoglyceride lipase in complex with an inhibitor at 1.35 A resolution. Protein Sci 2011 Apr;20(4):670-83.

[166] Labar G, Bauvois C, Borel F, Ferrer JL, Wouters J, Lambert DM. Crystal structure of the human monoacylglycerol lipase, a key actor in endocannabinoid signaling. Chembiochem 2010 Jan 25;11(2):218-27.

[167] Henderson R. Structure of crystalline alpha-chymotrypsin. IV. The structure of indoleacryloyl-alpha-chyotrypsin and its relevance to the hydrolytic mechanism of the enzyme. J Mol Biol 1970 Dec 14;54(2):341-54.

[168] Tamada T, Kinoshita T, Kurihara K, Adachi M, Ohhara T, Imai K, *et al*. Combined high-resolution neutron and X-ray analysis of inhibited elastase confirms the active-site oxyanion hole but rules against a low-barrier hydrogen bond. J Am Chem Soc 2009 Aug 12;131(31):11033-40.

[169] Di Marzo V, Melck D, Bisogno T, De Petrocellis L. Endocannabinoids: endogenous cannabinoid receptor ligands with neuromodulatory action. Trends Neurosci 1998 Dec;21(12):521-8.

[170] Piomelli D, Beltramo M, Giuffrida A, Stella N. Endogenous cannabinoid signaling. Neurobiol Dis 1998 Dec;5(6 Pt B):462-73.

[171] Giang DK, Cravatt BF. Molecular characterization of human and mouse fatty acid amide hydrolases. Proc Natl Acad Sci U S A 1997 Mar 18;94(6):2238-42.

[172] Arreaza G, Deutsch DG. Deletion of a Proline-Rich Region and a Transmembrane Domain in Fatty Acid Amide Hydrolase. FEBS Lett 1999;454:57-60.

[173] Goparaju SK, Ueda N, Yanaguchi H, Yamamoto S. Anandamide Amidohydrolase Reacting with 2-Arachidonylglycerol, Another Cannabinoid Receptor Ligand. FEBS Lett 1998;422:69-73.

[174] Lang W, Qin C, Lin S, Khanolkar AD, Goutopoulos A, Fan P, *et al*. Substrate specificity and stereoselectivity of rat brain microsomal anandamide amidohydrolase. J Med Chem 1999 Mar 11;42(5):896-902.

[175] Patricelli MP, Patterson JE, Boger DL, Cravatt BF. An endogenous sleep-inducing compound is a novel competitive inhibitor of fatty acid amide hydrolase. Bioorg Med Chem Lett 1998 Mar 17;8(6):613-8.

[176] Beltramo M, Piomelli D. Carrier-mediated transport and enzymatic hydrolysis of the endogenous cannabinoid 2-arachidonylglycerol. Neuroreport 2000 Apr 27;11(6):1231-5.

[177] Kathuria S, Gaetani S, Fegley D, Valino F, Duranti A, Tontini A, *et al*. Modulation of anxiety through blockade of anandamide hydrolysis. Nat Med 2003 Jan;9(1):76-81.

[178] Lichtman AH, Hawkins EG, Griffin G, Cravatt BF. Pharmacological activity of fatty acid amides is regulated, but not mediated, by fatty acid amide hydrolase *in vivo*. J Pharmacol Exp Ther 2002 Jul;302(1):73-9.

[179]   Patricelli MP, Lashuel HA, Giang DK, Kelly JW, Cravatt BF. Comparative characterization of a wild type and transmembrane domain-deleted fatty acid amide hydrolase: identification of the transmembrane domain as a site for oligomerization. Biochem 1998 Oct 27;37(43):15177-87.

[180]   Patricelli MP, Lovato MA, Cravatt BF. Chemical and mutagenic investigations of fatty acid amide hydrolase: evidence for a family of serine hydrolases with distinct catalytic properties. Biochem 1999 Aug 3;38(31):9804-12.

[181]   Patricelli MP, Cravatt BF. Fatty acid amide hydrolase competitively degrades bioactive amides and esters through a nonconventional catalytic mechanism. Biochem 1999 Oct 26;38(43):14125-30.

[182]   Patricelli MP, Cravatt BF. Characterization and manipulation of the acyl chain selectivity of fatty acid amide hydrolase. Biochem 2001 May 22;40(20):6107-15.

[183]   Wendt KU, Poralla K, Schulz GE. Structure and function of a squalene cyclase. Science 1997 Sep 19;277(5333):1811-5.

[184]   Picot D, Loll PJ, Garavito RM. The X-ray crystal structure of the membrane protein prostaglandin H2 synthase-1. Nature 1994 Jan 20;367(6460):243-9.

[185]   Kaczocha M, Glaser ST, Deutsch DG. Identification of intracellular carriers for the endocannabinoid anandamide. Proc Natl Acad Sci U S A 2009 Apr 14;106(15):6375-80.

[186]   Kaczocha M, Vivieca S, Sun J, Glaser ST, Deutsch DG. Fatty acid-binding proteins transport N-acylethanolamines to nuclear receptors and are targets of endocannabinoid transport inhibitors. J Biol Chem 2012 Jan 27;287(5):3415-24.

[187]   Fu J, Bottegoni G, Sasso O, Bertorelli R, Rocchia W, Masetti M, et al. A catalytically silent FAAH-1 variant drives anandamide transport in neurons. Nat Neurosci 2012 Jan;15(1):64-9.

[188]   Oddi S, Fezza F, Pasquariello N, D'Agostino A, Catanzaro G, De Simone C, et al. Molecular identification of albumin and Hsp70 as cytosolic anandamide-binding proteins. Chem Biol 2009 Jun 26;16(6):624-32.

[189]   Marcelino AM, Smock RG, Gierasch LM. Evolutionary coupling of structural and functional sequence information in the intracellular lipid-binding protein family. Proteins 2006 May 1;63(2):373-84.

[190]   Xu LZ, Sanchez R, Sali A, Heintz N. Ligand specificity of brain lipid-binding protein. J Biol Chem 1996 Oct 4;271(40):24711-9.

[191]   Howlett AC, Reggio PH, Childers SR, Hampson RE, Ulloa NM, Deutsch DG. Endocannabinoid tone *versus* constitutive activity of cannabinoid receptors. Br J Pharmacol 2011 Aug;163(7):1329-43.

[192]   Bisogno T, MacCarrone M, De Petrocellis L, Jarrahian A, Finazzi-Agro A, Hillard C, et al. The uptake by cells of 2-arachidonoylglycerol, an endogenous agonist of cannabinoid receptors. Eur J Biochem 2001 Apr;268(7):1982-9.

[193]   Hillard CJ, Jarrahian A. Cellular accumulation of anandamide: consensus and controversy. Br J Pharmacol 2003 Nov;140(5):802-8.

[194]   Hillard CJ, Jarrahian A. The movement of N-arachidonoylethanolamine (anandamide) across cellular membranes. Chem Phys Lipids 2000 Nov;108(1-2):123-34.

[195]   Di Marzo V, Bisogno T, De Petrocellis L, Melck D, Orlando P, Wagner JA, et al. Biosynthesis and inactivation of the endocannabinoid 2-arachidonoylglycerol in circulating and tumoral macrophages. Eur J Biochem 1999 Aug;264(1):258-67.

[196] Chicca A, Marazzi J, Nicolussi S, Gertsch J. Evidence for bidirectional endocannabinoid transport across cell membranes. J Biol Chem 2012 Oct 5;287(41):34660-82.

[197] Damborsky J, Petrek M, Banas P, Otyepka M. Identification of tunnels in proteins, nucleic acids, inorganic materials and molecular ensembles. Biotechnol J 2007 Jan;2(1):62-7.

CHAPTER 5

Dynamic Interactions Between Drugs of Abuse and the Endocannabinoid System: Molecular Mechanisms and Functional Outcome

Miriam Melis[1], Anna L. Muntoni[2] and Marco Pistis[1,2]*

[1]Department of Biomedical Sciences, [2]C.N.R. Neuroscience Institute-Cagliari, University of Cagliari, Monserrato (CA), Italy

Abstract: Regulation of motivated behavior toward both natural stimuli and drugs of abuse is among functions where the endocannabinoid system is deeply engaged. In fact, endocannabinoids and their receptors (CB1) are abundant in the limbic system and, particularly, they serve as retrograde signaling molecules at synapses onto midbrain dopamine (DA) neurons in the ventral tegmental area (VTA). These neurons are involved in neural processing contributing to drug addiction and DA plays a crucial role as learning signal, by changing the synaptic strength of neural circuits involved in action selection to optimize goal-directed behavior.

Endocannabinoids regulate different forms of synaptic plasticity in the VTA, exert a critical modulation of DA release and, ultimately, of the circuits within the limbic systems driving motivated behaviors. Hence, it is not surprising that drugs of abuse, namely alcohol, nicotine, opioids and psychostimulants exert wide arrays of effects on the endocannabinoid system, by affecting endocannabinoid release and catabolism as well as modulation of the functions and number of cannabinoid CB1 receptors. On the other hand, by genetic or pharmacological manipulation of the endocannabinoid system we can modulate neurochemical and neurophysiological effects of the drugs as well as their behavioral actions in experimental animals predictive of their addicting properties in humans. Accordingly, blockade of CB1 receptors was a promising therapeutic strategy against drug addiction, although rimonabant (the only clinically tested CB1 antagonist) was withdrawn due to serious side effects such as depression and suicide. These adverse effects though underscore the general role that the endocannabinoid system plays in the regulation of reward and motivation. Nevertheless, other drugs are emerging, *i.e.* the indirect cannabinoid agonists, which enhance endocannabinoids by blocking their catabolism or membrane transport, that are efficacious in animal model of relapse to drug addiction and that might prove beneficial in humans.

Keywords: Endocannabinoids, anandamide, 2-arachidonoylglycerol, dopamine neurons, synaptic plasticity, cannabinoid receptors, nicotine addiction, rimonabant, drug addiction, opiate addiction, morphine, alcohol, cocaine, psychostimulants, long-term synaptic plasticity, short-term synaptic plasticity, fatty acid amide hydrolase (FAAH), reward, relapse, oleoylethanolamide.

*****Address correspondence to Marco Pistis:** Department of Biomedical Sciences, University of Cagliari, Monserrato (CA), Italy; Tel: +390706754324; Fax: +390706754320; E-mail: mpistis@unica.it

Eric Murillo-Rodríguez, Emmanuel S. Onaivi, Nissar A. Darmani & Edward Wagner (Eds.)

INTRODUCTION

Among the functions in which the endocannabinoid system is engaged, the regulation of motivated behavior has a major impact on human disease, being behavioral and drug addiction a considerable burden for modern societies [1-3].

The neuroanatomical substrates of brain reward include neural circuits and mechanisms associated with the ventral limbic midbrain [4]. The midbrain dopamine (DA) system originating in the ventral tegmental area (VTA) and in the substantia nigra pars compacta (SNc) is involved in neural processing contributing to drug addiction and it is widely accepted that DA neurons process stimuli, such as food, sex, maternal care and addicting drugs, that are positively reinforcing and can elicit positive hedonic reactions [5-7] Hence, DA is deeply involved in reward learning, reinforcement and addiction and plays a crucial role as a learning signal, by changing the synaptic strength of neural circuits involved in action selection to optimize goal-directed behavior [8, 9] DA also functions as a signal for reverse learning: lack of expected reward, aversion, or punishment are encoded by DA neurons as pauses or reductions in their firing activity [10-12].

Axon terminals of VTA DA neurons project to forebrain areas such as the ventral striatum/nucleus accumbens (NAc) and the prefrontal cortex. Cannabinoid type 1 receptors (CB_1Rs) are abundantly expressed in these brain areas as well as in other structures related to motivation and reward, such the olfactory tubercle, the hippocampus and the amygdala, which strongly contribute to the motivational and addictive properties of cannabinoids [13, 14] These regions process distinct yet deeply intertwined functions that are among the hallmarks of reward-related behaviors: reinforcement (ventral striatum), declarative memory and learning (hippocampus), emotional memory (amygdala), habit forming (ventral and dorsal striatum), as well as executive functions and working memory (prefrontal and orbitofrontal cortex).

The endocannabinoid system plays a modulatory role on reward DA neurons [15-19] and this is corroborated by the expression of [20-22] CB_1Rs and the abundance of their endogenous ligands, the two major endocannabinoids anandamide and 2-arachidonoylglycerol (2-AG), within the VTA [23].

More than a decade ago, it was demonstrated that firing activity of mesencephalic DA neurons responds to exogenous cannabinoid agonist administration [24, 25] Both Δ^9-tetrahydrocannabinol (THC), the main psychoactive principle of *Cannabis sativa*, and synthetic CB_1R agonists dose-dependently enhance firing rate and burst activity of DA neurons in the VTA [24, 25] Enhanced firing and burst activity results in an increase in DA release in projecting regions, such as the shell of the NAc (ShNAc) [26, 27] and the prefrontal cortex [28, 29] Therefore, cannabinoids display effects analogous to those of other classes of drugs of abuse [30] Cannabinoids do not excite DA neurons directly, since CB_1Rs in the VTA and in the SNc are expressed on glutamate and GABA axon terminals impinging on DA neurons [20, 22, 31] where they can fine-tune the release of inhibitory and excitatory neurotransmitters and regulate DA neuron firing. An indirect (disinhibitory) effect of cannabinoid agonists on DA neurons is supported by the strong inhibitory effects of cannabinoids on firing activity and GABA release of rostromedial tegmental nucleus neurons, important inhibitory afferents to DA cells [32-34] The effect of exogenous cannabinoids on DA cells underscores the presence of a functional endogenous cannabinoid system in this brain region. Hence, the physiological role exerted by the endogenous cannabinoid system in the VTA is demonstrated by patch-clamp experiments which provided evidence that DA neurons release endocannabinoids as retrograde messengers. These messengers, synthetized in a Ca^{2+}-dependent manner, travel toward the presynaptic sites where they modulate inputs by acting at [35, 36] CB_1Rs.

Endocannabinoids are synthetized as needed (*on demand*) following depolarization of the DA neuron [37], stimulation of excitatory afferents and activation of metabotropic glutamate receptors [35], induction of burst firing *in vivo* [35] and *in vitro* [36]. These stimuli induce a cascade of intracellular events ultimately leading to increased intracellular Ca^{2+} concentration and release of endocannabinoids (Fig. **1**). Under these circumstances, released endocannabinoids transiently modulate presynaptic afferent activity and shape incoming inputs, thus inducing forms of short term synaptic plasticity such as depolarization-induced suppression of inhibition (DSI) or excitation (DSE) [36-38] (Fig. **1**).

Consistent with this mechanism, enzymes required for 2-AG synthesis and degradation have been identified in the VTA [22] which provide further support for its physiological role. In midbrain DA systems, in a fashion similar with other regions throughout the brain, 2-AG biosynthetic enzyme diacylglycerol (DAG) lipase is found postsynaptically in DA cells, whereas both CB_1Rs and the main degrading enzyme monoacylglycerol (MAG) lipase are localized at a presynaptic level [22] (Fig. **1**). In addition to MAG lipase, 2-AG can be hydrolyzed by a series of serine hydrolase α-β-hydrolase domain 6 or 12 (ABHD6, ABHD12) [39, 40] (Fig. **1**), their presence has not yet been demonstrated in the VTA. On the other hand, anatomical, behavioral and electrophysiological studies have provided convincing evidence that *N*-acylethanolamines, including anandamide, as well as the endocannabinoid/vanilloid *N*-arachidonoyl-dopamine (NADA) are also present within the VTA [20, 23, 41-46] but their role in the modulation synaptic inputs on DA cells is not clear yet. Anandamide is generated *via* a specific *n*-acylphosphatidylethanolamine phospholipase D (NAPE PLD)-dependent mechanism [47](, see also [48] for a recent excellent review), and its baseline levels are regulated by a family of hydrolyzing enzymes, the fatty acid amide hydrolases (FAAH) [49] (Fig. **1**). Besides FAAH, anandamide can be hydrolyzed by *N*-acylethanolamine-hydrolyzing acid amidase (NAAA) [50] and oxygenated by ciclooxygenase-2 (COX-2) [51], lipoxigenase isoenzymes (LOX) [52] and by cytochrome P-450 [53].

Besides short-term synaptic plasticity, endocannabinoids, specifically 2-AG, are mediators for long-term synaptic plasticity, namely long-term depression of inhibitory currents (LTD_{GABA}) on VTA DA neurons [54, 55] (Fig. **1**). This form of LTD is enhanced by DA D_2 receptor activation, either by cocaine or by direct DA agonists [54, 55]. Furthermore, Seif *et al.* [56] have described that 2-AG enables sub-threshold doses of DA D_1 and D_2 receptor agonists to increase firing activity of nucleus accumbens (NAc) neurons [56]. Taken together, these findings point to 2-AG as a neuromodulator involved in synaptic plasticity in the mesoaccumbens pathway.

The importance of short- or long-term forms of endocannabinoid-mediated synaptic plasticity relies in possibility that, by affecting the strength of incoming synaptic inputs, these molecules regulate firing activity of DA neurons. Hence, the firing pattern of DA neurons *in vivo* can switch from regular clock-like to bursting [57],

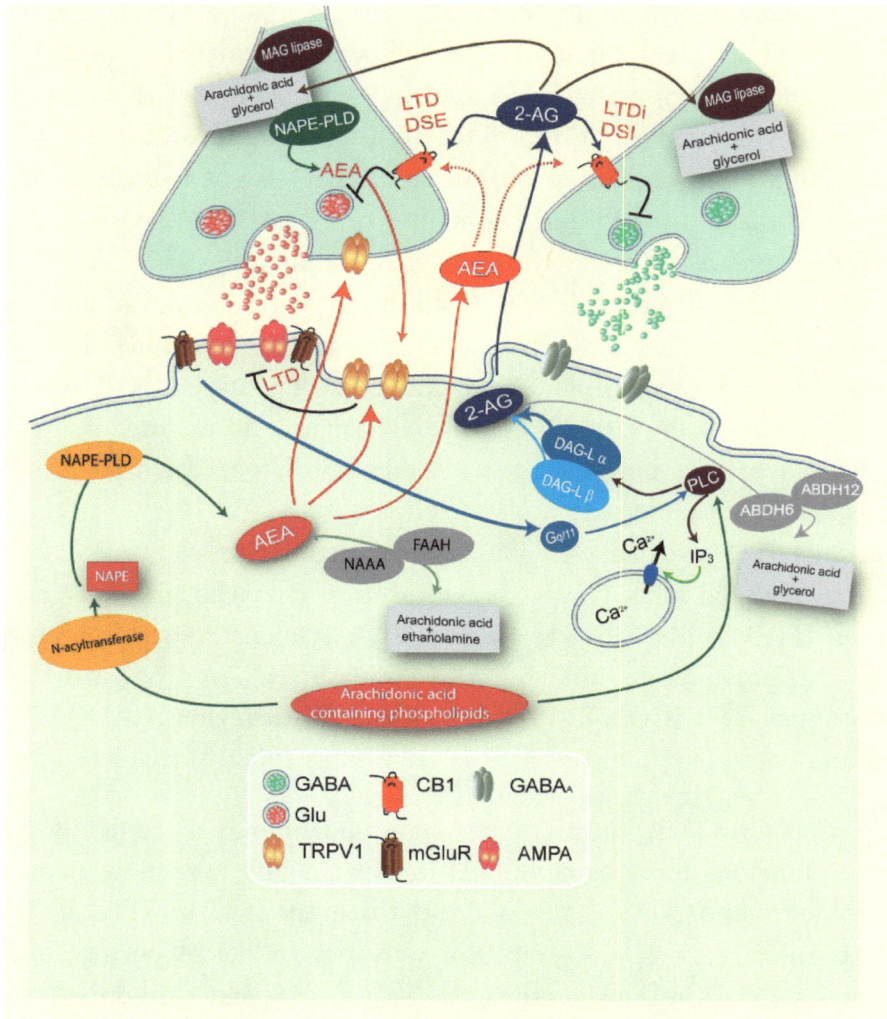

Figure 1: Synaptic mechanisms of action for anandamide (AEA) and 2-arachidonoylglycerol (2-AG). AEA is synthesized by postsynaptic NAPE-PLD and hydrolyzed by FAAH. NAPE-PLD is also expressed presynaptically and AEA might act at postsynaptic vanilloid (TRPV1) receptors. In addition, AEA might retrogradely activate presynaptic TRPV1, or in an autocrine-like fashion, postsynaptic TRPV1. In particular, postsynaptic activation of TRPV1 leads to LTD. AEA functions as a classical retrograde messenger at presynaptic CB₁R at specific synapses in the basolateral amygdala and in the dorsal raphe, where it evokes LTDi and DSE, respectively. Whether AEA exerts effects as a retrograde neurotransmitter at dopamine neurons is still uncertain. 2-AG is synthesized mainly by DAG-L α and β isoforms. Synthesis involves a rapid production of 2-AG which, in this example, is triggered by activation of metabotropic glutamate receptors (mGluRs) in the postsynaptic cell. mGluRs, *via* a $G_{q/11}$ protein, activate a phosholipase C-

(PLC) dependent increase in intracellular Ca^{2+} (mobilized from intracellular stores by IP_3) and DAG mobilization. This intracellular pathway leads to 2-AG-release. 2-AG activates CB_1Rs expressed on axon terminals, which ultimately suppress either GABA or glutamate release and trigger short- and long-term forms of synaptic plasticity (DSI, DSE, LTDi or LTD). 2-AG is then hydrolyzed by MAG lipase expressed in the presynaptic terminals or ABDH6, expressed postsynaptically.

Abbreviations: ABHD6, serine hydrolase α-β-hydrolase- 6; ABHD12, serine hydrolase α-β-hydrolase- 12; CB1, cannabinoid type-1 receptor; DAG, diacylglycerol; DSE, depolarization-induced suppression of excitation; DSI, depolarization-induced suppression of inhibition; FAAH, fatty acid amide hydrolase; Glu, glutamate; IP_3, inositol trisphosphate; LTD, long-term depression at excitatory synapses; LTDi, long-term depression at inhibitory synapses; MAG, monoacylglycerol; metabotropic glutamate receptors (mGluRs); NAPE-PLD, N-acylphosphatidylethanolamide phospholipase D; PLC, phopshplipase C; TRPV1, transient potential vanilloid receptor type 1.

This figure is courtesy of Antonio Luchicchi.

the former induces tonic release of DA in terminal regions, while the latter is responsible for the phasic elevation of synaptic DA [58]. DA neurons cannot regulate their own bursting, and this is demonstrated by the finding that *in vitro*, when all the afferent processes are severed, DA neurons fire in a regular pacemaker-like pattern [57]. In fact, firing pattern of DA neurons depends on the balance between excitatory and inhibitory inputs (see [59, 60] for a review), thus controling these inputs is crucial for normal functioning of DA neurons. Hence, an increase in glutamatergic or cholinergic transmission enhances DA neuronal activity and produces bursting pattern [61-64], whereas an increase in GABA drive reduces discharge rate and bursting, *via* both $GABA_A$ and $GABA_B$ receptors [65, 66].

Firing pattern of DA neurons is correlated with specific behavioral stimuli: these neurons fire in bursts and release phasic DA particularly in the NAc, in response to both drugs of abuse and non-pharmacological rewards. Under such circumstances, it was postulated that DA neurons encode reward prediction error: *i.e.* they display an enhanced firing rate and bursting when a reward is larger than expected and pause firing activity when no reward or punishment is delivered [10, 67-69] After training, DA neurons also fire in response to conditioned stimuli associated with reinforcers [68], highlighting the role of DA as a learning signal.

Thus, the finding that endocannabinoids are released during bursting events by DA neurons is particularly intriguing. These molecules may regulate DA neuron responses during emotional and sensory processing [70] and support the action of DA in learning tasks. Indeed, cannabinoids have been shown to perturb the emotional significance of sensory information [71, 72] and to affect emotional processing and sensory perceptions. Moreover, they perturb executive functions in which DA is involved, such as behavioral flexibility and reversal learning [73]. Consistently, endocannabinoid-dependent forms of synaptic plasticity occur both at afferents to DA neurons and at their terminal regions, such as the striatum, the amygdala and the prefrontal cortex [1].

ALCOHOL AND THE ENDOCANNABINOID SYSTEM

Early studies suggest interactions between cannabinoids and alcohol (see [74] for an excellent comprehensive review). Indeed, alcohol and marijuana are very often co-abused in western societies [74] due to subjectively similar effects on central nervous system functions, although alcohol affects a multiplicity of targets with low affinity, whereas THC has a very specific molecular target in the brain at least with regard to addiction.

The endocannabinoid system is affected by alcohol and, conversely, pharmacological manipulations of endocannabinoids and their receptors affect alcohol actions from molecular levels to behavior.

Alcohol triggers the release of endocannabinoids *in vitro* and *in vivo*. *In vitro* studies have demonstrated that acute alcohol incubation induces the release of endocannabinoids (anandamide and 2-AG) in a Ca^{2+}-dependent fashion [75]. Chronic exposure to alcohol induces a selective increase of endogenous cannabinoids anandamide and 2-AG in cultured SK-N-SH cells [76] or cerebellar granular neurons [77]. The same authors demonstrated that chronic alcohol downregulates CB_1R function and number in rodents, and suggested that this may result from the overstimulation of CB_1Rs by endocannabinoids [78]. Innate preference for alcohol might also be marked by altered endocannabinoid signaling, since decreased levels of CB_1Rs were also found in naive alcohol preferring rats [79].

Moreover, evidence suggests that endocannabinoid signaling may be involved in the modulation of alcohol reinforcing effects and alcohol drinking behavior.

Hence, the CB_1R antagonist/reverse agonist rimonabant (SR141716A) decreases alcohol intake in both alcohol preferring rats [80] and in C57BL/6 mice [81], and the motivation to consume alcohol in rats [82, 83]. Furthermore, deletion of CB_1R genes (in CB_1R knockout mice) reduces alcohol preference and intake [84-86], alcohol-induced conditioned place preference [87] and alcohol-induced increase of DA release in the NAc [86].

Alcohol-induced increases in anandamide and 2-AG depress presynaptic glutamate release from cultured hippocampal neurons [75]. Therefore, this finding supports the notion that some effects of alcohol might be induced by endocannabinoid-mediated regulation of neurotransmitter release. Consistently, we have found that blockade of CB_1Rs with rimonabant suppress alcohol-induced depression of basolateral amygdala projection neurons [88] and medium spiny neurons in the NAc or excitation of VTA DA cells [89]. In addition, rimonabant blocks alcohol-induced increase in DA transients in the NAc [90] and CB_1R knockout mice do not display alcohol-induced DA increase in the NAc, suggesting that CB_1R function is required for these alcohol-mediated effects and for voluntary alcohol intake [86]. In contrast to the studies mentioned above, other evidence suggests that alcohol may also decrease endocannabinoid levels in several brain regions [91, 92], and this decrease is not caused by an enhanced FAAH activity [91, 92]. Other studies highlighted that anandamide and 2-AG levels were decreased in the midbrain after chronic alcohol exposure [93].

The inhibitory effect of rimonabant on alcohol neurochemical, electrophysiological and behavioral effects suggest that pharmacological or genic manipulation of the endocannabinoid system affect alcohol actions, both at cellular and behavioral levels.

Studies by our group have shown that FAAH inhibition counteracted alcohol-induced responses in NAc medium spiny neurons [89], and Serrano *et al.* [94] reported that alcohol withdrawal in animals exposed to either acute or intermittent administration alters FAAH mRNA expression in the amygdala. Furthermore, in the latter study, changes in MAG lipase mRNA expression were described and the levels of this enzyme were more pronounced only during intermittent alcohol exposure, suggesting a prominent role of anandamide, rather than 2-AG, in the modulation of alcohol-induced responses. Anandamide might reduce alcohol intake by activating TRPV1 receptors, since TRPV1$^{-/-}$ mice show significantly higher preference for alcohol and consumed more alcohol in a two-bottle choice paradigm than wild type littermates [95]. Inhibition of endocannabinoid membrane transport (EMT) by AM404 was also reported to reduce alcohol intake in alcohol preferring rats [96], further supporting the idea that indirect endocannabinoid agonists might be useful as a treatment for drug addiction (see also below). The so-called EMT probably corresponds to the FAAH-like anandamide transporter (FLAT), which recently emerged as crucial element of anandamide transport in neural cells and whose activity is also blocked by AM404 [97].

Anandamide, increased by FAAH or EMT inhibition, might reduce alcohol effects, but it is less clear whether 2-AG is directly involved in the modulation of rewarding and addictive responses of alcohol. It was reported that dialysate levels of 2-AG in the NAc were increased after alcohol self-administration [98], supporting the role of 2-AG in early steps of alcohol dependence. This notion has been also confirmed by other studies showing that alcohol intake and preference was increased by chronic treatment with neurotoxic doses of the psychostimulant, methamphetamine [99]. In this case, the authors showed that seven days after methamphetamine administration, 2-AG levels were enhanced, whereas MAG lipase activity was reduced in the limbic forebrain and that MAG lipase inhibitors enhanced alcohol intake in treated and naïve mice [99]. In line with previous studies, Malinen *et al.* [100] found increased anandamide and 2-AG levels in specific brain regions of alcohol-preferring male and female rats (AA rats) compared with non-preferring counterparts. Anandamide and 2-AG changes were non-overlapping and showed differential occurrences in accordance with gender and alcohol exposure sessions, suggesting that anandamide and 2-AG might have a distinct modulatory role.

NICOTINE AND THE ENDOCANNABINOD SYSTEM

Tobacco and cannabis derivatives are among the most widely abused drugs, particularly by adolescents and young adults, being commonly smoked in combination (reviewed in [101]). Consistently, several lines of evidence support functional interactions between central nicotinic and endogenous cannabinoid systems with regard to addiction-related processes (see [101-105] for excellent reviews). The overlapping distribution of CB_1Rs and neuronal nicotinic acetylcholine receptors (nAChRs) in several brain regions related to motivation and reward, such as the VTA, the NAc, the prefrontal cortex, the hippocampus, and the amygdala [13, 14, 106] might provide the neurobiological substrate for these interactions.

Nicotine and cannabinoids reciprocally influence their rewarding and pharmacological effects (reviewed in [101, 102, 104, 105] and changes in endocannabinoid levels have been observed in different brain areas of rats chronically exposed to nicotine [93, 107, 108].

Acute nicotine potentiates several physiological and behavioral effects (*i.e.* hypothermia, antinociception, reduced locomotor activity) induced by acute administration of THC, the major psychoactive component of *Cannabis sativa* [109, 110]. Moreover, co-administration of non-effective doses of THC and nicotine induces significant anxiolytic-like responses, as well as a significant conditioned place preference in mice [110]. In the same study, co-treatment with both drugs strongly enhances c-Fos immunoreactivity in various limbic and cortical structures crucially implicated in the neuronal mechanisms of addictive substances (shell of the NAc, central and basolateral nucleus of amygdala, bed nucleus stria terminalis, cingular and piriform cortices, paraventricular nucleus of the hypothalamus) [110].

Acute THC exposure reduces the incidence of several precipitated nicotine withdrawal signs, ameliorates the aversive motivational state associated with nicotine abstinence in mice, and decreases anxiogenic-like effects of nicotine in rats [111, 112]. Accordingly, Cippitelli and coworkers [107] showed that pharmacological inhibition of FAAH by URB597, and the consequent increase in anandamide tone, suppresses anxiety symptoms associated with protracted nicotine withdrawal, but does not prevent the occurrence of somatic signs. Altogether these findings indicate that activation of CB_1Rs may be effective in counteracting the aversive aspects of nicotine withdrawal, which are critical for the maintenance of tobacco use. Conversely, the observed enhancement in the somatic expression of THC withdrawal in animals co-treated with nicotine and THC [110] suggests an unbalanced relationship between these two compounds. Finally, it should be mentioned that recent findings show that the synthetic CB_1R agonist WIN55212 increases the reinforcing effects of nicotine and precipitates relapse to nicotine-seeking in rats [113].

Converging preclinical and clinical evidence underline the importance of CB_1Rs in the interplay between the nicotinic and endocannabinoid systems and, consequently, in the etiology of nicotine addiction. Different studies demonstrated alterations in brain CB_1R expression and function in rats chronically exposed to nicotine [114-116], but see also [93, 112] On one hand, CB_1R knockout mice develop neither nicotine-induced increase in locomotor activity [117] nor nicotine-induced conditioned place preference [117, 118], suggesting that the rewarding effect of nicotine are blunted in CB_1R null mutant mice. On the other hand, Cossu and collaborators [119] reported that the absence of CB_1Rs does not modify nicotine self-administration, even though these discrepancies might be partially explained by methodological aspects such as the specific experimental protocol and the range of doses used.

Also, genetic investigations in humans indicate that CB_1R gene (CNR1) is associated with smoking initiation and nicotine addiction [120]. Intriguingly, given the reported associations of this gene with other substance abuse and dependence, an involvement of CNR1 in the manifestation of multiple substance abuse and dependence has been hypothesized (see [121] for a review).

Pharmacological blockade of the CB_1R is another approach that supports the role of endocannabinoid system in nicotine dependence (see [122] for an extensive review on this topic). In fact, administration of the CB_1R antagonists/reverse agonists rimonabant or AM251, blocks the acquisition of nicotine-induced conditioned place preference in rats [123, 124] and wild type mice [118]. Moreover, CB_1R antagonism dose-dependently reduces nicotine self-administration under a regular fixed ratio schedule or second-order reinforcement schedule in rats [125-129], blocks nicotine-induced increases in NAc DA levels in freely-moving rats [90], and decreases reinstatement of nicotine-seeking behavior in animal models of relapse [128]. The utility of CB_1R antagonists/reverse agonists (currently rimonabant and taranabant) has been tested also on several clinical trials in human smokers. Rimonabant showed efficacy not only as a treatment for smoking cessation, but also in moderating weight gain and decreasing relapse rate in abstinent smokers [130](; reviewed in [122]), even though its use was then suspended due to severe emotional side effects. Similarly, taranabant, while effective in controling weight gain, did not improve smoking cessation and was discontinued because of unacceptable psychiatric, gastrointestinal, and flushing adverse events [131]. Since the unwanted side effects of these compounds may be due, at least in part, to inverse agonism at the CB_1R (reviewed in [103]; see also [132]), the efficacy profile and reduced adverse event risk of CB_1R neutral antagonists make them a potential therapeutic option worth of translational study (reviewed in [133]).

While pharmacological blockade of CB_1Rs appears to reliably influence nicotine-seeking behavior, the direct involvement of the DA reward system in this effect is less clear. Indeed, despite evidence on nicotine-induced DA release, electrophysiological studies performed in our laboratory failed to demonstrate effects of CB_1R antagonists on drug-induced stimulation of mesolimbic DA neurons [44], leading us to hypothesize that endocannabinoids might modulate nicotine-evoked DA release at the synaptic level without affecting firing rate of DA cells. To add further complexity, Simonnet and coworkers [134] recently demonstrated that nicotine reinforcement is reduced by a selective blockade of CB_1Rs in the VTA, suggesting that in rats chronically exposed to nicotine intravenous self-administration the CB_1Rs located in the VTA rather than in the NAc specifically control nicotine reinforcement and, subsequently, nicotine-taking behavior.

Indirect cannabinoid agonists, like inhibitors of endogenous cannabinoid metabolism or uptake, emerged as promising alternative ways of modulating the endocannabinoid system.

For example, different studies investigated how pharmacological inhibition of FAAH, and the resulting increase in anandamide levels, modulates the effects of nicotine [42, 118, 128] In rats, inhibition of FAAH with URB597 blocks nicotine-induced conditioned place preference, acquisition of nicotine self-administration behavior, relapse to drug-seeking behavior, and DA increase in the shell of the NAc [42]. Accordingly, studies by our group [41, 44] demonstrate that FAAH inhibition prevents neuronal responses to nicotine administration predictive of its rewarding properties, *i.e.* stimulation of VTA DA cell firing rate [44] and inhibition of medium spiny neurons in the shell of the NAc [41]. Nevertheless, our results indicate that anandamide is probably not involved. In fact, FAAH inhibition not only raises anandamide levels, but also concentrations of other non-cannabinoid *N*-acylethanolamines, oleoylethanolamide (OEA) and palmitoylethanolamide (PEA). Unlike anandamide neither OEA nor PEA possess significant CB1-R affinity, but are endogenous ligands for nuclear peroxisome proliferator-activated receptor-α (PPAR-α). Likewise, we have observed that most URB597-mediated effects are indeed blocked by the PPAR-α antagonist, MK886 [41, 44]. Notably, the effects of PPAR-α activation on drug-induced DA cell excitation are selective for nicotine [41], and administration of the metabolically stable OEA analog, methOEA, and the selective PPAR-α agonist WY14643 selectively decrease nicotine, but not cocaine or food self-administration in both rats and monkeys [46].

Recent studies by Scherma *et al.* [135] and Gamaleddin *et al.* [136] with endocannabinoid uptake inhibitors shed light into the role of anandamide, and CB$_1$Rs, in nicotine rewarding and addictive behaviors. They found that the anandamide transport inhibitors, AM404 and VDM11, which enhance anandamide levels, but not those of OEA and PEA, suppress nicotine-induced conditioned place preferences and increase of DA levels in the ShNAc [135], and attenuate the reinstatement of seeking behavior induced by nicotine-associated cues and priming [136].

In addition, as already mentioned, Cippitelli *et al.* [107] show that anandamide levels in brain areas involved in nicotine rewarding responses are physiologically altered in nicotine-abstinent mice, providing evidence that FAAH inhibition may potentially offer therapeutic advantages to treat negative affective state associated with nicotine withdrawal. FAAH inhibitors represent suitable candidates for antismoking medications but other studies have reported contrasting results. For instance, Merritt *et al.* [118] report that both genetic (FAAH knockout mice) and pharmacological inhibition of FAAH (by URB597) enhances the rewarding effects of low nicotine doses in mice through a CB_1R mechanism, most likely due to elevated levels of anandamide. Despite an increasing amount of data suggesting that the endocannabinoid system is a component of the brain reward system and is involved in the modulation of nicotine-rewarding and nicotine-addictive properties, only few studies have yet evaluated changes in endocannabinoid content following nicotine exposure.

It has been demonstrated that rats chronically exposed to nicotine show an increase in endocannabinoid levels in certain brain regions [93]. In particular, AEA content augments in the limbic forebrain and the brainstem, whereas 2-AG levels increase only in the brainstem. In contrast, other regions such as the hippocampus, the striatum and the cerebral cortex exhibit a reduction in AEA and/or 2-AG levels [93]. More recently, an elegant paper from Buczynski and colleagues [108] compared the effects of volitional nicotine self-administration and forced nicotine exposure on levels of endocannabinoids and related neuroactive lipids in the VTA. Volitional nicotine self-administration, but not forced exposure, reduces baseline VTA OEA levels, and increases AEA release during nicotine intake. On the other hand, all nicotine administration protocols elevate VTA dialysate 2-AG levels. Altogether these results demonstrate that nicotine differentially affects brain lipid content, and these modulations are influenced by the voluntary nature of the drug exposure.

OPIOIDS AND THE ENDOCANNABINOID SYSTEM

Biochemical, pharmacological and anatomical evidence support the existence of a functional cross-talk between the endogenous cannabinoid and the endogenous opioid systems in discrete physiological functions including reward, motivation and reinforcement (for a review see [137, 138]). Additionally, consistent with the role of the endocannabinoid system in the modulation of the brain reward system [17], different studies reported the changes in endocannabinoid ligands and/or receptors in the brain of animals chronically exposed to opiates (for a review see [139]). However, the majority of the studies focused on the analysis of CB_1Rs, and not on the changes in the concentrations of the endogenous ligands. Though most of the studies focused on the analysis of CB_1Rs, the observations resulting led to contradictory findings showing mainly region-dependent differences among those areas directly or indirectly related to opiate dependence and addiction [140-144]. These discrepancies might be ascribed to both the animal species and the experimental protocols used to render animals opiate-dependent. For instance, specific modifications in the levels of endocannabinoids depending on the endocannabinoid examined (*e.g.* anandamide or 2-AG) and the brain region considered were observed at diverse phases of an opiate chronic regimen [141, 145]. In particular, anandamide levels did not change during chronic opiate treatment probably due to corresponding modifications in the activity of its main degrading enzyme, FAAH. On the other hand, 2-AG levels decreased during chronic opiate regimen when compared to baseline levels, and were further lowered long after opiate exposure [145].

Accordingly, Caillè *et al.* [98] observed that animals self-administering heroin display transient alterations in the levels of endocannabinoids in the shell of the NAc. In particular, anandamide levels increased, while 2-AG levels diminished. Remarkably, the changes in anandamide and 2-AG levels positively and negatively, respectively, correlated with the intake of heroin. Noteworthy, chronic passive opiate administration results in altered levels of anandamide and 2-AG in discrete postmortem rat brain regions [145], whereas when the whole brains were examined no changes were observed [146]. A possible explanation for such a discrepancy might be that changes in isolated areas might have been undetected due to a "dilution" effect by brain areas where no changes had occurred. As a result, the relative changes in each endocannabinoid within a certain brain region might have been washed out when the whole brain was examined.

Nonetheless, the above mentioned observations suggest that opiate treatment might influence the mechanisms regulating endocannabinoid homeostasis, and that these might eventually play a role in behavioral sensitization to opiates. Since behavioral sensitization is regarded as a model for investigating the incentive motivation underlying drug-seeking behavior [147], and because mesolimbic dopamine neurons display an increased sensitivity of opiate receptors that persists long after morphine withdrawal [148], these studies suggest that homeostatic adaptations of the endocannabinoid system triggered during exposure to opiates continue long after the drug is discontinued and, though opposite for each endocannabinoid examined, in the same direction for an acute exposure [145].

Mostly, the changes in anandamide levels appear to be part of the diverse mechanisms leading to a sensitized response, since its levels are enhanced not only during the withdrawal period [145], but also when its main degrading enzyme (*i.e.* FAAH) is pharmacologically blocked during acute withdrawal [149]. Moreover, 2-AG and anandamide in the NAc also appear to play a role in the reinforcing effects produced by opiates, given that both pharmacological blockade and genetic deletion of CB_1Rs is able to decrease heroin self-administration [119, 150-153].

Whether the endocannabinoid system has a causative role in opiate sensitization, or its levels change as a part of protective and adaptive responses during opiate exposure it remains to be elucidated yet.

PSYCHOSTIMULANTS AND THE ENDOCANNABINOID SYSTEM

Although many studies have associated the involvement of the endocannabinoid system in the mechanisms underlying drug dependence, both genetic deletion and pharmacological blockade of CB_1Rs have underplayed its role in psychostimulant reward, though disclosing its part in the persistence of the cycle of addiction to psychostimulants [154].

In fact, both cocaine self-administration and its rewarding properties are not sensitive to CB_1R inactivation [98, 119, 155, 156] but see [157-159]. The discrepancy between these studies has to be ascribed to the differences in the experimental settings used, where the progressive ratio schedule appears to be sensitive to CB1 antagonism [157, 158] but the fixed ratio does not. Remarkably, chronic exposure to cocaine produces a decrease in both 2-AG levels and CB_1R mRNA in brain areas related to addiction (*e.g.* cerebral cortex) [142]. However, both chronic passive administration and self-administration of cocaine did not change either endocannabinoid or CB_1R mRNA levels within the mesocorticolimbic system [98]. Notably, when the access to cocaine self-administration was modified from short to extended, some changes in the levels of endocannabinoids were observed within the NAc [160]. In particular, animals who had long access to cocaine self-administration displayed an increased endocannabinoidergic tone, as well as an upregulation of CB_1Rs in the NAc 24 h after last cocaine session, suggesting a dramatic increased activity of this system. Conversely, animals with short access to cocaine self-administration presented lower levels of endocannabinoids. Accordingly, both systemic or local (*i.e.* intra-NAc) blockade of CB_1Rs decreased the breakpoint for cocaine in animals with extended access to self-administration [160]. Thus, it appears that adaptations (*i.e.* increased tone) of the endocannabinoid system might take part in the increased motivation displayed under extended-access conditions.

In addition, the endocannabinoid system seems to play a crucial role in reinstatement of cocaine seeking behavior [161]. In fact, activation of CB_1Rs was able to reinstate cocaine seeking in rats, an effect that was abolished by blocking CB_1Rs, thus suggesting a role for CB_1Rs in triggering relapse to cocaine seeking. Accordingly, blockade of CB_1Rs prevented drug- and cue-, but not stress- induced reinstatement of cocaine seeking [154, 162, 163] Consistent with these findings, enhancement of the endocannabinoid tone significantly reduced drug- and cue-induced reinstatement [164], thus supporting the role that tonic activation of CB_1Rs plays a role in extinction/reinstatement of cocaine seeking-behavior, whereas it is not involved in the maintenance of cocaine self-administration.

Remarkably, CB_1Rs, but not CB_2Rs or TRPV1Rs, play the key role in reinstatement induced by conditioned stimuli (*i.e.* cocaine-associated cues) on cocaine-seeking behavior [165], since antagonism of either CB_2Rs and TRPV1Rs did not prevent cocaine-seeking behavior expressed as operant lever presses. Nonetheless, these latter seems to be involved in cocaine-seeking behavior [165], since CB_2R and TRPV1R antagonists have anti-reinstatement effects when unconditioned stimuli are presented. Altogether, these observations suggest the existence of independent neural pathways regulated by the endocannabinoid system through activation of discrete receptors aimed at modulating motivational and conditioned facets of goal-directed behaviors. This corroborates the evidence suggesting that dissociable neural mechanisms and anatomical substrates underlie diverse features of these behaviors [166-171].

In sharp contrast with cocaine, CB_1Rs are involved in the reinforcing properties of amphetamine-like drugs such as MDMA (*i.e.* ecstasy) [172-174], methamphetamine and amphetamine itself [175-178]. Notably, Thiemann *et al.*

[178] observed opposite effects on amphetamine-induced sensitization when CB1-R inactivation was achieved through either genetic or pharmacological manipulation. In particular, pharmacological blockade of CB_1Rs enhanced amphetamine sensitizing effects, whereas genetic deletion of CB_1Rs led to a reduction of the sensitizing effects of amphetamine. In addition, whether amphetamine was administered acutely or chronically resulted in opposite effects on anandamide and 2-AG levels depending on the brain region examined [178]. In the dorsal striatum, the levels of anandamide and 2-AG respectively increased and decreased, following the first exposure to amphetamine. The increased anandamide levels persisted in the dorsal striatum of sensitized animals, whereas 2-AG levels not only returned to baseline values but showed a positive trend. However, when the concentrations of the two endocannabinoids were measured in the ventral striatum a marked decrease was observed for both anandamide and 2-AG, the latter being further reduced in sensitized animals. Thus, it can be speculated that modifications of endocannabinoid levels contribute to amphetamine sensitization, especially those occurring in the ventral striatum. Altogether these observations point to a role of the endocannabinoid system in drug- and cue- induced relapse to psychostimulant seeking [154, 162, 163, 165, 175].

THERAPEUTIC PERSPECTIVES

The endocannabinoid system has been highlighted among other neurotransmitters/neuromodulators as a major player in the different phases of compulsive seeking of natural or drug-induced reward. Undeniably, pharmacological manipulation of endocannabinoids influences reward-seeking behavior. Among examples mentioned above, CB_1R blockade with rimonabant inhibits nicotine-induced DA release in the NAc, as measured by brain microdialysis, and nicotine self-administration [127]. Consistently, rimonabant suppresses nicotine-, alcohol- and cocaine induced phasic DA release in the ventral striatum measured with *in vivo* fast-scan voltammetry [90].

Endocannabinoids are involved in the effects of acute drug administration, but might also participate in long-term changes induced by chronic drug administration, by preferentially modulating multiple long-term, other than short-term, forms of synaptic plasticity, *i.e.* facilitating LTD$_{GABA}$ [54, 55, 179] or LTD on DA neurons [180] or inhibiting LTP [21].

Among behaviors consequent to chronic drug administration, reinstatement (equivalent to relapse in humans) is a major goal of therapies aimed to prevent binge drug use. Interestingly, reinstatement is very sensitive to CB1-R activation or blockade. Indeed, following extinction of drug-seeking behaviors such as drug self-administration, CB1-R antagonists have been consistently reported to block cue-induced or drug-induced reinstatement of drug-seeking behavior [2, 181-187] Conversely, primings with CB$_1$R agonists reinstate drug seeking behaviors [42, 113, 188].

How can these effects be explained according with synaptic plasticity events evoked by endocannabinoids? One hypothesis is that indiscriminate activation of CB$_1$Rs by exogenous cannabinoid agonists might desensitize or occlude 2-AG-mediated short- or long-term forms of synaptic plasticity predominantly on glutamatergic afferents to DA neurons (such as short-lasting suppression of excitation or LTD). Desensitization of CB$_1$Rs on excitatory synapses might render DA cells more responsive to priming with drugs or with drug-associated cues.

Cannabinoid antagonists were regarded as a promising therapy for drug addiction, due to their consistent blockade of reinstatement in animal models of addiction, and clinical trials with rimonabant for nicotine dependence demonstrated some efficacy [122, 130, 189-191] However, rimonabant was withdrawn from the market for increased risk of depression and suicide [192]. These side effects, in principle, would not have been completely unexpected, due to the role of the endocannabinoid system in the mechanisms of natural reward [3]. Hence, CB$_1$R blockade decreases the motivation to seek sources of reward, including natural ones [193] and induces states of anhedonia and enhanced sensitivity to aversive stimuli or punishment, that could lead vulnerable individuals to depression.

Indirect cannabinoid agonists, *i.e.* those compounds that enhance endogenous levels of endocannabinoids by inhibiting either their catabolic enzymes (*e.g.* FAAH or MAG lipase) or membrane uptake mechanisms (*e.g.* anandamide membrane transport inhibitors, such as AM404 or VDM11), are therapeutic avenues that theoretically would be more promising than CB_1R antagonists. As with CB_1R antagonists, these drugs suppress reinstatement of drug-seeking behavior in laboratory animals, including non-human primates (see [105] and references therein). The advantage over CB_1R antagonists is that a discriminate and localized activation of CB_1R might counteract DA neuron sensitization by selectively suppressing glutamate release from impinging excitatory axons. Accordingly, cue-induced reinstatement to nicotine self-administration is particularly sensitive to blockade by both FAAH inhibition, AM404 and VDM11 [42, 135, 136] It must be pointed out that FAAH inhibition enhances brain levels not only of anandamide but also of OEA and PEA, non-cannabinoid *N*-acylethanolamines, that could depress responses to nicotine by modulation of nAChRs through PPAR-α [16, 44, 45, 194] Studies with endocannabinoid uptake inhibitors do not rule out a role for CB_1Rs, since these drugs enhance brain anandamide levels without affecting those of OEA and PEA and suppress nicotine self-administration with a CB_1R dependent mechanism [135, 136]. FAAH and endocannabinoid uptake inhibitors do not show frank abuse liability in laboratory animals [136, 188], but see [195] for AM404. This advantage of CB_1R indirect agonists may pave the way for their clinical use.

In conclusion, after the failure of rimonabant, the road towards cannabinoid medications for drug addiction is not blocked. Further insights into the logic of endocannabinoid signaling are necessary, as it is a deeper knowledge of the interaction of this system with limbic circuits. Understanding these interactions might pave the road not only towards anti-addiction medications but also to drugs that might prove useful in treating anxiety or mood disorders, which are often comorbid with drug abuse. New hopes are relied upon the modulators of the endocannabinoid system, but the way to human use is still far away.

ACKNOWLEDGEMENTS

The authors wish to thank the Italian Ministry of University (MIUR) (grant PRIN 2009-200928EEX4 to Marco Pistis; grant PRIN 2009-2009HST9YF to Anna Lisa Muntoni), FIRE -AICE (Grant 2011 to Marco Pistis), Fondazione Banco di Sardegna (Grant 2012 to Marco Pistis) for research support.

CONFLICT OF INTEREST

The authors confirm that this chapter content has no conflicts interest.

REFERENCES

[1]   Fattore L, Fadda P, Spano MS, Pistis M, Fratta W. Neurobiological mechanisms of cannabinoid addiction. Mol Cell Endocrinol 2008;286:S97-S107.

[2]   Fattore L, Spano MS, Deiana S, *et al.* An endocannabinoid mechanism in relapse to drug seeking: a review of animal studies and clinical perspectives. Brain Res Rev 2007;53:1-16.

[3]   Fattore L, Melis M, Fadda P, Pistis M, Fratta W. The endocannabinoid system and nondrug rewarding behaviours. Exp Neurol 2010;224:23-36.

[4]   Koob GF, Volkow ND. Neurocircuitry of Addiction. Neuropsychopharmacology 2009;35:217-38.

[5]   Wise RA. Dopamine, learning and motivation. Nat Rev Neurosci 2004;5:483-94.

[6]   Wise RA, Rompre PP. Brain dopamine and reward. Annu Rev Psychol 1989;40:191-225.

[7]   Wise RA. Roles for nigrostriatal--not just mesocorticolimbic--dopamine in reward and addiction. Trends Neurosci 2009;32:517-24.

[8]   Hyman SE, Malenka RC, Nestler EJ. Neural mechanisms of addiction: the role of reward-related learning and memory. Annu Rev Neurosci 2006;29:565-98.

[9]   Kauer JA, Malenka RC. Synaptic plasticity and addiction. Nat Rev Neurosci 2007;8:844-58.

[10]   Schultz W. Predictive reward signal of dopamine neurons. J Neurophysiol 1998;80:1-27.

[11]   Ungless MA, Magill PJ, Bolam JP. Uniform inhibition of dopamine neurons in the ventral tegmental area by aversive stimuli. Science 2004;303:2040-2.

[12]   Jhou TC, Fields HL, Baxter MG, Saper CB, Holland PC. The rostromedial tegmental nucleus (RMTg), a GABAergic afferent to midbrain dopamine neurons, encodes aversive stimuli and inhibits motor responses. Neuron 2009;61:786-800.

[13]   Herkenham M, Lynn AB, Johnson MR, *et al.* Characterization and localization of cannabinoid receptors in rat brain: a quantitative *in vitro* autoradiographic study. J Neurosci 1991;11:563-83.

[14]   Matsuda LA, Bonner TI, Lolait SJ. Localization of cannabinoid receptor mRNA in rat brain. J Comp Neurol 1993;327:535-50.

[15]   Fernandez-Ruiz J, Hernandez M, Ramos JA. Cannabinoid-dopamine interaction in the pathophysiology and treatment of CNS disorders. CNS Neurosci Ther 2010;16:e72-91.

[16]   Melis M, Pistis M. Hub and switches: endocannabinoid signaling in midbrain dopamine neurons. Philos Trans R Soc Lond B Biol Sci 2012;367:3276-85.

[17]   Melis M, Muntoni AL, Pistis M. Endocannabinoids and the processing of value-related signals. Front Pharmacol 2012;3:7.

[18]   Luchicchi A, Pistis M. Anandamide and 2-arachidonoylglycerol: Pharmacological Properties, Functional Features, and Emerging Specificities of the Two Major Endocannabinoids. Mol Neurobiol 2012;46:374-92.

[19]   Melis M, Pistis M. Endocannabinoid Signaling in Midbrain Dopamine Neurons: More than Physiology? Current Neuropharmacology 2007;5:268-77.

[20]   Marinelli S, Di Marzo V, Florenzano F, *et al*. N-arachidonoyl-dopamine tunes synaptic transmission onto dopaminergic neurons by activating both cannabinoid and vanilloid receptors. Neuropsychopharmacology 2007;32:298-308.

[21]   Kortleven C, Fasano C, Thibault D, Lacaille JC, Trudeau LE. The endocannabinoid 2-arachidonoylglycerol inhibits long-term potentiation of glutamatergic synapses onto ventral tegmental area dopamine neurons in mice. Eur J Neurosci 2011;33:1751-60.

[22]   Mátyás F, Urbán GM, Watanabe M, *et al*. Identification of the sites of 2-arachidonoylglycerol synthesis and action imply retrograde endocannabinoid signaling at both GABAergic and glutamatergic synapses in the ventral tegmental area. Neuropharmacology 2008;54:95-107.

[23]   Melis M, Pillolla G, Bisogno T, *et al*. Protective activation of the endocannabinoid system during ischemia in dopamine neurons. Neurobiol Dis 2006;24:15-27.

[24]   French ED, Dillon K, Wu X. Cannabinoids excite dopamine neurons in the ventral tegmentum and substantia nigra. Neuroreport 1997;8:649-52.

[25]   Gessa GL, Melis M, Muntoni AL, Diana M. Cannabinoids activate mesolimbic dopamine neurons by an action on cannabinoid CB1 receptors. Eur J Pharmacol 1998;341:39-44.

[26]   Tanda G, Pontieri FE, Di Chiara G. Cannabinoid and heroin activation of mesolimbic dopamine transmission by a common mu1 opioid receptor mechanism. Science 1997;276:2048-50.

[27]   Cheer JF, Wassum KM, Heien ML, Phillips PE, Wightman RM. Cannabinoids enhance subsecond dopamine release in the nucleus accumbens of awake rats. J Neurosci 2004;24:4393-400.

[28]   Pistis M, Ferraro L, Pira L, *et al*. Delta(9)-tetrahydrocannabinol decreases extracellular GABA and increases extracellular glutamate and dopamine levels in the rat prefrontal cortex: an *in vivo* microdialysis study. Brain Res 2002;948:155-8.

[29]   Chen J, Paredes W, Lowinson JH, Gardner EL. Delta 9-tetrahydrocannabinol enhances presynaptic dopamine efflux in medial prefrontal cortex. Eur J Pharmacol 1990;190:259-62.

[30]   Di Chiara G, Imperato A. Drugs abused by humans preferentially increase synaptic dopamine concentrations in the mesolimbic system of freely moving rats. Proc Natl Acad Sci U S A 1988;85:5274-8.

[31]   Wenger T, Moldrich G, Furst S. Neuromorphological background of cannabis addiction. Brain Res Bull. 2003;61:125-8.

[32]   Lecca S, Melis M, Luchicchi A, *et al*. Effects of drugs of abuse on putative rostromedial tegmental neurons, inhibitory afferents to midbrain dopamine cells. Neuropsychopharmacology 2011;36:589-602.

[33]   Lecca S, Melis M, Luchicchi A, Muntoni AL, Pistis M. Inhibitory inputs from rostromedial tegmental neurons regulate spontaneous activity of midbrain dopamine cells and their responses to drugs of abuse. Neuropsychopharmacology 2012;37:1164-76.

[34]   Barrot M, Sesack SR, Georges F, *et al*. Braking Dopamine Systems: A New GABA Master Structure for Mesolimbic and Nigrostriatal Functions. J Neurosci 2012;32:14094-101.

[35]   Melis M, Perra S, Muntoni AL, *et al*. Prefrontal cortex stimulation induces 2-arachidonoyl-glycerol-mediated suppression of excitation in dopamine neurons. J Neurosci 2004;24:10707-15.

[36]   Riegel AC, Lupica CR. Independent presynaptic and postsynaptic mechanisms regulate endocannabinoid signaling at multiple synapses in the ventral tegmental area. J Neurosci 2004;24:11070-8.

[37] Melis M, Pistis M, Perra S, *et al*. Endocannabinoids mediate presynaptic inhibition of glutamatergic transmission in rat ventral tegmental area dopamine neurons through activation of CB1 receptors. J Neurosci 2004;24:53-62.

[38] Yanovsky Y, Mades S, Misgeld U. Retrograde signaling changes the venue of postsynaptic inhibition in rat substantia nigra. Neuroscience 2003;122:317-28.

[39] Marrs WR, Blankman JL, Horne EA, *et al*. The serine hydrolase ABHD6 controls the accumulation and efficacy of 2-AG at cannabinoid receptors. Nat Neurosci 2010;13:951-7.

[40] Savinainen JR, Saario SM, Laitinen JT. The serine hydrolases MAGL, ABHD6 and ABHD12 as guardians of 2-arachidonoylglycerol signaling through cannabinoid receptors. Acta Physiol (Oxf) 2012;204:267-76.

[41] Luchicchi A, Lecca S, Carta S, *et al*. Effects of fatty acid amide hydrolase inhibition on neuronal responses to nicotine, cocaine and morphine in the nucleus accumbens shell and ventral tegmental area: involvement of PPAR-alpha nuclear receptors. Addict Biol 2010;15:277-88.

[42] Scherma M, Panlilio LV, Fadda P, *et al*. Inhibition of anandamide hydrolysis by URB597 reverses abuse-related behavioral and neurochemical effects of nicotine in rats. J Pharmacol Exp Ther 2008.

[43] Egertova M, Simon GM, Cravatt BF, Elphick MR. Localization of N-acyl phosphatidylethanolamine phospholipase D (NAPE-PLD) expression in mouse brain: A new perspective on N-acylethanolamines as neural signaling molecules. J Comp Neurol 2008;506:604-15.

[44] Melis M, Pillolla G, Luchicchi A, *et al*. Endogenous Fatty Acid Ethanolamides Suppress Nicotine-Induced Activation of Mesolimbic Dopamine Neurons through Nuclear Receptors. J Neurosci 2008;28:13985-94.

[45] Melis M, Carta S, Fattore L, *et al*. Peroxisome proliferator-activated receptors-alpha modulate dopamine cell activity through nicotinic receptors. Biol Psychiatry 2010;68:256-64.

[46] Mascia P, Pistis M, Justinova Z, *et al*. Blockade of nicotine reward and reinstatement by activation of alpha-type peroxisome proliferator-activated receptors. Biol Psychiatry 2011;69:633-41.

[47] Okamoto Y, Morishita J, Tsuboi K, Tonai T, Ueda N. Molecular characterization of a phospholipase D generating anandamide and its congeners. J Biol Chem 2004;279:5298-305.

[48] Di Marzo V. Endocannabinoid signaling in the brain: biosynthetic mechanisms in the limelight. Nat Neurosci 2011;14:9-15.

[49] Vandevoorde S, Lambert DM. The multiple pathways of endocannabinoid metabolism: a zoom out. Chem Biodivers 2007;4:1858-81.

[50] Ueda N, Tsuboi K, Uyama T. N-acylethanolamine metabolism with special reference to N-acylethanolamine-hydrolyzing acid amidase (NAAA). Prog Lipid Res 2010;49:299-315.

[51] Yu M, Ives D, Ramesha CS. Synthesis of prostaglandin E2 ethanolamide from anandamide by cyclooxygenase-2. J Biol Chem 1997;272:21181-6.

[52] Ueda N, Yamamoto K, Yamamoto S, *et al*. Lipoxygenase-catalyzed oxygenation of arachidonylethanolamide, a cannabinoid receptor agonist. Biochim Biophys Acta 1995;1254:127-34.

[53] Bornheim LM, Kim KY, Chen B, Correia MA. The effect of cannabidiol on mouse hepatic microsomal cytochrome P450-dependent anandamide metabolism. Biochem Biophys Res Commun 1993;197:740-6.

[54]   Pan B, Hillard CJ, Liu QS. Endocannabinoid signaling mediates cocaine-induced inhibitory synaptic plasticity in midbrain dopamine neurons. J Neurosci 2008;28:1385-97.

[55]   Pan B, Hillard CJ, Liu QS. D2 dopamine receptor activation facilitates endocannabinoid-mediated long-term synaptic depression of GABAergic synaptic transmission in midbrain dopamine neurons *via* cAMP-protein kinase A signaling. J Neurosci 2008;28:14018-30.

[56]   Seif T, Makriyannis A, Kunos G, Bonci A, Hopf FW. The endocannabinoid 2-arachidonoylglycerol mediates D1 and D2 receptor cooperative enhancement of rat nucleus accumbens core neuron firing. Neuroscience 2011;193:21-33.

[57]   Grace AA, Bunney BS. Intracellular and extracellular electrophysiology of nigral dopaminergic neurons--1. Identification and characterization. Neuroscience 1983;10:301-15.

[58]   Gonon FG. Nonlinear relationship between impulse flow and dopamine released by rat midbrain dopaminergic neurons as studied by *in vivo* electrochemistry. Neuroscience 1988;24:19-28.

[59]   Marinelli M, Rudick CN, Hu XT, White FJ. Excitability of dopamine neurons: modulation and physiological consequences. CNS & neurological disorders drug targets. 2006;5:79-97.

[60]   Morikawa H, Paladini CA. Dynamic regulation of midbrain dopamine neuron activity: intrinsic, synaptic, and plasticity mechanisms. Neuroscience 2011;198:95-111.

[61]   Geisler S, Derst C, Veh RW, Zahm DS. Glutamatergic afferents of the ventral tegmental area in the rat. J Neurosci 2007;27:5730-43.

[62]   Maskos U. The cholinergic mesopontine tegmentum is a relatively neglected nicotinic master modulator of the dopaminergic system: relevance to drugs of abuse and pathology. Br J Pharmacol 2008;153 Suppl 1:S438-45.

[63]   Meltzer LT, Christoffersen CL, Serpa KA. Modulation of dopamine neuronal activity by glutamate receptor subtypes. Neurosci Biobehav Rev 1997;21:511-8.

[64]   Overton P, Clark D. Iontophoretically administered drugs acting at the N-methyl-D-aspartate receptor modulate burst firing in A9 dopamine neurons in the rat. Synapse 1992;10:131-40.

[65]   Suaud-Chagny MF, Chergui K, Chouvet G, Gonon F. Relationship between dopamine release in the rat nucleus accumbens and the discharge activity of dopaminergic neurons during local *in vivo* application of amino acids in the ventral tegmental area. Neuroscience 1992;49:63-72.

[66]   Erhardt S, Mathe JM, Chergui K, Engberg G, Svensson TH. GABA(B) receptor-mediated modulation of the firing pattern of ventral tegmental area dopamine neurons *in vivo*. Naunyn Schmiedebergs Arch Pharmacol 2002;365:173-80.

[67]   Schultz W. Getting formal with dopamine and reward. Neuron. 2002;36:241-63.

[68]   Schultz W. Behavioral theories and the neurophysiology of reward. Annu Rev Psychol 2006;57:87-115.

[69]   Schultz W, Dickinson A. Neuronal coding of prediction errors. Annu Rev Neurosci 2000;23:473-500.

[70]   Laviolette SR, Grace AA. The roles of cannabinoid and dopamine receptor systems in neural emotional learning circuits: implications for schizophrenia and addiction. Cell Mol Life Sci 2006;63:1597-613.

[71]   Green B, Kavanagh D, Young R. Being stoned: a review of self-reported cannabis effects. Drug Alcohol Rev 2003;22:453-60.

[72] Wachtel SR, ElSohly MA, Ross SA, Ambre J, de Wit H. Comparison of the subjective effects of Delta(9)-tetrahydrocannabinol and marijuana in humans. Psychopharmacology (Berl) 2002;161:331-9.

[73] Egerton A, Allison C, Brett RR, Pratt JA. Cannabinoids and prefrontal cortical function: insights from preclinical studies. Neurosci Biobehav Rev 2006;30:680-95.

[74] Pava MJ, Woodward JJ. A review of the interactions between alcohol and the endocannabinoid system: implications for alcohol dependence and future directions for research. Alcohol 2012;46:185-204.

[75] Basavarajappa BS, Ninan I, Arancio O. Acute ethanol suppresses glutamatergic neurotransmission through endocannabinoids in hippocampal neurons. J Neurochem 2008;107:1001-13.

[76] Basavarajappa BS, Hungund BL. Chronic ethanol increases the cannabinoid receptor agonist anandamide and its precursor N-arachidonoylphosphatidylethanolamine in SK-N-SH cells. J Neurochem 1999;72:522-8.

[77] Basavarajappa BS, Saito M, Cooper TB, Hungund BL. Stimulation of cannabinoid receptor agonist 2-arachidonylglycerol by chronic ethanol and its modulation by specific neuromodulators in cerebellar granule neurons. Biochim Biophys Acta 2000;1535:78-86.

[78] Basavarajappa BS, Hungund BL. Down-regulation of cannabinoid receptor agonist-stimulated [35S]GTP gamma S binding in synaptic plasma membrane from chronic ethanol exposed mouse. Brain Res 1999;815:89-97.

[79] Ortiz S, Oliva JM, Perez-Rial S, Palomo T, Manzanares J. Differences in basal cannabinoid CB1 receptor function in selective brain areas and vulnerability to voluntary alcohol consumption in Fawn Hooded and Wistar rats. Alcohol Alcohol 2004;39:297-302.

[80] Colombo G, Agabio R, Fa M, et al. Reduction of voluntary ethanol intake in ethanol-preferring sP rats by the cannabinoid antagonist SR-141716. Alcohol Alcohol 1998;33:126-30.

[81] Arnone M, Maruani J, Chaperon F, et al. Selective inhibition of sucrose and ethanol intake by SR 141716, an antagonist of central cannabinoid (CB1) receptors. Psychopharmacology (Berl) 1997;132:104-6.

[82] Gallate JE, McGregor IS. The motivation for beer in rats: effects of ritanserin, naloxone and SR 141716. Psychopharmacology (Berl) 1999;142:302-8.

[83] Gallate JE, Mallet PE, McGregor IS. Combined low dose treatment with opioid and cannabinoid receptor antagonists synergistically reduces the motivation to consume alcohol in rats. Psychopharmacology (Berl) 2004;173:210-6.

[84] Naassila M, Pierrefiche O, Ledent C, Daoust M. Decreased alcohol self-administration and increased alcohol sensitivity and withdrawal in CB1 receptor knockout mice. Neuropharmacology 2004;46:243-53.

[85] Poncelet M, Maruani J, Calassi R, Soubrie P. Overeating, alcohol and sucrose consumption decrease in CB1 receptor deleted mice. Neurosci Lett 2003;343:216-8.

[86] Hungund BL, Szakall I, Adam A, Basavarajappa BS, Vadasz C. Cannabinoid CB1 receptor knockout mice exhibit markedly reduced voluntary alcohol consumption and lack alcohol-induced dopamine release in the nucleus accumbens. J Neurochem 2003;84:698-704.

[87] Houchi H, Babovic D, Pierrefiche O, et al. CB1 receptor knockout mice display reduced ethanol-induced conditioned place preference and increased striatal dopamine D2 receptors. Neuropsychopharmacology 2005;30:339-49.

[88]   Perra S, Pillolla G, Luchicchi A, Pistis M. Alcohol inhibits spontaneous activity of basolateral amygdala projection neurons in the rat: involvement of the endocannabinoid system. Alcohol Clin Exp Res 2008;32:443-9.

[89]   Perra S, Pillolla G, Melis M, *et al*. Involvement of the endogenous cannabinoid system in the effects of alcohol in the mesolimbic reward circuit: electrophysiological evidence *in vivo*. Psychopharmacology (Berl) 2005;183:368-77.

[90]   Cheer JF, Wassum KM, Sombers LA, *et al*. Phasic Dopamine Release Evoked by Abused Substances Requires Cannabinoid Receptor Activation. J Neurosci 2007;27:791-5.

[91]   Ferrer B, Bermudez-Silva FJ, Bilbao A, *et al*. Regulation of brain anandamide by acute administration of ethanol. Biochem J 2007;404:97-104.

[92]   Rubio M, McHugh D, Fernandez-Ruiz J, Bradshaw H, Walker JM. Short-term exposure to alcohol in rats affects brain levels of anandamide, other N-acylethanolamines and 2-arachidonoyl-glycerol. Neurosci Lett 2007;421:270-4.

[93]   Gonzalez S, Cascio MG, Fernandez-Ruiz J, *et al*. Changes in endocannabinoid contents in the brain of rats chronically exposed to nicotine, ethanol or cocaine. Brain Res 2002;954:73-81.

[94]   Serrano A, Rivera P, Pavon FJ, *et al*. Differential Effects of Single *Versus* Repeated Alcohol Withdrawal on the Expression of Endocannabinoid System-Related Genes in the Rat Amygdala. Alcohol Clin Exp Res 2011.

[95]   Blednov YA, Harris RA. Deletion of vanilloid receptor (TRPV1) in mice alters behavioral effects of ethanol. Neuropharmacology 2009;56:814-20.

[96]   Cippitelli A, Bilbao A, Gorriti MA, *et al*. The anandamide transport inhibitor AM404 reduces ethanol self-administration. Eur J Neurosci 2007;26:476-86.

[97]   Fu J, Bottegoni G, Sasso O, *et al*. A catalytically silent FAAH-1 variant drives anandamide transport in neurons. Nature neuroscience 2012;15:64-9.

[98]   Caille S, Alvarez-Jaimes L, Polis I, Stouffer DG, Parsons LH. Specific Alterations of Extracellular Endocannabinoid Levels in the Nucleus Accumbens by Ethanol, Heroin, and Cocaine Self-Administration. J Neurosci 2007;27:3695-702.

[99]   Gutierrez-Lopez MD, Llopis N, Feng S, *et al*. Involvement of 2-arachidonoyl glycerol in the increased consumption of and preference for ethanol of mice treated with neurotoxic doses of methamphetamine. Br J Pharmacol 2010;160:772-83.

[100]   Malinen H, Lehtonen M, Hyytia P. Modulation of brain endocannabinoid levels by voluntary alcohol consumption in alcohol-preferring AA rats. Alcohol Clin Exp Res 2009;33:1711-20.

[101]   Viveros MP, Marco EM, File SE. Nicotine and cannabinoids: parallels, contrasts and interactions. Neurosci Biobehav Rev 2006;30:1161-81.

[102]   Castane A, Berrendero F, Maldonado R. The role of the cannabinoid system in nicotine addiction. Pharmacol Biochem Behav 2005;81:381-6.

[103]   Scherma M, Fadda P, Le Foll B, *et al*. The endocannabinoid system: a new molecular target for the treatment of tobacco addiction. CNS & neurological disorders drug targets 2008;7:468-81.

[104]   Maldonado R, Berrendero F. Endogenous cannabinoid and opioid systems and their role in nicotine addiction. Curr Drug Targets 2010;11:440-9.

[105]   Serrano A, Parsons LH. Endocannabinoid influence in drug reinforcement, dependence and addiction-related behaviors. Pharmacol Ther 2011;132:215-41.

[106] Picciotto MR, Caldarone BJ, King SL, Zachariou V. Nicotinic receptors in the brain. Links between molecular biology and behavior. Neuropsychopharmacology 2000;22:451-65.

[107] Cippitelli A, Astarita G, Duranti A, *et al*. Endocannabinoid regulation of acute and protracted nicotine withdrawal: effect of FAAH inhibition. PLoS One 2011;6:e28142.

[108] Buczynski MW, Polis IY, Parsons LH. The Volitional Nature of Nicotine Exposure Alters Anandamide and Oleoylethanolamide Levels in the Ventral Tegmental Area. Neuropsychopharmacology 2012.

[109] Pryor GT, Larsen FF, Husain S, Braude MC. Interactions of delta9-tetrahydrocannabinol with d-amphetamine, cocaine, and nicotine in rats. Pharmacol Biochem Behav 1978;8:295-318.

[110] Valjent E, Mitchell JM, Besson MJ, Caboche J, Maldonado R. Behavioural and biochemical evidence for interactions between Delta 9-tetrahydrocannabinol and nicotine. Br J Pharmacol 2002;135:564-78.

[111] Balerio GN, Aso E, Berrendero F, Murtra P, Maldonado R. Delta9-tetrahydrocannabinol decreases somatic and motivational manifestations of nicotine withdrawal in mice. Eur J Neurosci 2004;20:2737-48.

[112] Balerio GN, Aso E, Maldonado R. Role of the cannabinoid system in the effects induced by nicotine on anxiety-like behaviour in mice. Psychopharmacology 2006;184:504-13.

[113] Gamaleddin I, Wertheim C, Zhu AZ, *et al*. Cannabinoid receptor stimulation increases motivation for nicotine and nicotine seeking. Addict Biol 2012;17:47-61.

[114] Marco EM, Granstrem O, Moreno E, *et al*. Subchronic nicotine exposure in adolescence induces long-term effects on hippocampal and striatal cannabinoid-CB1 and mu-opioid receptors in rats. Eur J Pharmacol 2007;557:37-43.

[115] Werling LL, Reed SC, Wade D, Izenwasser S. Chronic nicotine alters cannabinoid-mediated locomotor activity and receptor density in periadolescent but not adult male rats. Int J Dev Neurosci 2009;27:263-9.

[116] Gerard N, Ceccarini J, Bormans G, *et al*. Influence of chronic nicotine administration on cerebral type 1 cannabinoid receptor binding: an *in vivo* micro-PET study in the rat using [18F]MK-9470. J Mol Neurosci 2010;42:162-7.

[117] Castane A, Valjent E, Ledent C, *et al*. Lack of CB1 cannabinoid receptors modifies nicotine behavioural responses, but not nicotine abstinence. Neuropharmacology 2002;43:857-67.

[118] Merritt LL, Martin BR, Walters C, Lichtman AH, Damaj MI. The Endogenous Cannabinoid System Modulates Nicotine Reward and Dependence. J Pharmacol Exp Ther 2008;326:483-92.

[119] Cossu G, Ledent C, Fattore L, *et al*. Cannabinoid CB1 receptor knockout mice fail to self-administer morphine but not other drugs of abuse. Behav Brain Res 2001;118:61-5.

[120] Chen X, Williamson VS, An SS, *et al*. Cannabinoid receptor 1 gene association with nicotine dependence. Arch Gen Psychiatry 2008;65:816-24.

[121] Lopez-Moreno JA, Echeverry-Alzate V, Buhler KM. The genetic basis of the endocannabinoid system and drug addiction in humans. J Psychopharmacol 2012;26:133-43.

[122] Le Foll B, Forget B, Aubin HJ, Goldberg SR. Blocking cannabinoid CB1 receptors for the treatment of nicotine dependence: insights from pre-clinical and clinical studies. Addict Biol 2008;13:239-52.

[123] Forget B, Hamon M, Thiebot MH. Cannabinoid CB1 receptors are involved in motivational effects of nicotine in rats. Psychopharmacology (Berl) 2005;181:722-34.

[124] Le Foll B, Goldberg SR. Rimonabant, a CB1 antagonist, blocks nicotine-conditioned place preferences. Neuroreport 2004;15:2139-43.

[125] Wing VC, Shoaib M. Second-order schedules of nicotine reinforcement in rats: effect of AM251. Addict Biol 2010;15:393-402.

[126] Cohen C, Perrault G, Griebel G, Soubrie P. Nicotine-associated cues maintain nicotine-seeking behavior in rats several weeks after nicotine withdrawal: reversal by the cannabinoid (CB1) receptor antagonist, rimonabant (SR141716). Neuropsychopharmacology 2005;30:145-55.

[127] Cohen C, Perrault G, Voltz C, Steinberg R, Soubrie P. SR141716, a central cannabinoid (CB(1)) receptor antagonist, blocks the motivational and dopamine-releasing effects of nicotine in rats. Behav Pharmacol 2002;13:451-63.

[128] Forget B, Coen KM, Le Foll B. Inhibition of fatty acid amide hydrolase reduces reinstatement of nicotine seeking but not break point for nicotine self-administration--comparison with CB(1) receptor blockade. Psychopharmacology 2009;205:613-24.

[129] Shoaib M. The cannabinoid antagonist AM251 attenuates nicotine self-administration and nicotine-seeking behaviour in rats. Neuropharmacology 2008;54:438-44.

[130] Cahill K, Ussher M. Cannabinoid type 1 receptor antagonists (rimonabant) for smoking cessation. Cochrane Database Syst Rev 2007:CD005353.

[131] Morrison MF, Ceesay P, Gantz I, Kaufman KD, Lines CR. Randomized, controlled, double-blind trial of taranabant for smoking cessation. Psychopharmacology 2010;209:245-53.

[132] Meye FJ, Trezza V, Vanderschuren LJ, Ramakers GM, Adan RA. Neutral antagonism at the cannabinoid 1 receptor: a safer treatment for obesity. Mol Psychiatry 2012.

[133] Janero DR. Cannabinoid-1 receptor (CB1R) blockers as medicines: beyond obesity and cardiometabolic disorders to substance abuse/drug addiction with CB1R neutral antagonists. Expert opinion on emerging drugs 2012;17:17-29.

[134] Simonnet A, Cador M, Caille S. Nicotine reinforcement is reduced by cannabinoid CB1 receptor blockade in the ventral tegmental area. Addict Biol 2012.

[135] Scherma M, Justinova Z, Zanettini C, *et al*. The anandamide transport inhibitor AM404 reduces the rewarding effects of nicotine and nicotine-induced dopamine elevations in the nucleus accumbens shell in rats. Br J Pharmacol 2012;165:2539-48.

[136] Gamaleddin I, Guranda M, Goldberg SR, Le Foll B. The selective anandamide transport inhibitor VDM11 attenuates reinstatement of nicotine seeking behaviour, but does not affect nicotine intake. Br J Pharmacol 2011;164:1652-60.

[137] Robledo P, Berrendero F, Ozaita A, Maldonado R. Advances in the field of cannabinoid--opioid cross-talk. Addict Biol 2008;13:213-24.

[138] Vigano D, Rubino T, Parolaro D. Molecular and cellular basis of cannabinoid and opioid interactions. Pharmacol Biochem Behav 2005;81:360-8.

[139] Fattore L, Deiana S, Spano SM, *et al*. Endocannabinoid system and opioid addiction: behavioural aspects. Pharmacology, biochemistry, and behavior 2005;81:343-59.

[140] Rubino T, Tizzoni L, Vigano D, Massi P, Parolaro D. Modulation of rat brain cannabinoid receptors after chronic morphine treatment. Neuroreport 1997;8:3219-23.

[141] Gonzalez S, Schmid PC, Fernandez-Ruiz J, *et al*. Region-dependent changes in endocannabinoid transmission in the brain of morphine-dependent rats. Addict Biol 2003;8:159-66.

[142] Gonzalez S, Fernandez-Ruiz J, Sparpaglione V, Parolaro D, Ramos JA. Chronic exposure to morphine, cocaine or ethanol in rats produced different effects in brain cannabinoid CB(1) receptor binding and mRNA levels. Drug Alcohol Depend 2002;66:77-84.

[143] Romero J, Fernandez-Ruiz JJ, Vela G, et al. Autoradiographic analysis of cannabinoid receptor binding and cannabinoid agonist-stimulated [35S]GTP gamma S binding in morphine-dependent mice. Drug Alcohol Depend 1998;50:241-9.

[144] Sim-Selley LJ, Selley DE, Vogt LJ, Childers SR, Martin TJ. Chronic heroin self-administration desensitizes mu opioid receptor-activated G-proteins in specific regions of rat brain. J Neurosci 2000;20:4555-62.

[145] Vigano D, Valenti M, Cascio MG, et al. Changes in endocannabinoid levels in a rat model of behavioural sensitization to morphine. Eur J Neurosci 2004;20:1849-57.

[146] Vigano D, Grazia Cascio M, Rubino T, et al. Chronic morphine modulates the contents of the endocannabinoid, 2-arachidonoyl glycerol, in rat brain. Neuropsychopharmacology 2003;28:1160-7.

[147] Steketee JD, Kalivas PW. Drug wanting: behavioral sensitization and relapse to drug-seeking behavior. Pharmacol Rev 2011;63:348-65.

[148] Diana M, Muntoni AL, Pistis M, Melis M, Gessa GL. Lasting reduction in mesolimbic dopamine neuronal activity after morphine withdrawal. Eur J Neurosci 1999;11:1037-41.

[149] Del Arco I, Navarro M, Bilbao A, et al. Attenuation of spontaneous opiate withdrawal in mice by the anandamide transport inhibitor AM404. Eur J Pharmacol 2002;454:103-4.

[150] Ledent C, Valverde O, Cossu G, et al. Unresponsiveness to cannabinoids and reduced addictive effects of opiates in CB1 receptor knockout mice. Science 1999;283:401-4.

[151] Caille S, Parsons LH. Cannabinoid modulation of opiate reinforcement through the ventral striatopallidal pathway. Neuropsychopharmacology 2006;31:804-13.

[152] Caille S, Parsons LH. SR141716A reduces the reinforcing properties of heroin but not heroin-induced increases in nucleus accumbens dopamine in rats. Eur J Neurosci 2003;18:3145-9.

[153] Solinas M, Panlilio LV, Antoniou K, Pappas LA, Goldberg SR. The cannabinoid CB1 antagonist N-piperidinyl-5-(4-chlorophenyl)-1-(2,4-dichlorophenyl) -4-methylpyrazole-3-carboxamide (SR-141716A) differentially alters the reinforcing effects of heroin under continuous reinforcement, fixed ratio, and progressive ratio schedules of drug self-administration in rats. J Pharmacol Exp Ther 2003;306:93-102.

[154] Wiskerke J, Pattij T, Schoffelmeer AN, De Vries TJ. The role of CB1 receptors in psychostimulant addiction. Addict Biol 2008;13:225-38.

[155] Martin M, Ledent C, Parmentier M, Maldonado R, Valverde O. Cocaine, but not morphine, induces conditioned place preference and sensitization to locomotor responses in CB1 knockout mice. Eur J Neurosci 2000;12:4038-46.

[156] Lesscher HM, Hoogveld E, Burbach JP, van Ree JM, Gerrits MA. Endogenous cannabinoids are not involved in cocaine reinforcement and development of cocaine-induced behavioural sensitization. Eur Neuropsychopharmacol 2005;15:31-7.

[157] Xi ZX, Spiller K, Pak AC, et al. Cannabinoid CB1 receptor antagonists attenuate cocaine's rewarding effects: experiments with self-administration and brain-stimulation reward in rats. Neuropsychopharmacology 2008;33:1735-45.

[158] Soria G, Mendizabal V, Tourino C, et al. Lack of CB1 cannabinoid receptor impairs cocaine self-administration. Neuropsychopharmacology 2005;30:1670-80.

[159] Corbille AG, Valjent E, Marsicano G, *et al.* Role of cannabinoid type 1 receptors in locomotor activity and striatal signaling in response to psychostimulants. J Neurosci 2007;27:6937-47.

[160] Orio L, Edwards S, George O, Parsons LH, Koob GF. A role for the endocannabinoid system in the increased motivation for cocaine in extended-access conditions. J Neurosci 2009;29:4846-57.

[161] De Vries TJ, Shaham Y, Homberg JR, *et al.* A cannabinoid mechanism in relapse to cocaine seeking. Nat Med 2001;7:1151-4.

[162] Xi ZX, Gilbert JG, Peng XQ, *et al.* Cannabinoid CB1 receptor antagonist AM251 inhibits cocaine-primed relapse in rats: role of glutamate in the nucleus accumbens. J Neurosci 2006;26:8531-6.

[163] Filip M, Golda A, Zaniewska M, *et al.* Involvement of cannabinoid CB1 receptors in drug addiction: effects of rimonabant on behavioral responses induced by cocaine. Pharmacol Rep 2006;58:806-19.

[164] Adamczyk P, McCreary AC, Przegalinski E, *et al.* The effects of fatty acid amide hydrolase inhibitors on maintenance of cocaine and food self-administration and on reinstatement of cocaine-seeking and food-taking behavior in rats. J Physiol Pharmacol 2009;60:119-25.

[165] Adamczyk P, Miszkiel J, McCreary AC, *et al.* The effects of cannabinoid CB1, CB2 and vanilloid TRPV1 receptor antagonists on cocaine addictive behavior in rats. Brain Res 2012;1444:45-54.

[166] Pilla M, Perachon S, Sautel F, *et al.* Selective inhibition of cocaine-seeking behaviour by a partial dopamine D3 receptor agonist. Nature 1999;400:371-5.

[167] Grimm JW, See RE. Dissociation of primary and secondary reward-relevant limbic nuclei in an animal model of relapse. Neuropsychopharmacology 2000;22:473-9.

[168] McFarland K, Davidge SB, Lapish CC, Kalivas PW. Limbic and motor circuitry underlying footshock-induced reinstatement of cocaine-seeking behavior. J Neurosci 2004;24:1551-60.

[169] Shaham Y, Shalev U, Lu L, De Wit H, Stewart J. The reinstatement model of drug relapse: history, methodology and major findings. Psychopharmacology (Berl) 2003;168:3-20.

[170] Schmidt HD, Anderson SM, Famous KR, Kumaresan V, Pierce RC. Anatomy and pharmacology of cocaine priming-induced reinstatement of drug seeking. Eur J Pharmacol 2005;526:65-76.

[171] See RE. Neural substrates of conditioned-cued relapse to drug-seeking behavior. Pharmacol Biochem Behav 2002;71:517-29.

[172] Braida D, Sala M. Role of the endocannabinoid system in MDMA intracerebral self-administration in rats. Br J Pharmacol 2002;136:1089-92.

[173] Braida D, Iosue S, Pegorini S, Sala M. 3,4 Methylenedioxymethamphetamine-induced conditioned place preference (CPP) is mediated by endocannabinoid system. Pharmacol Res 2005;51:177-82.

[174] Tourino C, Ledent C, Maldonado R, Valverde O. CB1 cannabinoid receptor modulates 3,4-methylenedioxymethamphetamine acute responses and reinforcement. Biol Psychiatry 2008;63:1030-8.

[175] Anggadiredja K, Nakamichi M, Hiranita T, *et al.* Endocannabinoid system modulates relapse to methamphetamine seeking: possible mediation by the arachidonic acid cascade. Neuropsychopharmacology 2004;29:1470-8.

[176] Vinklerova J, Novakova J, Sulcova A. Inhibition of methamphetamine self-administration in rats by cannabinoid receptor antagonist AM 251. J Psychopharmacol 2002;16:139-43.

[177] Rodriguez JS, Boctor SY, Flores LC, Phelix CF, Martinez JL, Jr. Local pretreatment with the cannabinoid CB1 receptor antagonist AM251 attenuates methamphetamine intra-accumbens self-administration. Neurosci Lett 2011;489:187-91.

[178] Thiemann G, Di Marzo V, Molleman A, Hasenohrl RU. The CB(1) cannabinoid receptor antagonist AM251 attenuates amphetamine-induced behavioural sensitization while causing monoamine changes in nucleus accumbens and hippocampus. Pharmacol Biochem Behav 2008;89:384-91.

[179] Pan B, Zhong P, Sun D, Liu QS. Extracellular signal-regulated kinase signaling in the ventral tegmental area mediates cocaine-induced synaptic plasticity and rewarding effects. J Neurosci 2011;31:11244-55.

[180] Haj-Dahmane S, Shen RY. Regulation of plasticity of glutamate synapses by endocannabinoids and the cyclic-AMP/protein kinase A pathway in midbrain dopamine neurons. J Physiol 2010;588:2589-604.

[181] Le Foll B, Goldberg SR. Cannabinoid CB1 receptor antagonists as promising new medications for drug dependence. J Pharmacol Exp Ther 2005;312:875-83.

[182] Schindler CW, Panlilio LV, Gilman JP, et al. Effects of cannabinoid receptor antagonists on maintenance and reinstatement of methamphetamine self-administration in rhesus monkeys. Eur J Pharmacol 2011;633:44-9.

[183] Yu LL, Zhou SJ, Wang XY, et al. Effects of cannabinoid CB receptor antagonist rimonabant on acquisition and reinstatement of psychostimulant reward memory in mice. Behav Brain Res 2011;217:111-6.

[184] Ward SJ, Rosenberg M, Dykstra LA, Walker EA. The CB1 antagonist rimonabant (SR141716) blocks cue-induced reinstatement of cocaine seeking and other context and extinction phenomena predictive of relapse. Drug Alcohol Depend 2009;105:248-55.

[185] Fattore L, Spano M, Melis V, Fadda P, Fratta W. Differential effect of opioid and cannabinoid receptor blockade on heroin-seeking reinstatement and cannabinoid substitution in heroin-abstinent rats. Br J Pharmacol 2011;163:1550-62.

[186] Fattore L, Spano MS, Cossu G, Deiana S, Fratta W. Cannabinoid mechanism in reinstatement of heroin-seeking after a long period of abstinence in rats. Eur J Neurosci 2003;17:1723-6.

[187] Fattore L, Spano S, Cossu G, et al. Cannabinoid CB(1) antagonist SR 141716A attenuates reinstatement of heroin self-administration in heroin-abstinent rats. Neuropharmacology 2005;48:1097-104.

[188] Justinova Z, Mangieri RA, Bortolato M, et al. Fatty acid amide hydrolase inhibition heightens anandamide signaling without producing reinforcing effects in primates. Biol Psychiatry 2008;64:930-7.

[189] Lancaster T, Stead L, Cahill K. An update on therapeutics for tobacco dependence. Expert Opin Pharmacother 2008;9:15-22.

[190] Cohen C, Kodas E, Griebel G. CB1 receptor antagonists for the treatment of nicotine addiction. Pharmacol Biochem Behav 2005;81:387-95.

[191] Carai MA, Colombo G, Gessa GL. Rimonabant: the first therapeutically relevant cannabinoid antagonist. Life Sci 2005;77:2339-50.

[192] Christensen R, Kristensen PK, Bartels EM, Bliddal H, Astrup A. Efficacy and safety of the weight-loss drug rimonabant: a meta-analysis of randomised trials. Lancet 2007;370:1706-13.

[193] Horder J, Harmer CJ, Cowen PJ, McCabe C. Reduced neural response to reward following 7 days treatment with the cannabinoid CB1 antagonist rimonabant in healthy volunteers. Int J Neuropsychopharmacol 2010;13:1103-13.

[194] Melis M, Carta G, Pistis M, Banni S. Physiological Role of Peroxisome Proliferator-Activated Receptors Type Alpha on Dopamine Systems. CNS & Neurological Disorders - Drug Targets 2012:in press.

[195] Bortolato M, Campolongo P, Mangieri RA, *et al.* Anxiolytic-like properties of the anandamide transport inhibitor AM404. Neuropsychopharmacology 2006;31:2652-9.

Send Orders for Reprints at reprints@benthamscience.net

CHAPTER 6

The Development of Cannabinoid Based Therapies for Epilepsy

Andrew J. Hill, Thomas D.M. Hill and Benjamin J. Whalley[*]

The School of Chemistry, Food and Nutritional Sciences and Pharmacy, The University of Reading, Whiteknights, Reading, Berkshire, RG53SA, UK

Abstract: Epilepsy is a chronic, progressive, neurological disorder affecting ~0.5-1% of the population for which there is no cure. Furthermore, efficacious seizure suppression is yet to be achieved for all patients; ~35% of people with epilepsy (PWE) have seizures pharmacoresistant to existing drugs. In this regard, the endocannabinoid system (ECS) is an attractive therapeutic target as it can limit synaptic transmission to oppose hyperexcitability in addition to central cannabinoid type-2 receptor (CB2R) modulation potentially limiting neuronal death associated with epilepsy. Postsynaptic endocannabinoid (eCB) synthesis is stimulated by excitatory neurotransmission, eCBs then act retrogradely *via* presynaptic cannabinoid type-1 receptors (CB1R) to suppress subsequent excitatory (glutamatergic) and inhibitory (GABAergic) synaptic activity close to the synthetic locus. Thus, eCBs can limit excessive excitation but also hinder inhibitory processes such that their effects on epileptic foci and the spread of seizure activity is dependent on the relative proportions of excitatory and inhibitory synapses, and their organisation into local and global circuits within the CNS. Cannabis has a history of antiepileptic use that continues to the present day in medical marijuana programmes, and CB1R receptor agonism, either by medical marijuana, pure Δ^9-tetrahydrocannabinol (Δ^9-THC) or synthetic CB1R ligands, can be anticonvulsant in humans and in *in vitro* and *in vivo* seizure models, but paradoxically can cause seizures in healthy rodents. Furthermore, it is clear that other cannabis constituents are anti-epileptic, and, whilst the mechanisms by which they act remain undetermined, they certainly extend beyond ECS modulation. Moreover, whilst CB1R agonism can control seizures in some patients and many animal seizure models, it is unlikely to represent a widely exploitable target for seizure control due to its psychoactive sequelae. Conversely, many non-Δ^9-THC plant cannabinoids are inactive at CB1R or CB2R at therapeutically relevant concentrations and a subset of these (*e.g.* cannabidiol) exert significant anticonvulsant effects in numerous animal models of seizure at clinically promising doses.

Keywords: Cannabis, endocannabinoids, epilepsy, seizures, tetrahydrocannabinol, cannabidiol, cannabidavarin, tetrahydrocannabivarin, drug resistance, 2-arachidonoyl glycerol, anandamide, hyperexcitability, pharmacology, marijuana.

---

[*]**Address correspondence to Benjamin J. Whalley:** The School of Chemistry, Food and Nutritional Sciences and Pharmacy, The University of Reading, Whiteknights, Reading, Berkshire, RG6 6AP, UK; Tel: +44 (0) 118 378 4745; Mob: +44 (0) 797 424 9607; Fax: +44 (0) 118 378 4703; E-mail: b.j.whalley@reading.ac.uk

Eric Murillo-Rodríguez, Emmanuel S. Onaivi, Nissar A. Darmani & Edward Wagner (Eds.)

INTRODUCTION

Epilepsy is a chronic neurological disorder characterised by spontaneous recurrent high-frequency synchronous electrical discharges in the brain that manifest as periodic seizures [1]. Seizures, defined as abnormal electrical activity in the brain, are often symptomatically characterised by convulsions, but are not necessarily defined by their presence (*i.e.* non-convulsive epileptic episodes result in seizures, but not convulsions [2]). It is also possible to have convulsions without seizures (*e.g.* motor tics in Tourette syndrome [3]).

The word epilepsy is derived from the Greek meaning to be seized or attacked, as historically, it was believed that supernatural forces attacked a person due to their misdeeds; some ancient civilisations believed that seizures arose from demonic possession. Fortunately, societal and clinical views of epilepsy have changed over the centuries where Hippocrates was first credited with indicating that epilepsy was a disease of the brain, not a result of possession [4]. In the early 19th century, epilepsy was considered a psychiatric disorder and people were treated for epilepsy in psychiatric units. By the 1850s epilepsy was redefined as a neurological disease although it was still considered to be a psychiatric illness [5]. Epilepsy is no longer regarded as a psychiatric illness but rather as a chronic neurological condition [6].

It is estimated that there are >50 million people with epilepsy (PWE) worldwide [7, 8] which equates to ~0.7% of the world's population and 0.5% of the total disease burden [9]. However the incidence of epilepsy is not evenly distributed throughout the population, with increased incidence in people aged <20 or >60 years [10], as well as people in developing countries [9, 10]. The greater incidence in developing countries, combined with the lack of resources available for treatments, produces 90% of the epilepsy disease burden [11], this is largely a result of 90% of PWE in Africa not receiving appropriate treatment (according to Margaret Chan, the Director General of WHO, News release WHO/4 27/01/2007) [12]. In addition, the widespread use of phenobarbital as an anti-epileptic drug (AED) in developing countries which causes cognitive deficits, dependency and thus an increase in care requirements [13, 14].

The process by which non-idiopathic epileptic syndromes manifest typically follows a three stage process; an initial insult begins the process (*e.g.* traumatic brain injury, CNS infection) which is then followed by a symptomatically and behaviourally latent period before the onset of seizures, the principal symptom [15]. During the apparent latent period a process termed epileptogenesis occurs, which is characterised by the reorganisation of neurons and results in discord between GABAergic inhibition and glutamatergic excitability, creating a brain that is hyperexcitable and prone to seizures [15]. At the time of writing, there are no drugs available that either retard or prevent epileptogenesis although many currently available AEDs have been examined in this regard as they are known to reduce excitotoxicity [16], which may be beneficial. Whilst is has been postulated that neuroprotective drugs are likely to represent the best candidates to prevent epileptogenesis, any drug showing antiepileptogenetic efficacy would represent a highly desirable 'first in class' [15, 17]. Such drugs could be given prophylactically following an event that is likely to cause epilepsy, if they do not have a severe side effect profile.

In 1981, the International League Against Epilepsy (ILAE) proposed a classification scheme for epileptic seizures with the intent to unify internationally disparate classification systems and so enable clinicians to better understand and treat epilepsy and its many complicated facets. Here, seizures were placed in two broad categories: generalised seizures where epileptiform activity occurs in both brain hemispheres and partial seizures which involve a discrete brain region. It is notable that partial seizures can spread ("generalise") across the whole brain in a process known as secondary generalisation. Partial seizures were further subcategorised into complex, characterised by a total or partial loss of consciousness, and simple, where there is no loss in consciousness. In this context consciousness was defined as the individual being fully aware of his surroundings and responsive to external stimuli [18].

Generalised seizures were also subcategorised to distinguish between convulsive and nonconvulsive epilepsies. Convulsive epilepsies include myoclonic (contraction of a specific body region or muscle group), tonic (tetanoid symptoms) and clonic (rhythmic contraction of all muscles) convulsions, with tonic and clonic convulsions accompanied by unconsciousness. Some epilepsies exhibit tonic-clonic convulsions where the individual first enters the tonic phase, which is soon followed by the clonic phase (formerly known as 'grand mal' seizures). Nonconvulsive seizures are not associated with visible convulsions, however EEG recordings show epileptiform activity and include absence seizures and atypical absence seizures [18].

In 1989, the ILAE recognised that epilepsy is too complex a disease state to be classified solely by convulsion type alone and led to a new classification system based on the totality of the disease rather than solely by seizure type. The initial classification into generalised and partial seizure types remained although the epilepsies were aetiologically defined further into three different major classes: idiopathic, symptomatic and cryptogenic [19]. Idiopathic epilepsies exhibit no underlying cause other than a familial or genetic predisposition, often manifest in childhood with a natural regression in later life and are frequently pharmacologically tractable; as a result, they are often erroneously thought to be benign [17]. Symptomatic epilepsies arise from a known structural or functional abnormality, whilst the cryptogenic epilepsies are defined by the absence of an obvious genetic or functional abnormality; notably, the latter are diminishing due to modern diagnostic (EEG and brain imaging) tools [19].

Such significant advances in neuroimaging have led to more recent updates to the ILAE classification system. Between 2005 and 2009, the ILAE Commission on Classification and Terminology introduced a revised terminology for epilepsy classification that is based upon new neuroimaging approaches to allow better understanding of the disease between researchers and clinicians [20, 21]. Generalised seizures are now defined as seizures that rapidly distribute to both hemispheres of the brain, whereas focal epilepsies have been redefined as affecting either a discrete region or single hemisphere of the brain. The changes also better define different epilepsy subcategories within the generalised seizure category, replacing the terms idiopathic, symptomatic and cryptogenic with genetic, structural/metabolic and unknown, respectively [20]. These changes are in part to allow easier translation of disease type between epilepsy experts and general practitioners ('family doctors' in the USA) as the archaic terms previously used could be confusing. The genetic category has largely replaced the idiopathic category, with an emphasis on epilepsies with a known genetic component. The structural/metabolic subcategory has largely replaced symptomatic classifications, with more recognition given to the underlying cause of the epilepsy. The unknown category has replaced the cryptogenic category and includes all epilepsies that may either result from as yet unknown genetic defect or from another undiagnosed disorder. The system of definition for partial seizures has relinquished its reliance upon strict terminology and now employs a more descriptive series of categories that better describe exhibited symptoms (*e.g.* "with/without consciousness" instead of "simple" or "complex") [20].

Pharmacoresistance in Epilepsy

Approximately 30% of PWE have refractory seizures despite optimised pharmacological treatment [22, 23]. There is currently no unified definition of pharmacoresistant epilepsy however, if two separate drugs fail to adequately control seizures, PWE are referred to a specialist unit for further evaluation [24]. Despite the increase in the number of available AEDs, there has not been an appreciable decrease in the proportion of PWE whose seizures are fully controlled [25]. This leads to two separate hypotheses proposed to explain such pharmacoresistance: the transporter hypothesis and the target hypothesis [26]. The transporter hypothesis asserts that upregulation of multidrug transporters in the blood-brain or blood-CSF barriers produces a greater efflux of AEDs from the cerebral parenchyma [27]. This hypothesis is supported by human studies which reported an increase of MDR1 (multidrug resistance protein 1) mRNA (which encodes P-glycoprotein) [28], as well as MRP1/2 [29, 30], in people with pharmacoresistant epilepsy. The target hypothesis puts forward the idea that there are modifications in the AED's primary targets, including sodium channels [26] and the GABAergic system [31]. These modifications can manifest as differential expression of subunits of ion channels, with the up regulation of subunits that are insensitive to AEDs and down regulation of subunits that act as binding sites for AEDs [32, 33]. The main targets for AEDs are sodium channels [34], with the β_1 and β_2 subunits being the primary targets within the channel [35, 36]. Down regulation or mutation of these subunits has been observed in phenytoin and carbamazepine resistant chronic epilepsy models [37, 38], which supports the target hypothesis for this subgroup of epilepsies.

Side-Effects and Co-Morbidities in Epilepsy

When treating any disease state, there is a risk to benefit assessment required in order to determine the best course of treatment in order to improve the welfare of the patient [39, 40]. The ultimate aim of AEDs is to stop seizure activity [41], however as this is not always being possible, the advantages of reducing seizure frequency and associated co-morbidities must be counterbalanced with the detrimental side effects arising from a more aggressive (*i.e.* polypharmacy and/or high dose) treatment regime [40]. This is particularly pertinent in PWE since all currently available treatments have significant side effects [42-44]. The commonly reported side effects of currently available AEDs include dizziness, mental fatigue, tremors and ataxia. There are also idiosyncratic side effects reported for various AEDs including dermatitis and rashes, Steven-Johnson syndrome, hepatic failure and bone marrow damage [43, 45]. Some side effects can be fatal which not only makes treatment judgements in the clinic more complicated but can also affect the choice and order of AED selected for use (*i.e.* felbamate has a severe side effect profile, however it is used in some countries for severe, previously uncontrolled, seizures [46]).

However, there are co-morbidities with epilepsy that are often worsened by uncontrolled seizures [40, 47]. These include cognitive impairment [47] and psychiatric disorders, including depression and schizophrenia [48-50]. There is also an increase in mortality reported in PWE [51] that can be directly associated with seizures (*i.e.* injury as a result of a seizure event), or indirectly associated with epilepsy (*i.e.* suicide following epilepsy induced depression). Sudden unexplained death in epilepsy (SUDEP) is the most common cause of death directly caused by epilepsy, however the reasons for it are not fully understood [52-54]. The leading theories for SUDEP are respiratory or cardiovascular dysfunction although some genetic factors have also been reported [52]. Mortality-associated seizures can be reduced by effective AED treatment, however the underlying cause of the epilepsy (*e.g.* brain damage), even if known, remains unaffected which in itself may be fatal [40].

Anti-Epileptic Drug Development

Antiepileptic drug discovery is usually separated into three different eras; that of charlatanism (pre-1857), serendipity (1957–1980) and rational drug design (1980–

present day) [15]. Three main classes of AED (benzodiazepines and, carbamazepine- and valproic acid-like substances) were discovered through serendipitous means, with valproic acid originally being used as the vehicle into which prospective anti-epileptic compounds under investigation were dissolved [15]. Despite the aspirational ethos behind the modern era of rational drug design, there remains no established cascade for developing AEDs [55]. However, in order for a new drug to make it successfully through development it has to fulfil one of the following clinical requirements; efficacy in refractory seizures, prevention or retardation of epileptogenesis, greater tolerability/fewer side effects, improved pharmacokinetic profile or use in other CNS disorders [41]. The National Institute of Health (NIH) has created the Anticonvulsant Drug Development (ADD) program [55] in order to help develop new AEDs in collaborating with pharmaceutical or academic sponsors, using screening cascades to evaluate potential compounds. This newer generation of AEDs have increased the quality of life for PWE, as they are better tolerated with fewer side effects than the older generation of AEDs [56].

There are two modern approaches to AED development; mechanistic and non-mechanistic methods [55]. These use a number of different *in vitro* and *in vivo* models of epileptiform activity, seizure and epilepsy [57-59]. Non-mechanistic methods use *in vivo* screening models (*e.g.* pentylenetetrazole model of acute seizure) to evaluate the ability of compounds to prevent or reduce seizures [55, 57]. These models allow investigation and preclinical assessment of efficacy, but do not determine mechanisms of action [57]. There are a number of well-established and characterised acute models of seizure that involve chemical or electrical insults in otherwise healthy animals that result in the production of seizures. These models have helped develop a large number of currently available AEDs, however they are not infallible and have failed to pick up compounds that have subsequently proved to be useful anticonvulsants. One notable example is levetiracetam, which does not prevent seizures in the acute pentylenetetrazole model of acute seizure [19, 60]. There are also genetic models of seizure which can give insight into the clinical indication of AEDs; however these models can often give a false positive for anticonvulsant activity [15]. Compounds that show efficacy in the acute models are then tested in chronic models (*e.g.* lithium-pilocarpine and chemical or electrical kindling models), which are more labour and time intensive, but allow for investigation of animals with brain activity permanently modified to better reflect the chronic disease state and its pharmacological responsiveness [61]. Mechanistic methods initially employ high throughput *in vitro* screening in order to evaluate the ability of a large number of compounds to interact with a target known to be anticonvulsant [55, 62], before being tested in the above models. This has the potential to produce many new AEDs, however they may not have a novel mechanism of action since the assay process is weighted towards identifying compound activity at existing targets (*e.g.* voltage-gated sodium channels), drugs for which already exist but fail to control seizures in >30% of PWE.

THE ENDOCANNABINOID SYSTEM AND EPILEPSY

Relevance of the Endocannabinoid System to Epilepsy as a Drug Target

Epileptic seizures result from dysfunctions that cause an imbalance between excitatory and inhibitory activity in the CNS, allowing ascendancy of excessive excitatory neurotransmission. As understanding about how the endocannabinoid system works to suppress synaptic transmission in the CNS has developed, a significant body of research has focussed on whether CB1R and the synthetic and degradative enzymes of endocannabinoids can be targeted to limit, suppress or prevent seizure activity.

As described elsewhere in this eBook, activation of the presynaptic G protein-coupled CB1R modulates voltage-gated Ca^{2+} channels and enhances K^+ channels at the presynapse, limiting vesicular release of neurotransmitter within the CNS. The principal endogenous CB1R agonists are the endocannabinoids, 2-arachidonoylglycerol (2-AG) and anandamide (AEA). Endocannabinoids are synthesised postsynaptically in an on-demand manner, in response to depolarisation of the postsynaptic cell [63]. In brief, 2-AG and anandamide are synthesised by diacylglycerol lipase alpha (DAGLα) [64] and *N*-acylphosphatidyl-ethanolamine specific phospholipase D (NAPE-PLD) [65] respectively; other synthetic enzymes have also been reported [63], and these are degraded by fatty acid amide hydrolase (FAAH) and monoacylglycerol lipase (MAGL) [66-68]. The method of endocannabinoid transport across biological membranes is still not entirely clear [63]. In addition to being a potential drug target to modulate hyperexcitability in the CNS, there is also strong evidence that the endocannabinoid system undergoes changes in both human and experimental epilepsies and seizures. In this section, we discuss the evidence that targeting or altering the endocannabinoid system can affect seizure susceptibility or incidence, and describe data regarding the changes that can occur in the endocannabinoid system during epilepsy.

The Endocannabinoid System: Role in Endogenous Suppression of Seizures

Both the role of the endocannabinoid system in hyperexcitable states and its potential as a drug target in epilepsy have been widely studied. A seminal and elegant series of studies by Lutz and colleagues in which CB1R expression levels were genetically manipulated in mice indicate that this receptor plays a pivotal reactive role during seizures, counteracting hyperexcitability and excitotoxicity. In their first study [69], mice lacking CB1R (CB1$^{-/-}$) exhibited significantly more severe seizures in response to systemic kainic acid (KA; 30 mg/kg) administration than CB1$^{+/+}$ littermates. Systemic kainic acid administration in rodents induces seizures with a limbic focus (*e.g.* hippocampus, entorhinal cortex, amygdala), and is therefore considered a model of temporal lobe seizure. Seizure behaviour is repetitive and causes significant limbic excitotoxicity resulting in significant neuronal death in the hippocampus [70]. Furthermore, seizure behaviour did not differ between CB1$^{-/-}$ mice and another line lacking CB1R expression solely in principal forebrain neurons, indicating that CB1R in this neuronal population may be crucial in the endogenous, endocannabinoid-mediated defence against seizure activity. A further study using more selective conditional CB1R deletions showed that seizure severity was worsened by CB1R deletion from principal cells of the hippocampus, neocortex and amygdala, but not cortical GABAergic cells [71]. To further highlight the importance of hippocampal CB1R, virally-induced deletion of CB1R significantly exacerbated seizure severity when applied focally to the hippocampus (dentate gyrus, CA1 and CA3 CB1R expression decreased, surrounding cortical regions were unaffected). In a final study, the same researchers conditionally overexpressed CB1R *via* a similar focally-applied viral method to increase CB1R expression in hippocampal pyramidal cells alone [72]. This overexpression was demonstrated functionally as well as histologically, and, after application of 30 mg/kg KA, significantly protected against seizure severity compared to control mice.

These studies elegantly demonstrate that hippocampal CB1R expression can be protective against acutely-induced seizures. There is also evidence that activation of CB1R by endocannabinoids is an important part of the endogenous defence against acute seizures. Several studies have investigated the effect of artificially raised endocannabinoid levels on seizure behaviour by blocking either their degradation or reuptake. Karanian [73] showed that the severity of KA-induced seizures in rats (10 mg/kg) was significantly decreased by the FAAH inhibitor, AM374 ($\geq$5 mg/kg; I.P.). Further evidence that inhibition of endocannabinoid metabolism can decrease the severity of seizures has been reported by Naidoo and co-workers where AM5206, a potent FAAH inhibitor (IC_{50}: 42nM *in vitro*), reduced the severity of KA-induced seizures in rat when administered directly after KA [74]. A further study [75] compared the degree of seizure suppression produced by the administration of AM6701 and AM6702 directly after KA in rat. Both compounds inhibit anandamide and 2-AG degradation by targeting FAAH and MAGL respectively. AM6701 which blocks anandamide and 2-AG degradation equipotently (*in vitro* IC_{50} of 1.2 nM for both enzymes), suppressed seizures more effectively than AM6702, which inhibits FAAH activity 44 times more potently than it does MAGL (*in vitro* IC_{50} for FAAH: 0.65 nM). This suggests that both 2-AG and anandamide play a role in endogenous defence against acute seizures. Marsicano [69] also reported that pharmacological blockade of endocannabinoid reuptake by pretreatment with UCM707 (3 mg/kg) – predicted to maintain endocannabinoid levels after release in the brain - was protective against KA-induced seizures in mice. There is evidence that pharmacological approaches to block 2-AG and anandamide metabolism do, as designed, increase endocannabinoid levels and CB1R activity *in vivo*; administration of AM374 [73] enhances endocannabinoid function, as demonstrated by significantly increased hippocampal anandamide levels and enhanced activation of signaling pathways associated with CB1R agonism. Furthermore, in an *in vitro* model of *status epilepticus*-like activity, application of methanandamide (EC_{50}: 145 nM) and 2-AG (EC_{50}: 1.68 μM) suppressed *status epilepticus*-like activity induced in cultured hippocampal neurons by treatment with Mg^{2+}-free media [76]. This effect was blocked by the CB1R antagonist, AM251 (1 μM) which had no effect when applied alone.

Finally, there are *in vivo* data indicating that brain endocannabinoid levels rise during seizures. Further data from the Lutz study [69] discussed above revealed that anandamide (but not 2-AG) levels in the brain increased significantly after KA administration, peaking at 20 minutes and returning to basal levels one hour after KA. Anandamide but not 2-AG levels were also increased by an excitotoxic NMDA insult applied intrastriatally in rat brains, measured up to 24 hours after administration of NMDA [77]. Similarly, Naidoo and co-workers [74] found anandamide levels to be higher in brain tissue two hours after KA treatment than KA vehicle controls. Systemic administration of high doses of the muscarinic receptor agonist, pilocarpine, induces acute *status epilepticus* in rodents [78]; Wallace [79] found 2-AG levels to be significantly elevated in the hippocampus of rats 15 minutes after *status* started, compared to sham-treated controls. In contrast to the above findings, there is some limited evidence that anandamide may also be proconvulsant in some conditions; FAAH$^{-/-}$, but not wild type, mice exhibit more severe KA-induced seizures after administration of anandamide ($\geq$12.5 mg/kg), an effect blocked by the CB1R antagonist, SR141716A [80]. More recently an interesting study suggested that anandamide's proconvulsant properties are seen only at higher doses and are due to the agonistic properties of anandamide at TRPV1 channels [81]. Here, at lower doses, pentylenetetazole-induced (PTZ) seizures in mice were attenuated by anandamide application into the right lateral cerebral ventricle at doses up to 40 μg; an anticonvulsant effect that was blocked by AM251 administration. Conversely, higher anandamide doses (80-100 μg) potentiated PTZ seizures, a proconvulsant effect facilitated by AM251 but reversed by the TRPV1 antagonist, capsaicin, rendering anandamide anticonvulsant at the higher doses that were previously proconvulsant.

One obvious pharmacological intervention that has not been discussed above is the administration of CB1R ligands (including Δ^9-THC) to alter seizure activity *in vivo*. A summary of this extensive literature is presented and discussed hereafter in the section **EFFECTS OF CANNABINOID TYPE 1 RECEPTOR LIGANDS IN EPILEPSY**; although, as would be expected from the above discussion of CB1R and endocannabinoids, the majority of studies concluded that

CB1R agonists are anticonvulsant *in vivo* and suppress "epileptiform" activity *in vitro* in slice and culture models of neuronal epileptic activity (see below). These effects are blocked by CB1R antagonists which can, although not consistently, exert their own proconvulsant effects when administered alone. One study concerned with the effects of CB1R ligands on seizure activity is worthy of discussion in this section as it points to a more complex role for CB1R activity in opposing seizure activity than a simple suppression of excessive synaptic activity [82]. Seizure activity is characterised by highly synchronous neuronal activity, in this study anaesthetised rats were treated with KA (10 mg/kg) which caused randomly firing hippocampal neurons (simultaneously recorded from using intra-hippocampal electrodes) to develop highly synchronous bursting activity. This synchrony was reversed by administration of the CBR agonist HU210 [83], an effect that was blocked by the CB1R antagonist, SR141716A. This suggests that the anticonvulsant effects of CB1R activity can be ascribed, at least in part, by preventing or destabilising the pathologically synchronous states that characterise seizure activity.

The above studies indicate that CB1R expression and artificially increased endocannabinoid levels (particularly anandamide) are both positively correlated with limiting seizure severity. These data, together with reports that endocannabinoid levels increase in response to administration of pharmacological convulsants, provide strong evidence that the endocannabinoid system opposes hyperexcitability in an on-demand manner by synthesis of endocannabinoids that act *via* CB1R agonism. However, as a dynamic and responsive system, one must also consider the extent of the endocannabinoid system's propensity to change as a consequence of pathophysiological insults which is discussed in detail in **Changes to the Endocannabinoid System in Epilepsy**.

Neuroprotection by the Endocannabinoid System During Seizures and in Epilepsy

A corollary of the endocannabinoid system's ability to limit the hyperexcitability symptomatic of seizure activity in the brain is that the excitotoxicity and neuronal death associated with seizures and epilepsy can also be mitigated. In addition to inducing seizures, KA administration causes significant excitotoxic injury to the brain, with emphasis on the hippocampus and related brain regions [84]. Several of the above studies demonstrating the anti-seizure properties of the endocannabinoid system in the KA model also show that enhancement or activation of the endocannabinoid system can limit the effects of this excitotoxic insult. Marsicano [69] reported that, 4 days after KA administration, animals lacking forebrain CB1R expression showed a greater number of apoptotic cells (as assessed by TUNEL staining) in the CA1/3 regions of the hippocampus than wild type animals. Further analysis showed that animals lacking CB1R were unable to activate protective mechanisms including *c-fos*, in direct contrast to wild type littermates; gliosis was also seen to a higher degree in mutants (determined by GFAP staining). Additionally, neurons in hippocampal slices from forebrain CB1R knockout mice were excited significantly by low-concentration KA (150 nM), with increased excitatory postsynaptic current (EPSC) frequency observed in whole-cell voltage clamp recordings. This effect was absent in hippocampal slices from wild type animals, indicating that the functional ECS in wild type mice prevented this KA-induced excitation. In a further study [72], neuronal death in the CA3 region induced by KA administration in wild type animals was prevented by virally-induced CB1R overexpression in the hippocampus (other brain regions unaffected). Studies investigating the effects of endocannabinoid metabolism inhibitors have found that AM5206 (see above; [74]) protected hippocampal neurons from KA-induced excitotoxicity both *in vitro* in brain slices and *in vivo* after systemic KA administration. 48 hours after KA administration it was shown that concurrent treatment with AM374 (see above, [73]) also protected CA1 neurons, this effect was prevented by the CB1R antagonist, AM251.

Systemic administration of pilocarpine induces acute *status epilepticus*, if halted pharmacologically (*e.g.* by diazepam), animals latterly develop spontaneous recurrent seizures (SRS) in the following weeks [78] which is considered a model of temporal lobe epilepsy. The pilocarpine insult models the initial (often physical) trauma that is frequently the underlying cause of human temporal lobe epilepsy where a "latent period" of several days or weeks (analogous to the delay between initial trauma and the development of human temporal lobe seizures) is seen before SRS develop. The use of a model of epilepsy (the disease as compared to acute seizure, the symptom) allows more direct parallels between human epilepsy and animal models to be drawn. Using this model in rat, the CB1R agonists WINN55,212 (5 mg/kg) and Δ^9-THC (10 mg/kg) both completely abolished the appearance of SRS in rats previously treated with pilocarpine, outperforming the clinically-licensed AEDs phenytoin and phenobarbital [79]. Conversely, administration of the CB1R antagonist, SR141716A (10 mg/kg), exacerbated seizures, increasing both their duration and incidence.

The studies discussed above show that the endocannabinoid system can limit the damage done to CNS neurons – particularly in the hippocampus, a highly epileptogenic region of the brain – by seizures and their associated excitotoxicity. This is an important finding, as epilepsy is a chronic disease in which continuing progressive neurodegeneration stimulated by seizures in turn increases the likelihood of further seizure activity. Beyond the above seizure- and epilepsy-specific data, there is a large body of literature showing that activation of CB1R is neuroprotective [85]. It is also worthy of note that the CB2 receptor, which is expressed in the CNS primarily in immune cells (*e.g.* microglia; [86]). CB2R activation tends to limit inflammation and the CNS immune response, acting to decrease microglia and astrocytic activation [85, 86]. In the context of a chronic progressive disease, although continual suppression of the CNS immune system should be met with caution, enhanced CB2R signaling may protect neurons and slow or halt disease progression. A detailed discussion of the potential of the endocannabinoid system as a neuroprotective mechanism can be found in.

Changes to the Endocannabinoid System in Epilepsy

The endocannabinoid system changes in both animal models of epilepsy and in the human condition. The greatest body of work focuses upon changes in hippocampal CB1R expression and there is also evidence that endocannabinoid levels vary. In treatment-naïve patients with newly-diagnosed temporal lobe epilepsy, anandamide but not 2-AG cerebrospinal fluid levels were reduced compared to healthy control individuals [87]; importantly levels were assessed in patients who had been seizure-free for over 24 hours, suggesting that these results were not due to acute changes in response to seizure activity. This may also explain why findings in acute models of seizure in animal models (*e.g.* KA, see above) indicate increases in anandamide levels, in contrast to the decreases seen here. In another study, the function of FAAH in neocortical tissue surgically removed from patients with mesial temporal lobe epilepsy was found to be no different to that taken from patients with non-epileptogenic brain tumours [88]. Whilst this patient population was necessarily different from the study above in which CSF alone was taken, and age, treatment and time since diagnosis varied, the absence of a difference between epileptic and non-epileptic tissue in anandamide hydrolysis by FAAH could suggest that variation in anandamide levels is due to changes in levels of synthesis and not metabolism.

To our knowledge, only two studies have examined CB1R expression in human patients with epilepsy. In 2008, Ludanyi [89] used quantitative polymerase chain reaction experiments (qPCR) to assess differences in the expression levels of endocannabinoid system proteins in the hippocampus between healthy (post mortem) tissue and epileptic tissue (taken surgically from people with intractable temporal lobe epilepsy). They found that CB1R mRNA levels in epileptic tissues were significantly less abundant, with only a third of the amount found in healthy tissue, a finding confirmed at the protein level by immunohistochemistry. Additionally they found that levels of the CB1R interacting protein 1a (CRIP1a; [90]) and DAGLα was lower in epileptic tissue. In contrast, CRIP1b and MAGL levels were consistent between healthy and epileptic tissues. Similarly and consistently with the findings of Steffens *et al.* [88], the proteins responsible for degradation of anandamide (*e.g.* FAAH) were not expressed at different levels in healthy and epileptic tissues. A second study [91] investigating CB1R expression in sclerotic human hippocampus from PWE demonstrated that CB1R expression in GABAergic interneurons was maintained in the dentate gyrus (DG) and CA1 regions, whilst it was enhanced compared to healthy controls in the dentate molecular layer. These findings were mirrored in mice previously treated with pilocarpine to induce SRS with a temporal lobe focus and hippocampal sclerosis. All other available data regarding CB1R expression also come from models of pilocarpine-induced SRS and hippocampal remodeling/sclerosis in rodents. Karlocai and co-workers [92] separated pilocarpine-treated mice into "weakly" and "strongly" epileptic based on the severity of their initial pilocarpine-induced acute seizure activity. They found that in weakly epileptic mice no change in CB1R expression occurred compared to control animals. In strongly epileptic animals a significant decrease in CB1R expression across the hippocampus was observed in the acute phase of the model (2-24 hours after pilocarpine; hypothesised to be due to receptor internalisation). A recovery in expression levels was observed in the latent period (3 days post pilocarpine), and during the chronic phase, in which SRS start to manifest and sclerosis of the hippocampus occurs, DG CB1R expression had increased, as had CB1R staining on GABAergic terminals. DeLorenzo and co-workers have performed similar investigations in rat after pilocarpine treatment [93-95]. In their initial study, they found that CB1R decreased in the chronic phase compared to healthy control animals in the pyramidal cell layers of CA1-3 and the DG inner molecular layer, whilst it increased in the strata oriens and radiatum of CA1-3 [93]. This broadly represents an increase in presynaptic CB1R expression at glutamatergic synapses and a decrease at GABAergic synapses across the DG and CA regions. In a further study [94], the same group showed broadly similar results to [92] in the early stages of the pilocarpine model of SRS, with significant decreases in CB1R expression across the hippocampus but with interneuronal expression maintained; after one month expression levels were as described in [93]. In a third study [95] looking at CB1R expression in brain regions outside the hippocampus in the chronic phase of the model in rat, CB1R binding and activity increased in the cortex, selected thalamic nuclei, the caudate-putamen and the septum, but remained the same as control animals in substantia nigra and cerebellum; findings that were confirmed by immunohistochemistry.

Whilst these human and rodent studies all point to the endocannabinoid system changing during epilepsy, the differences in findings in the experimental animal models of epilepsy and the variation in the method of SRS induction make a unifying hypothesis of CB1R changes in epilepsy elusive. Combined with the obvious issues in investigating CB1R expression at the ultrastructural level in human hippocampi (and the wider brain) as human epilepsy is caused and then develops, as well as the underlying uncertainty as to whether changes in (particularly human) hippocampal CB1R expression are part of the pathology of epilepsy or a response to it, it is clear that significant further investigation of this area is required.

EFFECTS OF CANNABINOID TYPE 1 RECEPTOR LIGANDS IN EPILEPSY

The role of the endocannabinoid system in seizures and epilepsy remains difficult to fully generalise, not least because of the near ubiquitous presence of CB1R upon inhibitory and excitatory synaptic terminals and its reactive and compensatory nature in response to sustained changes in neuronal activity such as highly heterogenous (by patient) seizure events. However, the preceding section does demonstrate that an overall effect of global increases in endocannabinoid system function in the CNS is to mitigate seizure severity and/or events. It is these findings, together with the longstanding historical and anecdotal use of herbal cannabis for the control of epileptic seizures [96], which continues to the present day, that has driven investigation of the effects of exogenous CB1 receptor ligands upon seizures and epilepsy.

However, the well known psychoactive effects of the archetypal CB1R agonist, Δ^9-THC [97], a property common to all CB1R agonists, presents a serious complicating factor when considering either the utility of synthetic CB1R agonist drug development programmes in epilepsy or the continued use of cannabis as part of medical marijuana programmes in countries such as the USA and Canada. The debate surrounding the negative implications of an adverse psychoactive profile is a complex one, made more so by the extent of recreational use of cannabis (~147 million recreational cannabis users worldwide [98]) wherein the pharmacological actions defined as side effects in therapeutic contexts represent the desired recreational effects. Given that such considerations exceed the scope of this review, a definitive conclusion regarding the side-effect risk *vs* anticonvulsant benefit of CB1R agonist use by pharmacoresistant PWE cannot be reached and so remains an important factor for consideration by scientists, the pharmaceutical industry, regulatory bodies, PWE and society as a whole when the clinical development of any cannabis or cannabinoid-based medicine is considered.

Despite this specific limitation, considerable preclinical research has been conducted to investigate the usefulness of CB1R agonism in the control of seizures and epilepsy which is presented and discussed in detail hereafter. The evidence presented is divided into categories describing the effects of synthetic CB1R ligands, modulators of endocannabinoid synthesis and degradation (see **The Endocannabinoid System: Role in Endogenous Suppression of Seizures**) and, finally, due to the extent of the evidence base in the literature, the plant cannabinoid, Δ^9-THC. Evidence describing the effects of non-Δ^9-THC plant cannabinoids, despite rarely being endocannabinoid system modulators, is provided thereafter. Since epilepsy is a disease state that involves the whole organism, not solely the CNS, the evidence summarised here focuses largely upon the effects of these agents in whole animal (*in vivo*) models of disease unless specific *in vitro* evidence casts additional light upon the specific manner in which a given agent exerts its anticonvulsant effects.

The identification of a specific G-protein coupled receptor target for the exogenous cannabinoid, Δ^9-THC, immediately provided opportunities for the development of synthetic ligands, including agonists, antagonists and allosteric modulators [99], the profiles of many of which have been investigated in models of seizure and epilepsy. Synthetic CB1R ligands can be pharmacologically distinguished by virtue of their agonistic or antagonistic properties at the target receptor.

Synthetic Cannabinoid Type-1 Receptor Agonists and Modulators Of Endocannabinoid (AEA and 2-AG) Synthesis And Degradation

On the above basis, our systematic review of the available literature describing CB1R agonist and endocannabinoid modulator effects in whole animal models of seizure and epilepsy (Table **1**) revealed that investigations have thus far only been conducted in murine species (c.f. Δ^9-THC below). Of the models used, the majority represented generalised seizures (employing 9 different chemical, electrical or auditory insults or stimuli) with individual instances of studies examining effects upon temporal lobe epilepsy, generalised epilepsy, absence epilepsy and partial seizures with a secondary generalisation comprising the remainder.

A total of 55 independent conditions, models or experimental designs have been examined to date with 10 (18%) that reported no significant effect of drug, 4 (7%)

reported mixed effects (*e.g.* decreased severity with decreased latency), a single study reporting a proconvulsant (2%) effect whilst a notable majority (40; 73%) reported significant anticonvulsant effects. The critical measures described in these reports are summarised in Table **1** and include details of route and timing of administration in addition to dose used. This information is relevant particularly as some reports describing an absence of drug effect may result from early investigations of new compounds for which bioavailability or other pharmacokinetic data was not yet available; particularly given the highly lipophilic nature of many CB1R ligands (see also Δ^9-**Tetrahydrocannabinol**). Moreover, a number of the reports shown in Table **1** also reported observable motor side effects of CB1R agonist administration (see [100, 101] for exemplar instances where this was investigated in parallel with ligand effects upon seizures), consistent with the known side-effect profile of such agents but, in the context of epilepsy, potential confounders of behavioural assessments of drug effects upon seizure, the principal symptom. Finally, whilst not models of seizure *per se*, the CB1R agonists, Δ^9-THC and HU210 when administered to R6/1 Huntington's Disease model mice over a period of eight weeks both increased the incidence of handling-induced seizures although its significance in the wider context of epilepsy remains unknown at present [102].

Overall, whilst limited by the well known motor and psychoactive side-effects caused by CB1R activation, the widespread reproducibility of anticonvulsant effects between studies, compounds and models provides compeling evidence for – at least in largely acute treatment paradigms - significant anticonvulsant efficacy for synthetic CB1R agonists. Given the reactive and compensatory properties of the endocannabinoid system, whether such effects translate to chronic treatment situations remains to be seen.

Table1: Summary of synthetic CB1R agonist effects upon whole animal models of seizure and epil anticonvulsant, ■; proconvulsant, ■; mixed effect, ■; no effect. MES: maximal electroshock, PTZ: pentylene chloroethylamide-2'-chloro-AEA, AEA: anandamide. Note: URB597 is a FAAH inhibitor and not a CB1R ag table where investigations of CB1R agonists were concurrently performed.

Species	Strain	Age	Model	Symptom/disease	Inducing agent	Treatment	Dose range	Administr
Mouse	Swiss	Adult	Acute	Generalised seizure	PTZ	WIN55,212 plus clonazepam	5-15 mg/kg	15 mins before t
						WIN55,212 plus ethosuximide		45 mins before t
						WIN55,212 plus valproate		30 mins before t
						WIN55,212 plus phenobarbital		60 mins before t
		Adult	Acute	Generalised seizure	MES	WIN55,212 plus valproate	10 mg/kg and AED dose-response	30 mins before t
						WIN55,212 plus carbamazepine		30 mins before t
						WIN55,212 plus phenobarbitone		60 mins before t
						WIN55,212 plus phenytoin		120 mins before
						WIN55,212	2.5-15 mg/kg	20 mins before
Rat	Wistar	Juvenile	Acute	Generalised seizure	Kainic acid	WIN55,212	0.5-5 mg/kg	90 mins before
Mouse	Swiss	Adult	Acute	Generalised seizure	MES	ACEA	1.25-15 mg/kg	10 mins prior to
						ACEA plus 30 mg/kg valproate	1.25-2.5 mg/kg	
Rat	Long-Evans	Adult	Acute	Generalised seizure	PTZ	N-palmitoylethanolamide	40 mg/kg	2 hours prior to
Rat		Adult	Chronic	Generalised seizure	Amygdala kindling		1, 10 & 100 mg/kg	2 hours prior to
Mouse	OF1	Adult	Acute	Generalised seizure	PTZ		25 mg/kg	2 hours prior to
					3-mercaptopropionic acid			
					Bicuculline			
					Strychnine			

Species	Strain	Age	Duration	Seizure type	Model	Drug	Dose	Timing
					Picrotoxin			
					NMDA			
					MES		50 & 100 mg/kg	
					MES	Anandamide	50 mg/kg	0.5 to 4 hours
Mouse	NMRI	Adult	Acute	Generalised seizure	MES	WIN55,212	0.5-4 mg/kg	30 mins before
						WIN55,212 plus diazepam	0-4 mg/kg of each in mixed ratios	
						AM404	0.125-4 mg/kg	
						AM404 plus diazepam	0-4 mg/kg of each in mixed ratios	
						URB597	0.05-1 mg/kg	
						URB597 plus diazepam	0-2 mg/kg of each in mixed ratios	
Rat	Wistar	Adult	Acute	Generalised seizure	PTZ	WIN55,212	1-100 µg	5 mins before t
						WIN55,212 plus isoguvacine	1-100 µg and 5-5 µg respectively	
						URB597	10-100 µg	
						URB597 plus isoguvacine	10-100 µg plus 5-50 µg respectively	
						URB602	10-500 µg	
Mouse	Swiss	Adult	Acute	Generalised seizure	MES	ACEA plus carbamazepine	2.5 mg/kg	10 mins prior t
						ACEA plus lamotrigine		
						ACEA plus oxcarbazepine		
						ACEA phenobarbitone		
						ACEA plus phenytoin		
						ACEA plus topiramate		
Rat	WAG/Rij	Adult	Chronic	Absence	Genetic	WIN55,212	3-12 mg/kg	2 hours prior to
Rat	Wistar	Adult	Acute	Partial with secondary generalisation	Penicillin (i.c.v.)	ACEA	0.25 µg	45 mins after e epileptiform ac
						ACEA plus memantine	0.25 µg and 1-20 mg/kg respectively	Memantine 30 mins after estab epileptiform ac

Rat	Wistar	Adult	Acute	Partial seizure	Maximal dentate gyrus activation	WIN55,212	1-21 mg/kg	Monitored for u administration
Rat	Not stated	Adult	Acute	Partial with secondary generalisation	Penicillin (i.c.v.)	ACEA	2.5-15 µg	Monitored for u administration
Mouse	NMRI	Adult	Acute	Generalised seizure	PTZ	ACEA	0.1-8 mg/kg	Up to 60 mins b
						ACEA plus naltrexone	0.1-8 mg/kg and 1-500 pg/kg respectively	Up to 60 mins b
Mouse	NMRI	Adult	Acute	Generalised seizure	PTZ	ACEA	0.1-4 mg/kg	60 mins before
Mouse	NMRI	Adult	Acute	Generalised seizure	PTZ	ACEA	0.1-8 mg/kg	15 mins before
Mouse	NMRI	Adult	Acute	Generalised seizure	PTZ	ACPA	0.5-2 mg/kg	60 mins before
Rat	Sprague-Dawley	Adult	Chronic	Temporal lobe epilepsy	Pilocarpine-induced SRS	WIN55,212	5 mg/kg	Single dose imr EEG and behav
Mouse	CF-1	Adult	Acute	Generalised seizure	MES	WIN55,212	1-100 mg/kg	120 mins befor
Mouse	NMRI	Adult	Chronic	Generalised seizure	Amygdala kindling	WIN55,212	2.5 & 4 mg/kg	30 or 60 mins b
								30 mins before
						URB597	1 & 3 mg/kg	30 or 60 mins b
								30 mins before

Synthetic Cannabinoid Type-1 Receptor Antagonists

Given the consistent and reproducible cases where CB1R activation exerts anticonvulsant effects in whole animal models of seizure that are summarised above, one would predict that CB1R antagonism, if not seizuregenic *per se*, would potentiate the effects of convulsant agents and stimuli. Consequently, whether it is an effect of this strong hypothesis or a manifestation of positive reporting bias within the literature, the number of extant studies reporting CB1R antagonist effects upon seizure and epilepsy models is much more limited yet nonetheless provides an important context for the preceding information reporting predominantly positive effects of CB1R agonists in models of seizure and epilepsy. Readers interested in CB1R antagonist effects in epilepsy are also referred to the evidence of effects of the plant cannabinoid and propyl analogue of Δ^9-THC, Δ^9-THCV (see **EFFECTS OF NON-Δ^9-THC PLANT CANNABINOIDS IN EPILEPSY**) which is a well characterised neutral antagonist at CB1R.

The detailed summary of CB1R antagonist effects in these models is provided hereafter (Table **2**) although, briefly, effects have again been limited to murine models of seizure and epilepsy, comprising individual instances of temporal lobe epilepsy, generalised seizure, generalised epilepsy, absence epilepsy and partial seizures with secondary generalisation and predominantly using the i.p. route for cannabinoid administration. Summary statistics from these studies reveal that of the 13 separate conditions, models and/or experimental design investigated, the majority (8; 62%) revealed no effect of drug on seizure measures whilst, consistent with the above starting hypothesis, 4 (31%) instances of proconvulsant effects exist and one (8%) of anticonvulsant effects (see also Δ^9-THCV).

Consequently, whilst initial concerns of widespread proconvulsant effects of CB1R antagonism do not seem wholly substantiated in the face of this evidence, the effect of such modulation is clearly non-trivial and, where beneficial effects are seen, effect sizes remain small and so offer little potential for clinical development.

Table 2: Summary of synthetic CB1R antagonist effects upon whole animal models of seizure and epi anticonvulsant, ■; proconvulsant, ■; mixed effect, ■; no effect. MES: maximal electroshock, PTZ: pentyler THCV below.

Species	Strain	Age	Model	Symptom/disease	Inducing agent	Treatment	Dose range	Administr
Rat	Wistar	Adult	Acute	Generalised seizure	Audiogenic	SR141716A	30 mg/kg	o.d. for 5 days
Mouse	NMRI	Adult	Acute	Generalised seizure	MES	AM251	0.25-5 mg/kg	30 mins before
						AM251 plus diazepam	0-4 mg/kg of each in mixed ratios	
Rat	WAG/Rij	Adult	Chronic	Absence	Genetic	AM251	6-12 mg/kg	2 hours prior to
Rat	Wistar	Adult	Acute	Partial with secondary generalisation	Penicillin (i.c.v.)	AM251	7.5ug	45 mins after es epileptiform act
						AM251 plus memantine	7.5 ug and 1-20 mg/kg respectively	Memantine 30 m 45 mins after es epileptiform act
Rat	Wistar	Adult	Acute	Partial seizure	Maximal dentate gyrus activation	AM251	1 mg/kg	EEG monitored after AM251 ad (includes period
Rat	Not stated	Adult	Acute	Partial with secondary generalisation	Penicillin (i.c.v.)	AM251	0.125-1 ug	induction and co
Mouse	NMRI	Adult	Acute	Generalised seizure	PTZ	AM251	0.01-1 mg/kg	15 mins before
Rat	Sprague-Dawley	Adult	Chronic	Epileptogenesis	Kainic acid	SR141716A	10 mg/kg	Once at first sig acid-induced sei
Rat	Wistar	Adult/Immature	Chronic	Juvenile head trauma followed by acute proconvulsant challenge 6 weeks later	Kainic acid	SR141716A	1 & 10 mg/kg	Immediately fol trauma
Mouse	NMRI	Adult	Acute	Generalised seizure	PTZ	AM251	1 fg/kg-1 mg/kg	45 mins before
Mouse	NMRI	Adult	Acute	Generalised seizure	PTZ	AM251	0.5-3 mg/kg	60 mins before

Δ^9-Tetrahydrocannabinol (Δ^9-THC)

Δ^9-THC is the primary cannabinoid constituent of cannabis, however there are several additional phytocannabinoids with potential or proven anticonvulsant actions in humans (see **EFFECTS OF NON-Δ^9-THC PLANT CANNABINOIDS IN EPILEPSY**).

One of the earliest reports regarding the effect of Δ^9-THC described the effect of two analogues of the cannabinoid on institutionalised children with epilepsy refractory to treatment with phenobarbital or phenytoin [123]. Two of five children had their epilepsy controlled by Δ^9-THC treatment, with three experiencing no effects on seizure occurrence. Beyond this single study, investigations of the anticonvulsant properties of Δ^9-THC have largely been limited to preclinical investigations in animals.

The effects of Δ^9-THC in animal models of seizure are summarised in Table **3**. Δ^9-THC has been investigated in what may be considered commonly-used murine models of seizure, and also in unusual species such as cat and baboon. Taking all preclinical data as a whole, Δ^9-THC has been tested in 31 different experimental conditions (taking into account species, seizure model and experimental design). In 19 experimental paradigms (61% of total) Δ^9-THC was found to be significantly anticonvulsant, whilst no effect was observed in nine studies (29%). In a further three studies (10%), Δ^9-THC exerted proconvulsant effects. Δ^9-THC was proconvulsant when administered orally to mice at 20-75 mg/kg 30 minutes before MES, increasing hindlimb extension [124]; in contrast at $160 - 200$ mg/kg Δ^9-THC was anticonvulsant. This finding appears to be in contrast to other studies using MES in mouse (Table **3**). In the 60 Hz electroshock model of generalised seizure, 100 mg/kg Δ^9-THC administered i.p. once a day for three to four days reduced seizure threshold in a proconvulsant manner [125], whether this represents a genuine proconvulsant effect of Δ^9-THC or that treatment with Δ^9-THC affected CB1R expression levels prior to the seizure insult leading to a reduced protective endocannabinoid response is not clear. The final study in which Δ^9-THC was proconvulsant utilised a spontaneously epileptic gerbil strain, in which 50 mg/kg (but not 20 mg/kg) Δ^9-THC significantly decreased latency to seizure [126]. In those studies in which Δ^9-THC had no effect on seizure, three of nine utilised low doses (<4 mg/kg), three were in unusual species (cat, baboon and chicken) and three used dosing times of 30 minutes, which is a relatively short time compared to other studies (see Table **3**). Interestingly, Δ^9-THC, when combined with CBD and CBN (all at 50 mg/kg *via* oral gavage) reversed the proconvulsant effect of THC in the MES model of seizure in mouse [124], producing instead a significant anticonvulsant effect. This could underlie the variability in responsiveness seen in PWE using cannabis since phytocannabinoid proportions can vary significantly dependent on strain, storage and consumption process. This study also demonstrated a significant reduction in phenytoin ED_{50} by Δ^9-THC (50 mg/kg *via* oral gavage) co-administration which was further reduced by co-administration of Δ^9-THC plus CBD (each 50 mg/kg *via* oral gavage). Δ^9-THC (50 mg/kg) also potentiated the effect of phenytoin [124] and phenobarbitone [127] in the MES model in mouse.

EFFECTS OF NON-Δ^9-THC PLANT CANNABINOIDS IN EPILEPSY

Cannabidiol (CBD)

CBD, the non-psychoactive and usually second most abundant cannabinoid in the cannabis plant (after Δ^9-THC), has also been extensively tested for anticonvulsant properties in murine species, with some promising results. CBD has been reported to be a low affinity but high potency CB1R antagonist *in vitro* at high concentrations [136], however the anticonvulsant profile of CBD makes unlikely that that its mechanism of action in this regard arises *via* antagonism of the CB1 receptor (*c.f.* **Synthetic Cannabinoid Type-1 Receptor Antagonists**). Whilst CBD's mechanism of anticonvulsant does remain to be definitively elucidated, the cellular and molecular targets at which CBD is known to act are numerous and not limited to the endocannabinoid system itself (for extensive reviews see [85, 137]).

The effects of CBD have been investigated in a total of 21 different conditions, models or experimental designs. The vast majority (17; 81%) reported anticonvulsant effects, a small proportion (4; 19%) reported no effect and, importantly, none reported any overall proconvulsant effects. These data are summarised in Table **4**, along with the main parameters including route of administration, time to challenge following CBD administration, species and strain. It is of note that some studies administered seizure inducing agents prior to the now known brain T_{max} (60-120 mins following i.p. administration) for CBD [138] had elapsed, potentially underestimating CBD's anticonvulsant potency.

Table 3: Summary of Δ^9-THC effects upon whole animal models of seizure and epilepsy. **Key:** Summ proconvulsant, ■; mixed effect, ■; no effect. MES: maximal electroshock, PTZ: pentylenetetrazole.

Species	Strain	Age	Model	Symptom/disease	Inducing agent	Treatment	Dose range	Administration ti
Mouse	C57BL/6	Adult	Acute	Generalised seizure	Audiogenic priming	Δ^9-THC	10 mg/kg	5-135 mins before t
							1.25-10 mg/kg	15 mins before test
							10 mg/kg	15 -90 mins before stimulus
							10-50 mg/kg	15 -90 mins after p stimulus
Mouse	QS	Adult	Acute	Generalised seizure	PTZ	Δ^9-THC	1-80 mg/kg	30 mins before test
				Generalised seizure	MES		160 – 200 mg/kg	30 mins before test
							20-75 mg/kg	30 mins before test
							20 mg/kg	30 mins before test
						Δ^9-THC plus CBD plus CBN	50 mg/kg Δ^9-THC, 50mg/kg CBD, 50 mg/kg CBN	30 mins before test
Mouse	QS	Adult	Acute	Generalised seizure	MES	Δ^9-THC plus PHN	50mg/kg Δ^9-THC (with a range on phenytoin doses)	30 mins before test
						Δ^9-THC plus PHN plus CBD	50 mg/kg Δ^9-THC, 50 mg/kg CBD (with a range of phenytoin doses)	30 mins before testi
Mouse	CF-1	Adult	Acute	Generalised seizure	MES	Δ^9-THC	1-100mg/kg	120 mins before tes
Mouse	QS	Adult	Acute	Generalised seizure	MES	Δ^9-THC plus PBL	25-50 mg/kg Δ^9-THC plus 9.3-40 mg/kg PBL	Δ^9-THC: 120 mins; mins before testing
						Δ^9-THC plus CBD plus PBL	25 mg/kg Δ^9-THC, 25 mg/kg CBD, 9.3-40 mg/kg phenobarbitone	Δ^9-THC & CBD: 1. PBL: 60 mins befor
Mouse	Not stated	Adult	Acute	Generalised seizure	MES	Δ^9-THC	100 mg/kg	Once daily for 3-4 testing
					6Hz electroshock			
					60Hz			

					electroshock				
Mouse	Not stated	Adult	Acute	Generalised seizure	MES	Δ^9-THC	up to 80 mg/kg	15 mins to 24 hours testing
					PTZ			30 mins before test
					Nicotine			
					Strychnine			
Gerbil	*Meriones unguiculatus*	Adult	Chronic	Generalised seizure	Spontaneously epileptic	Δ^9-THC	20 & 50 mg/kg	Single dose
								o.d. for 6 days befo
Cat	Not stated	Adult	Chronic	Generalised seizure	Amygdala kindling (electrical)	Δ^9-THC	0.25 mg/kg	At onset of kindlin
							0.25 - 4 mg/kg	At stage 3 (head no
								At stage 5 (clonic j
								At kindling endpoi
Rat	Sprague-Dawley	Adult	Chronic	Temporal lobe epilepsy	Pilocarpine-induced SRS	Δ^9-THC	0.5-30mg/kg	Single dose immed before EEG and be monitoring
Rat	Not stated	Adult	Acute	Generalised seizure	PTZ	Δ^9-THC	15-200 mg/kg	45 mins before test
Baboon	*Papio papio*	Adult	Chronic	Generalised seizure	Photogenic	Δ^9-THC	0.25-1 mg/kg	~60 minutes before
					Amygdala kindling (electrical)			
Chicken	*Gallus domesticus*	Adult	Acute	Generalised seizure	Photogenic	Δ^9-THC	0.25-1 mg/kg	0.5 or 2 hours befo
					PTZ (35 mg/kg in epileptic fowl)			
					PTZ (80 mg/kg in non-epileptic fowl)			

Table 4: Summary of cannabidiol effects upon whole animal models of seizure and epilepsy. **Key:** Sum proconvulsant, ■; mixed effect, ■; no effect. MES: maximal electroshock, PTZ: pentylenetetrazole.

Species	Strain	Age	Model	Symptom/disease	Inducing agent	Treatment	Dose range	Administrat
Mouse	QS	Adult	Acute	Generalised seizure	MES	CBD plus PBL	50 mg/kg CBD plus 9.3-40 mg/kg phenobarbitone	CBD: 2 hours, before testing
Mouse	CF-1	Adult	Acute	Generalised seizure	MES	CBD	1-100 mg/kg	120 mins befor
Mouse	Not stated	Adult	Acute	Generalised seizure	MES / 6 Hz electroshock / 60 Hz electroshock		100 mg/kg	o.d. for 3-4 day testing
Rat	Not stated	Adult	Acute	Generalised seizure	MES		1.5-12 mg/kg	1 hour before te
Mouse	Not stated	Adult	Acute	Generalised seizure	PTZ / MES		50-200 mg/kg	30 mins before
Mouse	ICR	Adult	Acute	Generalised seizure	MES		120 mg/kg (ED$_{50}$)	0.5-6 hours bef
Rat	Sprague-Dawley	Adult	Chronic	Generalised seizure	Limbic kindling (electrical)		0.3-3 mg/kg	15-300 minutes
Rat	Not stated	Adult	Chronic	Partial seizure with secondary generalisation	Cortical implantation of cobalt		60 mg/kg	Twice daily aft implantation
Mouse	Not stated	Adult	Acute	Generalised seizure	MES / 3-mercaptoproprionic acid / Picrotoxin / Isonicotinic acid / Bicuculline / Hydrazine / PTZ / Strychnine	CBD	5-400 mg/kg	60 minutes bef
Rat	Wistar-Kyoto	Adult	Acute	Generalised seizure	PTZ		1, 10 & 100 mg/kg	1 hour before te
Rat	Wistar-Kyoto	Adult	Acute	Temporal lobe seizure	Pilocarpine (acute)			
Rat	Wistar-Kyoto	Adult	Acute	Partial seizure with secondary generalisation	Penicillin			

In addition to these non-clinical studies, a small human trial was reported in 1980, where CBD was used as an adjunctive therapy in patients exhibiting seizures refractory to conventional treatment. Fifteen people took part in the study, initially seven of whom received CBD and eight received a placebo. From a group receiving 200-300 mg/kg/day CBD; 4/8 obtained full seizure control, 1/8 improved markedly, 2/8 improved somewhat and 1/8 showed no improvement; compared to the placebo (glucose capsules) group where 7/8 showed no improvement and 1/8 showed improvements. It is also noted that one patient in the placebo group, who showed no improvement, was transferred to the CBD group and subsequently markedly improved [139].

Whilst the above clinical trial was performed in a small population, significant positive results were yielded in a pharmacoresistant population and the scale of study required for Phase IIa exploratory randomised trials in epilepsy do not employ significantly greater number of participants. This, combined with the uniformly positive preclinical data gathered over several decades and highly favourable tolerability of CBD, strongly mandates the resumption of clinical exploration of CBD in the clinic although the extent of the evidence base for anticonvulsant efficacy that lies in the public domain may explain why this has not yet been undertaken.

OTHER NON-Δ^9-THC PLANT CANNABINOIDS IN EPILEPSY

Finally, the anticonvulsant activity of two further plant cannabinoids, CBN and Δ^9-THCV, have also been reported. CBN was tested in the mouse MES model of seizure, using i.p. administration and reported to have an ED_{50} of 230 mg/kg [141], higher than either Δ^9-THC or CBD and has not been pursued further. Δ^9-THCV was tested in the rat acute PTZ model of seizure, using i.p. administration and reported to reduce the incidence of seizures (0.25 mg/kg) [147] although efficacy was lost at higher concentrations. There is also evidence to suggest that co-administration of CBN with Δ^9-THC and CBD increases the anticonvulsant effects of the individual cannabinoids [124], and therefore could contribute to the anticonvulsant effects reported by PWE in medical marijuana programmes.

Most recently, anti-epileptiform and anticonvulsant effects of cannabidivarin (CBDV), the propyl variant of CBD have been reported [148], although understanding of its pharmacology remains very limited. Here, CBDV exerted significant effects in two *in vitro* models of epileptiform activity and four *in vivo* models of seizure, in addition to showing good tolerability in motor function tests. CBDV attenuated *status epilepticus*-like epileptiform LFPs at ≥ 10 μM *in vitro*. Moreover, in the MES model, tonic hindlimb extension (100-200 mg/kg) and tonic convulsions (50-200 mg/kg) were reduced whilst the number of animals remaining free from any sign of seizure increased (200 mg/kg) and all seizure-related deaths were ablated (100-200 mg/kg). In the PTZ model of acute generalized seizure in rat, CBDV significantly reduced seizure severity (200 mg/kg) and mortality (100-200 mg/kg) whilst significantly increasing both the number of animals remaining free from any sign of seizure (100-200 mg/kg) and the latency to first sign of seizure (200 mg/kg); effects that were retained when the oral route of administration was also used. CBDV was also shown to be well tolerated in co-administration with conventional anticonvulsants (sodium valproate or ethosuximide). Whilst CBDV's possible mechanism(s) of anticonvulsant action remains unknown, to date two reports have described differential effects of CBDV at transient receptor potential (TRP) channels (the role of TRP channels in epilepsy is unknown) and to inhibit diacylglycerol lipase-α (a role for which in epilepsy also remains undetermined) [149, 150]. However, given the diversity of cellular systems targeted by plant cannabinoids, it would be misleading to conclude that CBDV exerts significant and broad anticonvulsant effects *via* TRP or DAGLα modulation and, as such, further research in this area is required.

CONCLUSIONS

In this chapter we have highlighted the continued and pressing need for new, novel AEDs to combat epileptogenesis, pharmacoresistant epilepsy and, if possible, improve on the frequently debilitating side effect profile of currently-used AEDs; all previously identified and leading ILAE research priorities [151]. It is clear that the preclinical research discussed above strongly supports enhancement of endocannabinoid function as a rational strategy for treatment of epilepsy and suppression of seizures; whether the anti-seizure properties of the endocannabinoid system outweigh the undesirable side effects of, for example, exogenous CB1R agonism, is a debate that continues and could limit clinical investigation of this therapeutic avenue for the foreseeable future. The potential of the endocannabinoid system to limit neuronal damage *via* CB2R activation in this chronic disease is also worthy of investigation, although long-term suppression of the CNS immune system and protective systems comes with its own associated risks. One consistently attractive alternative is cannabidiol, a non-psychoactive plant cannabinoid with a history of safe use that has been shown to limit seizure activity in preclinical and clinical investigations over what is now a forty year period, and is likely to have its effects *via* one or more mechanisms outside of the endocannabinoid system. Finally, whilst many plant cannabinoids do not exert their pharmacological effects exclusively *via* the endocannabinoid system modulation, the broad anticonvulsant effects exhibited by those thus far studied and the large number that remain to be investigated supports a continuation of their study in this area; either as clinical development candidates, mechanistic probes or prototypical anticonvulsants for subsequent structure-activity and synthetic chemistry approaches.

ACKNOWLEDGEMENT

Declared None.

CONFLICT OF INTEREST

The authors have no conflict of interest.

REFERENCES

[1]   Rang HP, Dale MM, Ritter JM, Flower RJ, Henderson G. Rang & Dale's Pharmacology. 7th edition ed: Churchill Livingstone; 2011.
[2]   Walker M, Cross H, Smith S, Young C, Aicardi J, Appleton R, *et al*. Nonconvulsive status epilepticus: Epilepsy Research Foundation workshop reports. Epileptic Disord 2005;7(3):253-96.
[3]   Karp BI, Porter S, Toro C, Hallett M. Simple motor tics may be preceded by a premotor potential. Journal of Neurology, Neurosurgery & Psychiatry 1996;61(1):103-6.
[4]   Page TE, Capps E, Rouse WHD, Post LA, Warmington EH. Hippocrates: The sacred disease. 1967.
[5]   Berrios GE. Epilepsy and Insanity During the Early 19th Century: A Conceptual History. Archives of neurology 1984;41(9):978.
[6]   Bell G, Sander J. CPD--Education and self-assessment The epidemiology of epilepsy: the size of the problem. Seizure 2001;10(4):306-16.
[7]   CAD P. International classification of functioning, disability and health (ICF). 2001.

[8]   Leonardi M, Ustun TB. The global burden of epilepsy. Epilepsia 2002;43:21-5.

[9]   De Boer HM. "Out of the Shadows": A Global Campaign Against Epilepsy. Epilepsia 2002;43:7-8.

[10]   Sander JW. The epidemiology of epilepsy revisited. Current opinion in neurology 2003;16(2):165.

[11]   ILAE. Proposal for Revised Classification of Epilepsies and Epileptic Syndromes. Epilepsia 1989;30(4):389-99.

[12]   MacDonald B, Cockerell O, Sander J, Shorvon S. The incidence and lifetime prevalence of neurological disorders in a prospective community-based study in the UK. Brain 2000;123(4):665-76.

[13]   Engel Jr J. A proposed diagnostic scheme for people with epileptic seizures and with epilepsy: report of the ILAE Task Force on Classification and Terminology. Epilepsia 2001;42(6):796-803.

[14]   Forsgren L, Beghi E, Oun A, Sillanpää M. The epidemiology of epilepsy in Europe–a systematic review. European Journal of Neurology 2005;12(4):245-53.

[15]   Engel J, Pedley TA, Aicardi J. Epilepsy: a comprehensive textbook: Lippincott Williams & Wilkins; 2008.

[16]   Walker M, White H, Sander J. Disease modification in partial epilepsy. Brain 2002;125(9):1937-50.

[17]   Sasa M. A new frontier in epilepsy: novel antiepileptogenic drugs. Journal of pharmacological sciences 2006;100(5):487-94.

[18]   Angeles DKF. Proposal for revised clinical and electroencephalographic classification of epileptic seizures. Epilepsia 1981;22489(501).

[19]   Klitgaard H, Pitkanen A. Antiepileptogenesis, neuroprotection, and disease modification in the treatment of epilepsy: focus on levetiracetam. Epileptic disorders 2003;5:9-16.

[20]   Berg AT, Berkovic SF, Brodie MJ, Buchhalter J, Cross JH, Van Emde Boas W, *et al*. Revised terminology and concepts for organization of seizures and epilepsies: report of the ILAE Commission on Classification and Terminology, 2005–2009. Epilepsia 2010;51(4):676-85.

[21]   Fisher RS, Boas WE, Blume W, Elger C, Genton P, Lee P, *et al*. Epileptic seizures and epilepsy: definitions proposed by the International League Against Epilepsy (ILAE) and the International Bureau for Epilepsy (IBE). Epilepsia 2005;46(4):470-2.

[22]   Hitiris N, Mohanraj R, Norrie J, Sills GJ, Brodie MJ. Predictors of pharmacoresistant epilepsy. Epilepsy research 2007;75(2):192-6.

[23]   Regesta G, Tanganelli P. Clinical aspects and biological bases of drug-resistant epilepsies. Epilepsy research 1999;34(2):109-22.

[24]   Berg AT. Identification of pharmacoresistant epilepsy. Neurologic clinics 2009;27(4):1003.

[25]   Pati S, Alexopoulos AV. Pharmacoresistant epilepsy: From pathogenesis to current and emerging therapies. Cleveland Clinic journal of medicine 2010;77(7):457.

[26]   Remy S, Beck H. Molecular and cellular mechanisms of pharmacoresistance in epilepsy. Brain 2006;129(1):18-35.

[27]   Löscher W, Potschka H. Role of multidrug transporters in pharmacoresistance to antiepileptic drugs. Journal of Pharmacology and Experimental Therapeutics 2002;301(1):7-14.

[28]   Leveille-Webster C, Arias I. The biology of the P-glycoproteins. Journal of Membrane Biology 1995;143(2):89-102.

[29]   Abbott NJ, Khan EU, Rollinson C, Reichel A, Janigro D, Dombrowski SM, *et al*. Drug resistance in epilepsy: the role of the blood–brain barrier. Mechanisms of Drug Resistance in Epilepsy 2002:38-53.

[30]   Sisodiya S, Lin WR, Harding B, Squier M, Thom M. Drug resistance in epilepsy: expression of drug resistance proteins in common causes of refractory epilepsy. Brain 2002;125(1):22-31.

[31]   Naylor DE, Liu H, Wasterlain CG. Trafficking of GABAA receptors, loss of inhibition, and a mechanism for pharmacoresistance in status epilepticus. The Journal of neuroscience 2005;25(34):7724-33.

[32]   Bartolomei F, Gastaldi M, Massacrier A, Planells R, Nicolas S, Cau P. Changes in the mRNAs encoding subtypes I, II and III sodium channel alpha subunits following kainate-induced seizures in rat brain. Journal of neurocytology 1997;26(10):667-78.

[33]   Whitaker W, Faull R, Dragunow M, Mee E, Emson P, Clare J. Changes in the mRNAs encoding voltage-gated sodium channel types II and III in human epileptic hippocampus. Neuroscience 2001;106(2):275-85.

[34]   Kwan P, Sills GJ, Brodie MJ. The mechanisms of action of commonly used antiepileptic drugs. Pharmacology & therapeutics 2001;90(1):21-34.

[35]   Ellerkmann R, Remy S, Chen J, Sochivko D, Elger C, Urban B, *et al*. Molecular and functional changes in voltage-dependent Na+ channels following pilocarpine-induced status epilepticus in rat dentate granule cells. Neuroscience 2003;119(2):323-33.

[36]   Gastaldi M, Robaglia-Schlupp A, Massacrier A, Planells R, Cau P. mRNA coding for voltage-gated sodium channel [beta] 2 subunit in rat central nervous system: cellular distribution and changes following kainate-induced seizures. Neuroscience letters 1998;249(1):53-6.

[37]   Remy S, Gabriel S, Urban BW, Dietrich D, Lehmann TN, Elger CE, *et al*. A novel mechanism underlying drug resistance in chronic epilepsy. Annals of neurology 2003;53(4):469-79.

[38]   Lucas PT, Meadows LS, Nicholls J, Ragsdale DS. An epilepsy mutation in the β1 subunit of the voltage-gated sodium channel results in reduced channel sensitivity to phenytoin. Epilepsy research 2005;64(3):77-84.

[39]   Edwards IR, Wiholm BE, Martinez C. Concepts in risk-benefit assessment. Drug safety 1996;15(1):1-7.

[40]   Perucca E, Beghi E, Dulac O, Shorvon S, Tomson T. Assessing risk to benefit ratio in antiepileptic drug therapy. Epilepsy research 2000;41(2):107-39.

[41]   EMEA. European Medicines Agency, Guideline on clinical investigation of medicinal products in the treatment of epileptic disorders 2010.

[42]   Ortinski P, Meador KJ. Cognitive side effects of antiepileptic drugs. Epilepsy & Behavior 2004;5:60-5.

[43]   Schachter SC. Currently available antiepileptic drugs. Neurotherapeutics 2007;4(1):4-11.

[44]   Schachter SC. Quality of life for patients with epilepsy is determined by more than seizure control: the role of psychosocial factors. Expert review of neurotherapeutics 2006;6(1):111-8.

[45]   BNF. British National Formulary, 61st edition. Committee JF, editor. London: British Medical Association and Royal Pharmaceutical Society of Great Britain; 2011.

[46]   William JC, David LK, Milton S. Newer antiepileptic drugs: gabapentin, lamotrigine, felbamate, topiramate and fosphenytoin. Am Fam Physician 1998;57(3):513-20.

[47] Hermann BP, Seidenberg M, Bell B, Woodard A, Rutecki P, Sheth R. Comorbid psychiatric symptoms in temporal lobe epilepsy: association with chronicity of epilepsy and impact on quality of life. Epilepsy & Behavior 2000;1(3):184-90.

[48] Tellez-Zenteno JF, Patten SB, Jetté N, Williams J, Wiebe S. Psychiatric comorbidity in epilepsy: a population-based analysis. Epilepsia 2007;48(12):2336-44.

[49] Gaitatzis A, Trimble M, Sander JW. The psychiatric comorbidity of epilepsy. Acta Neurologica Scandinavica 2004;110(4):207-20.

[50] de Boer HM, Mula M, Sander JW. The global burden and stigma of epilepsy. Epilepsy & Behavior 2008;12(4):540-6.

[51] Cockerell O, Hart Y, Sander J, Goodridge D, Shorvon S, Johnson A. Mortality from epilepsy: results from a prospective population-based study. The Lancet 1994;344(8927):918-21.

[52] Johnston A, Smith P. Sudden unexpected death in epilepsy. Expert review of neurotherapeutics 2007;7(12):1751-61.

[53] Langan Y, Nashef L, Sander J. Sudden unexpected death in epilepsy: a series of witnessed deaths. Journal of Neurology, Neurosurgery & Psychiatry 2000;68(2):211-3.

[54] Lhatoo S, Langan Y, Sander J. Sudden unexpected death in epilepsy. Postgraduate medical journal 1999;75(890):706-9.

[55] Stables JP, Kupferberg HJ. The NIH Anticonvulsant Drug Development (ADD) Program: preclinical anticonvulsant. Molecular and cellular targets for anti-epileptic drugs 1997;12:191.

[56] Perucca E. The new generation of antiepileptic drugs: advantages and disadvantages. British journal of clinical pharmacology 1996;42(5):531-43.

[57] Löscher W. Critical review of current animal models of seizures and epilepsy used in the discovery and development of new antiepileptic drugs. Seizure: the journal of the British Epilepsy Association 2011.

[58] White HS. Preclinical development of antiepileptic drugs: past, present, and future directions. Epilepsia 2003;44:2-8.

[59] Mody I, Lambert J, Heinemann U. Low extracellular magnesium induces epileptiform activity and spreading depression in rat hippocampal slices. Journal of neurophysiology 1987;57(3):869-88.

[60] Klitgaard H. Levetiracetam: the preclinical profile of a new class of antiepileptic drugs? Epilepsia 2001;42:13-8.

[61] Cavalheiro E. The pilocarpine model of epilepsy. The Italian Journal of Neurological Sciences 1995;16(1):33-7.

[62] Meldrum BS, Rogawski MA. Molecular targets for antiepileptic drug development. Neurotherapeutics 2007;4(1):18-61.

[63] Di Marzo V. The endocannabinoid system: its general strategy of action, tools for its pharmacological manipulation and potential therapeutic exploitation. Pharmacol Res 2009;60(2):77-84. Epub 2009/06/30.

[64] Bisogno T, Howell F, Williams G, Minassi A, Cascio MG, Ligresti A, *et al.* Cloning of the first sn1-DAG lipases points to the spatial and temporal regulation of endocannabinoid signaling in the brain. The Journal of cell biology 2003;163(3):463-8. Epub 2003/11/12.

[65] Okamoto Y, Morishita J, Tsuboi K, Tonai T, Ueda N. Molecular characterization of a phospholipase D generating anandamide and its congeners. J Biol Chem 2004;279(7):5298-305. Epub 2003/11/25.

[66]   Cravatt BF, Giang DK, Mayfield SP, Boger DL, Lerner RA, Gilula NB. Molecular characterization of an enzyme that degrades neuromodulatory fatty-acid amides. Nature 1996;384(6604):83-7. Epub 1996/11/07.

[67]   Dinh TP, Carpenter D, Leslie FM, Freund TF, Katona I, Sensi SL, *et al*. Brain monoglyceride lipase participating in endocannabinoid inactivation. Proc Natl Acad Sci U S A 2002;99(16):10819-24. Epub 2002/07/24.

[68]   Karlsson M, Contreras JA, Hellman U, Tornqvist H, Holm C. cDNA cloning, tissue distribution, and identification of the catalytic triad of monoglyceride lipase. Evolutionary relationship to esterases, lysophospholipases, and haloperoxidases. J Biol Chem 1997;272(43):27218-23. Epub 1997/10/27.

[69]   Marsicano G, Goodenough S, Monory K, Hermann H, Eder M, Cannich A, *et al*. CB1 cannabinoid receptors and on-demand defense against excitotoxicity. Science 2003;302(5642):84-8. Epub 2003/10/04.

[70]   Leite JP, Garcia-Cairasco N, Cavalheiro EA. New insights from the use of pilocarpine and kainate models. Epilepsy Res 2002;50(1-2):93-103. Epub 2002/08/02.

[71]   Monory K, Massa F, Egertova M, Eder M, Blaudzun H, Westenbroek R, *et al*. The endocannabinoid system controls key epileptogenic circuits in the hippocampus. Neuron 2006;51(4):455-66.

[72]   Guggenhuber S, Monory K, Lutz B, Klugmann M. AAV vector-mediated overexpression of CB1 cannabinoid receptor in pyramidal neurons of the hippocampus protects against seizure-induced excitoxicity. PloS one 2010;5(12):e15707. Epub 2011/01/05.

[73]   Karanian DA, Karim SL, Wood JT, Williams JS, Lin S, Makriyannis A, *et al*. Endocannabinoid enhancement protects against kainic acid-induced seizures and associated brain damage. J Pharmacol Exp Ther 2007;322(3):1059-66. Epub 2007/06/05.

[74]   Naidoo V, Nikas SP, Karanian DA, Hwang J, Zhao J, Wood JT, *et al*. A new generation fatty acid amide hydrolase inhibitor protects against kainate-induced excitotoxicity. Journal of molecular neuroscience: MN. 2011;43(3):493-502. Epub 2010/11/12.

[75]   Naidoo V, Karanian DA, Vadivel SK, Locklear JR, Wood JT, Nasr M, *et al*. Equipotent Inhibition of Fatty Acid Amide Hydrolase and Monoacylglycerol Lipase - Dual Targets of the Endocannabinoid System to Protect against Seizure Pathology. Neurotherapeutics 2012. Epub 2012/01/25.

[76]   Deshpande LS, Blair RE, Ziobro JM, Sombati S, Martin BR, DeLorenzo RJ. Endocannabinoids block status epilepticus in cultured hippocampal neurons. Eur J Pharmacol 2007;558(1-3):52-9. Epub 2006/12/19.

[77]   Hansen HH, Schmid PC, Bittigau P, Lastres-Becker I, Berrendero F, Manzanares J, *et al*. Anandamide, but not 2-arachidonoylglycerol, accumulates during *in vivo* neurodegeneration. Journal of neurochemistry 2001;78(6):1415-27. Epub 2001/10/02.

[78]   Curia G, Longo D, Biagini G, Jones RS, Avoli M. The pilocarpine model of temporal lobe epilepsy. Journal of neuroscience methods 2008;172(2):143-57. Epub 2008/06/14.

[79]   Wallace MJ, Blair RE, Falenski KW, Martin BR, DeLorenzo RJ. The endogenous cannabinoid system regulates seizure frequency and duration in a model of temporal lobe epilepsy. J Pharmacol Exp Ther 2003;307(1):129-37. Epub 2003/09/05.

[80]   Clement AB, Hawkins EG, Lichtman AH, Cravatt BF. Increased seizure susceptibility and proconvulsant activity of anandamide in mice lacking fatty acid amide hydrolase. J Neurosci 2003;23(9):3916-23. Epub 2003/05/09.

[81]   Manna SS, Umathe SN. Involvement of transient receptor potential vanilloid type 1 channels in the pro-convulsant effect of anandamide in pentylenetetrazole-induced seizures. Epilepsy Res 2012;100(1-2):113-24. Epub 2012/03/06.

[82]   Mason R, Cheer JF. Cannabinoid receptor activation reverses kainate-induced synchronized population burst firing in rat hippocampus. Frontiers in integrative neuroscience 2009;3:13. Epub 2009/06/30.

[83]   Titishov N, Mechoulam R, Zimmerman AM. Stereospecific effects of (-)- and (+)-7-hydroxy-delta-6-tetrahydrocannabinol-dimethylheptyl on the immune system of mice. Pharmacology 1989;39(6):337-49. Epub 1989/01/01.

[84]   Vincent P, Mulle C. Kainate receptors in epilepsy and excitotoxicity. Neuroscience 2009;158(1):309-23. Epub 2008/04/11.

[85]   Hill AJ, Williams CM, Whalley BJ, Stephens GJ. Phytocannabinoids as novel therapeutic agents in CNS disorders. Pharmacol Ther 2012;133(1):79-97. Epub 2011/09/20.

[86]   Stella N. Cannabinoid and cannabinoid-like receptors in microglia, astrocytes, and astrocytomas. Glia 2010;58(9):1017-30. Epub 2010/05/15.

[87]   Romigi A, Bari M, Placidi F, Marciani MG, Malaponti M, Torelli F, et al. Cerebrospinal fluid levels of the endocannabinoid anandamide are reduced in patients with untreated newly diagnosed temporal lobe epilepsy. Epilepsia 2010;51(5):768-72. Epub 2009/10/13.

[88]   Steffens M, Huppertz HJ, Zentner J, Chauzit E, Feuerstein TJ. Unchanged glutamine synthetase activity and increased NMDA receptor density in epileptic human neocortex: implications for the pathophysiology of epilepsy. Neurochemistry international 2005;47(6):379-84. Epub 2005/08/13.

[89]   Ludanyi A, Eross L, Czirjak S, Vajda J, Halasz P, Watanabe M, et al. Downregulation of the CB1 cannabinoid receptor and related molecular elements of the endocannabinoid system in epileptic human hippocampus. J Neurosci 2008;28(12):2976-90. Epub 2008/03/21.

[90]   Niehaus JL, Liu Y, Wallis KT, Egertova M, Bhartur SG, Mukhopadhyay S, et al. CB1 cannabinoid receptor activity is modulated by the cannabinoid receptor interacting protein CRIP 1a. Mol Pharmacol 2007;72(6):1557-66. Epub 2007/09/27.

[91]   Magloczky Z, Toth K, Karlocai R, Nagy S, Eross L, Czirjak S, et al. Dynamic changes of CB1-receptor expression in hippocampi of epileptic mice and humans. Epilepsia 2010;51 Suppl 3:115-20. Epub 2010/07/22.

[92]   Karlocai MR, Toth K, Watanabe M, Ledent C, Juhasz G, Freund TF, et al. Redistribution of CB1 cannabinoid receptors in the acute and chronic phases of pilocarpine-induced epilepsy. PloS one 2011;6(11):e27196. Epub 2011/11/15.

[93]   Falenski KW, Blair RE, Sim-Selley LJ, Martin BR, DeLorenzo RJ. Status epilepticus causes a long-lasting redistribution of hippocampal cannabinoid type 1 receptor expression and function in the rat pilocarpine model of acquired epilepsy. Neuroscience 2007;146(3):1232-44. Epub 2007/04/17.

[94]   Falenski KW, Carter DS, Harrison AJ, Martin BR, Blair RE, DeLorenzo RJ. Temporal characterization of changes in hippocampal cannabinoid CB(1) receptor expression following pilocarpine-induced status epilepticus. Brain research 2009;1262:64-72. Epub 2009/04/17.

[95]   Sayers KW, Nguyen PT, Blair RE, Sim-Selley LJ, DeLorenzo RJ. Statistical parametric mapping reveals regional alterations in cannabinoid CB1 receptor distribution and G-

protein activation in the 3D reconstructed epileptic rat brain. Epilepsia 2012;53(5):897-907. Epub 2012/04/19.

[96]   O'Shaughnessy WB. On the preparations of the Indian hemp, or gunjah (Cannabis indica). Transactions of the Medical and Physical Society of Bengal 1840:71-102.

[97]   Seely KA, Prather PL, James LP, Moran JH. Marijuana-based drugs: innovative therapeutics or designer drugs of abuse? Mol Interv 2011;11(1):36-51. Epub 2011/03/29.

[98]   WHO. 2012; Available from: http://www.who.int/substance_abuse/facts/cannabis/en/.

[99]   Pertwee RG. The therapeutic potential of drugs that target cannabinoid receptors or modulate the tissue levels or actions of endocannabinoids. Aaps J 2005;7(3):E625-54.

[100] Luszczki JJ, Andres-Mach M, Barcicka-Klosowska B, Florek-Luszczki M, Haratym-Maj A, Czuczwar SJ. Effects of WIN 55,212-2 mesylate (a synthetic cannabinoid) on the protective action of clonazepam, ethosuximide, phenobarbital and valproate against pentylenetetrazole-induced clonic seizures in mice. Prog Neuropsychopharmacol Biol Psychiatry 2011;35(8):1870-6. Epub 2011/07/23.

[101] Luszczki JJ, Misiuta-Krzesinska M, Florek M, Tutka P, Czuczwar SJ. Synthetic cannabinoid WIN 55,212-2 mesylate enhances the protective action of four classical antiepileptic drugs against maximal electroshock-induced seizures in mice. Pharmacol Biochem Behav 2011;98(2):261-7. Epub 2011/01/18.

[102] Dowie MJ, Howard ML, Nicholson LF, Faull RL, Hannan AJ, Glass M. Behavioural and molecular consequences of chronic cannabinoid treatment in Huntington's disease transgenic mice. Neuroscience 2010;170(1):324-36. Epub 2010/07/06.

[103] Rudenko V, Rafiuddin A, Leheste JR, Friedman LK. Inverse relationship of cannabimimetic (R+)WIN 55, 212 on behavior and seizure threshold during the juvenile period. Pharmacol Biochem Behav 2012;100(3):474-84. Epub 2011/10/25.

[104] Luszczki JJ, Czuczwar P, Cioczek-Czuczwar A, Czuczwar SJ. Arachidonyl-2'-chloroethylamide, a highly selective cannabinoid CB1 receptor agonist, enhances the anticonvulsant action of valproate in the mouse maximal electroshock-induced seizure model. Eur J Pharmacol 2006;547(1-3):65-74. Epub 2006/08/26.

[105] Sheerin AH, Zhang X, Saucier DM, Corcoran ME. Selective antiepileptic effects of N-palmitoylethanolamide, a putative endocannabinoid. Epilepsia 2004;45(10):1184-8. Epub 2004/10/06.

[106] Lambert DM, Vandevoorde S, Diependaele G, Govaerts SJ, Robert AR. Anticonvulsant activity of N-palmitoylethanolamide, a putative endocannabinoid, in mice. Epilepsia 2001;42(3):321-7. Epub 2001/07/10.

[107] Naderi N, Haghparast A, Saber-Tehrani A, Rezaii N, Alizadeh AM, Khani A, et al. Interaction between cannabinoid compounds and diazepam on anxiety-like behaviour of mice. Pharmacol Biochem Behav 2008;89(1):64-75. Epub 2007/12/22.

[108] Naderi N, Ahmad-Molaei L, Aziz Ahari F, Motamedi F. Modulation of anticonvulsant effects of cannabinoid compounds by GABA-A receptor agonist in acute pentylenetetrazole model of seizure in rat. Neurochem Res 2011;36(8):1520-5. Epub 2011/04/26.

[109] Luszczki JJ, Czuczwar P, Cioczek-Czuczwar A, Dudra-Jastrzebska M, Andres-Mach M, Czuczwar SJ. Effect of arachidonyl-2'-chloroethylamide, a selective cannabinoid CB1 receptor agonist, on the protective action of the various antiepileptic drugs in the mouse maximal electroshock-induced seizure model. Prog Neuropsychopharmacol Biol Psychiatry 2010;34(1):18-25. Epub 2009/09/16.

[110] van Rijn CM, Gaetani S, Santolini I, Badura A, Gabova A, Fu J, *et al*. WAG/Rij rats show a reduced expression of CB(1) receptors in thalamic nuclei and respond to the CB(1) receptor agonist, R(+)WIN55,212-2, with a reduced incidence of spike-wave discharges. Epilepsia 2010;51(8):1511-21. Epub 2010/02/06.

[111] Cakil D, Yildirim M, Ayyildiz M, Agar E. The effect of co-administration of the NMDA blocker with agonist and antagonist of CB1-receptor on penicillin-induced epileptiform activity in rats. Epilepsy Res 2011;93(2-3):128-37. Epub 2010/12/24.

[112] Rizzo V, Ferraro G, Carletti F, Lonobile G, Cannizzaro C, Sardo P. Evidences of cannabinoids-induced modulation of paroxysmal events in an experimental model of partial epilepsy in the rat. Neurosci Lett 2009;462(2):135-9. Epub 2009/07/15.

[113] Kozan R, Ayyildiz M, Agar E. The effects of intracerebroventricular AM-251, a CB1-receptor antagonist, and ACEA, a CB1-receptor agonist, on penicillin-induced epileptiform activity in rats. Epilepsia 2009;50(7):1760-7. Epub 2009/05/21.

[114] Bahremand A, Shafaroodi H, Ghasemi M, Nasrabady SE, Gholizadeh S, Dehpour AR. The cannabinoid anticonvulsant effect on pentylenetetrazole-induced seizure is potentiated by ultra-low dose naltrexone in mice. Epilepsy Res 2008;81(1):44-51. Epub 2008/05/27.

[115] Bahremand A, Nasrabady SE, Shafaroodi H, Ghasemi M, Dehpour AR. Involvement of nitrergic system in the anticonvulsant effect of the cannabinoid CB(1) agonist ACEA in the pentylenetetrazole-induced seizure in mice. Epilepsy Res 2009;84(2-3):110-9. Epub 2009/02/19.

[116] Gholizadeh S, Shafaroodi H, Ghasemi M, Bahremand A, Sharifzadeh M, Dehpour AR. Ultra-low dose cannabinoid antagonist AM251 enhances cannabinoid anticonvulsant effects in the pentylenetetrazole-induced seizure in mice. Neuropharmacology 2007;53(6):763-70. Epub 2007/09/18.

[117] Shafaroodi H, Samini M, Moezi L, Homayoun H, Sadeghipour H, Tavakoli S, *et al*. The interaction of cannabinoids and opioids on pentylenetetrazole-induced seizure threshold in mice. Neuropharmacology 2004;47(3):390-400. Epub 2004/07/28.

[118] Wallace MJ, Martin BR, DeLorenzo RJ. Evidence for a physiological role of endocannabinoids in the modulation of seizure threshold and severity. Eur J Pharmacol 2002;452(3):295-301. Epub 2002/10/03.

[119] Wendt H, Soerensen J, Wotjak CT, Potschka H. Targeting the endocannabinoid system in the amygdala kindling model of temporal lobe epilepsy in mice. Epilepsia 2011;52(7):e62-5. Epub 2011/06/02.

[120] Vinogradova LV, Shatskova AB, van Rijn CM. Pro-epileptic effects of the cannabinoid receptor antagonist SR141716 in a model of audiogenic epilepsy. Epilepsy Res 2011;96(3):250-6. Epub 2011/07/08.

[121] Dudek FE, Pouliot WA, Rossi CA, Staley KJ. The effect of the cannabinoid-receptor antagonist, SR141716, on the early stage of kainate-induced epileptogenesis in the adult rat. Epilepsia 2010;51 Suppl 3:126-30. Epub 2010/07/22.

[122] Echegoyen J, Armstrong C, Morgan RJ, Soltesz I. Single application of a CB1 receptor antagonist rapidly following head injury prevents long-term hyperexcitability in a rat model. Epilepsy Res 2009;85(1):123-7. Epub 2009/04/17.

[123] Davis JP, H. RH. Antiepileptic action of marijuana-active substances. Federation proceedings, Baltimore. 1949;8:284-5.

[124] Chesher GB, Jackson DM. Anticonvulsant effects of cannabinoids in mice: drug interactions within cannabinoids and cannabinoid interactions with phenytoin. Psychopharmacologia 1974;37(3):255-64. Epub 1974/07/11.

[125] Karler R, Turkanis SA. Subacute cannabinoid treatment: anticonvulsant activity and withdrawal excitability in mice. Br J Pharmacol 1980;68(3):479-84. Epub 1980/03/01.

[126] Loskota WJ, Lomax P. The Mongolian gerbil (Meriones unguiculatus) as a model for the study of the epilepsies: EEG records of seizures. Electroencephalogr Clin Neurophysiol 1975;38(6):597-604. Epub 1975/06/01.

[127] Chesher GB, Jackson DM, Malor RM. Interaction of delta9-tetrahydrocannabinol and cannabidiol with phenobarbitone in protecting mice from electrically induced convulsions. J Pharm Pharmacol 1975;27(8):608-9. Epub 1975/08/01.

[128] Boggan WO, Steele RA, Freedman DX. 9 -Tetrahydrocannabinol effect on audiogenic seizure susceptibility. Psychopharmacologia 1973;29(2):101-6. Epub 1973/03/16.

[129] Wallace MJ, Wiley JL, Martin BR, DeLorenzo RJ. Assessment of the role of CB1 receptors in cannabinoid anticonvulsant effects. Eur J Pharmacol 2001;428(1):51-7. Epub 2002/01/10.

[130] Sofia RD, Kubena RK, Barry H, 3rd. Comparison among four vehicles and four routes for administering delta9-tetrahydrocannabinol. J Pharm Sci 1974;63(6):939-41. Epub 1974/06/01.

[131] Wada JA, Wake A, Sato M, Corcoran ME. Antiepileptic and prophylactic effects of tetrahydrocannabinols in amygdaloid kindled cats. Epilepsia 1975;16(3):503-10. Epub 1975/09/01.

[132] Corcoran ME, McCaughran JA, Jr., Wada JA. Acute antiepileptic effects of 9-tetrahydrocannabinol in rats with kindled seizures. Experimental neurology 1973;40(2):471-83. Epub 1973/08/01.

[133] Fried PA, McIntyre DC. Electrical and behavioral attenuation of the anti-convulsant properties of delta 9-TNC following chronic administrations. Psychopharmacologia 1973;31(3):215-27. Epub 1973/07/19.

[134] Wada JA, Osawa T, Corcoran ME. Effects of tetrahydrocannabinols on kindled amygdaloid seizures and photogenic seizures in Senegalese baboons, Papio papio. Epilepsia 1975;16(3):439-48. Epub 1975/09/01.

[135] Johnson DD, McNeill JR, Crawford RD, Wilcox WC. Epileptiform seizures in domestic fowl. V. The anticonvulsant activity of delta9-tetrahydrocannabinol. Can J Physiol Pharmacol 1975;53(6):1007-13. Epub 1975/12/01.

[136] Thomas A, Baillie G, Phillips A, Razdan R, Ross R, Pertwee R. Cannabidiol displays unexpectedly high potency as an antagonist of CB1 and CB2 receptor agonists *in vitro*. British journal of pharmacology 2007;150(5):613-23.

[137] Izzo AA, Borrelli F, Capasso R, Di Marzo V, Mechoulam R. Non-psychotropic plant cannabinoids: new therapeutic opportunities from an ancient herb. Trends in pharmacological sciences 2009;30(10):515-27. Epub 2009/09/05.

[138] Deiana S, Watanabe A, Yamasaki Y, Amada N, Arthur M, Fleming S, *et al.* Plasma and brain pharmacokinetic profile of cannabidiol (CBD), cannabidivarine (CBDV), Δ 9-tetrahydrocannabivarin (THCV) and cannabigerol (CBG) in rats and mice following oral and intraperitoneal administration and CBD action on obsessive–compulsive behaviour. Psychopharmacology 2012:1-15.

[139] Cunha JM, Carlini EA, Pereira AE, Ramos OL, Pimentel C, Gagliardi R, *et al.* Chronic administration of cannabidiol to healthy volunteers and epileptic patients. Pharmacology 1980;21(3):175-85. Epub 1980/01/01.

[140] Izquierdo I, Tannhauser M. Letter: The effect of cannabidiol on maximal electroshock seizures in rats. J Pharm Pharmacol 1973;25(11):916-7. Epub 1973/11/01.

[141] Karler R, Turkanis SA. Cannabis and epilepsy. Adv Biosci 1978;22-23:619-41. Epub 1978/07/22.

[142] Turkanis SA, Smiley KA, Borys HK, Olsen DM, Karler R. An electrophysiological analysis of the anticonvulsant action of cannabidiol on limbic seizures in conscious rats. Epilepsia 1979;20(4):351-63. Epub 1979/08/01.

[143] Colasanti BK, Lindamood C, 3rd, Craig CR. Effects of marihuana cannabinoids on seizure activity in cobalt-epileptic rats. Pharmacol Biochem Behav 1982;16(4):573-8. Epub 1982/04/01.

[144] Consroe P, Benedito MA, Leite JR, Carlini EA, Mechoulam R. Effects of cannabidiol on behavioral seizures caused by convulsant drugs or current in mice. Eur J Pharmacol 1982;83(3-4):293-8. Epub 1982/09/24.

[145] Jones NA, Hill AJ, Smith I, Bevan SA, Williams CM, Whalley BJ, *et al.* Cannabidiol displays antiepileptiform and antiseizure properties *in vitro* and *in vivo*. J Pharmacol Exp Ther 2010;332(2):569-77. Epub 2009/11/13.

[146] Jones NA, Glyn SE, Akiyama S, Hill TDM, Hill AJ, Weston SE, *et al.* Cannabidiol exerts anti-convulsant effects in animal models of temporal lobe and partial seizures. Seizure 2012;21(5):344-52.

[147] Hill AJ, Weston SE, Jones NA, Smith I, Bevan SA, Williamson EM, *et al.* 9 Tetrahydrocannabivarin suppresses *in vitro* epileptiform and *in vivo* seizure activity in adult rats. Epilepsia 2010;51(8):1522-32.

[148] Hill A, Mercier M, Hill T, Glyn S, Jones N, Yamasaki Y, *et al.* Cannabidivarin is anticonvulsant in mouse and rat *in vitro* and in seizure models. British journal of pharmacology 2012.

[149] De Petrocellis L, Ligresti A, Moriello AS, Allarà M, Bisogno T, Petrosino S, *et al.* Effects of cannabinoids and cannabinoid-enriched Cannabis extracts on TRP channels and endocannabinoid metabolic enzymes. British journal of pharmacology 2011;163(7):1479-94.

[150] De Petrocellis L, Orlando P, Moriello AS, Aviello G, Stott C, Izzo A, *et al.* Cannabinoid actions at TRPV channels: effects on TRPV3 and TRPV4 and their potential relevance to gastrointestinal inflammation. Acta Physiologica 2011;204(2):255-66.

[151] Baulac M, Pitkanen A. Research Priorities in Epilepsy for the Next Decade-A Representative View of the European Scientific Community. Epilepsia 2008. Epub 2008/09/25.

Index

2-AG 93, 94

2-Arachidonoyl Glycerol 136, 164

20-HETE 28, 49

20-Hydroxy- ProstaglandinE$_2$ 26

9-THC 27-28, 36

A

ACEA 43, 51

Alcohol 149

Anandamide 112, 135, 171

Appetite 68, 74

Arachidonic Acid 93

Area Postrema 58

B

Body Temperature 77

Brain Stem 60

C

Cannabidavarin 164

Cannabidiol 189

Cannabinoid Receptor Genes 6

Cannabinoid Receptors 4, 5, 152

Cannabinoid 4, 27, 62, 103, 104

Cannabis 14, 180

CB$_1$ 104, 105

CB$_2$ 105, 106

CNR1 6, 8

CNR2 6

Cnvs 12

Cocaine 135, 144

Contraction 34, 166

www.ingramcontent.com/pod-product-compliance
Lightning Source LLC
Chambersburg PA
CBHW050839220326
41598CB00006B/402